THE ENCYCLOPEDIA OF
LEARNING DISABILITIES

Second Edition

THE ENCYCLOPEDIA OF

LEARNING DISABILITIES

Second Edition

Carol Turkington
Joseph R. Harris, Ph.D.
American Bookworks

Facts On File

An imprint of Infobase Publishing

The Encyclopedia of Learning Disabilities, Second Edition

Copyright © 2006, 2002 by Carol Turkington

Facts On File, Inc.
An imprint of Infobase Publishing
132 West 31st Street
New York NY 10001

Library of Congress Cataloging-in-Publication Data

Turkington, Carol.
The encyclopedia of learning disabilities / Carol Turkington, Joseph R. Harris ; American Bookworks.—2nd ed.
p. cm.
Includes bibliographical references and index.
ISBN 0-8160-6399-0 (hc: alk. paper)
1. Learning disabilities—Encyclopedias. 2. Learning disabled—Education—United States—Encyclopedias. I. Harris, Joseph, 1951 Dec. 20–II. American BookWorks Corporation. III. Title.
LC4704.5.T86 2006

371.9′03—dc22   2005053045

Text and cover design by Cathy Rincon

Printed in the United States of America

VB Hermitage 10 9 8 7 6 5 4 3 2 1

This book is printed on acid-free paper.

CONTENTS

Foreword   vii

Introduction   xi

Entries A–Z   1

Appendixes   249

Glossary   277

Bibliography   279

Index   289

FOREWORD

Dr. Sam Kirk may have coined the term *learning disabilities* in 1963, but problems in learning ability have been a part of the human condition for centuries. Indeed, there is evidence that as early as 3000 B.C.E., the Chinese recognized differences in learning ability among individuals and administered standardized tests to differentiate those candidates who were able to train for trades from those who were not.

Differences in the ability to learn became critically important to educators in the West at the beginning of the Industrial Revolution. Families left their farms and came to the cities in search of better lives and sent their children to school in hopes that they could eventually obtain the best jobs. Schools, no longer the exclusive privilege of the middle and upper classes, began to see their enrollments swell. Educators recognized that not all students could learn with the same degree of success. At the beginning of the 20th century, the first modern tests were developed to identify students with learning problems who needed different educational services.

The presence of learning disabilities among prominent historical and contemporary figures has helped raise public awareness about learning disorders and also helped remove some of the stigma associated with them. For example, the gifted French sculptor Auguste Rodin's teachers informed his parents that he was uneducable. In shame, his parents withdrew him from school and put him to work. President Woodrow Wilson was nine before he learned the alphabet and did not learn to read until age 11. Thomas Edison's teachers referred to him as "addled," "abnormal," and "mentally deficient." Albert Einstein did not learn to speak until the age of three and was considered by his teachers of possessing "subnormal intelligence." Even as an adult, Einstein continued to struggle with what we today would most likely be diagnosed as learning disabilities. Finally, the late vice president Nelson Rockefeller had such severe dyslexia that he was not able to even read his own speeches: He had to commit them to memory.

Before Kirk, there were as many theories about learning disorders as there were practitioners. Physicians emphasized learning disabilities as the result of neurological disorders and nervous system damage and advised medical treatment. Indeed, recent discoveries in the Human Genome Project have identified possible genetic links to attention deficit and hyperactivity disorder (ADHD) and several learning disabilities. Advances in imaging now allow researchers to view the living brains while their owners engage in different tasks, allowing them to determine more precisely which areas of the brain are important to understanding learning and learning disorders. In the past, optometrists saw learning disabilities as deficits in visual perception of written symbols and recommended corrective lenses or ocular training. Speech and language pathologists defined learning disabilities as language-based and recommended language therapy. Psychologists assumed that learning disabilities were caused by emotional problems or faulty learning and emphasized psychotherapy or behavioral retraining. Finally, educators saw learning disabilities as the result of faulty learning abilities or mismatches between instruction and students' learning styles and recommended diagnostic-prescriptive teaching that would match instruction with students' learning styles.

Kirk emphasized the role of information-processing abilities in learning disabilities, and his views on learning disabilities continue to be among the more influential in the field nearly 40 years after he introduced them. His term *learning disabilities* replaced more antiquated terms, reflecting more obsolete views of learning, such as:

- word blindness
- reading (or math or spelling) retardation
- Strauss Syndrome
- brain dysfunction
- hard-of-learning
- six-hour retardation
- backwardness

In fact, until recently, there were still pockets in the country where school districts had not come to identify children as learning disabled: If they had adequate intelligence but still had learning problems, these schools labeled them *"brain damaged"* whether or not there was any evidence of neurological disorders.

Problems with identification were not the only obstacle affected individuals faced. Even if they were able to obtain a diagnosis of "learning disabled," there were few public schools in the country before the 1970s that provided any sort of special education, much less related services such as physical or occupational therapy. Individuals with learning disabilities had few of today's rights or avenues to appeal schools' decisions regarding their education if they disagreed.

Even as of the early 1970s, in many places in the country, only the largest school districts had any classes for students with learning disabilities, and those were frequently where schools dumped their worst troublemakers. Even if children with learning disabilities were fortunate to reside in an area in which special education services were available, there were typically long waiting lists for classes that did not always provide the degree of individualized educational programs that students with disabilities enjoy today.

American education changed radically for children with learning disabilities and other types of handicaps in the mid-1970s. In 1975, President Gerald Ford signed Public Law 94-142 (since reauthorized as the Individuals with Disabilities Education Act, or IDEA). The law provided a legal definition of learning disabilities that emphasized a "severe discrepancy between potential and achievement" in specific academic areas. (The recent reauthorization of IDEA has done away with the discrepancy model in favor of a more process-oriented identification model.) At the ceremony at which he signed the bill into law, President Ford made a prophetic comment that Congress would probably never authorize enough money to states to fully implement the new requirements. He was right. Since that time, many parents seeking the range of services they believe their children need have found themselves at odds with school district administrators who do not always have sufficient funding to implement the law. Advocates for students with handicaps, who foresaw an era when schools and families would work together to provide meaningful special education to children who needed it, saw an adversarial process in which parents must fight funding-strapped school administrators for the very services they consider essential to their children's success.

Politicians frequently fiddle with laws regarding special education because of their ideologies or to satisfy special interests to whom they feel some sort of allegiance. For example, No Child Left Behind has drastically limited the rights of Individualized Educational Program teams to provide standardized testing accommodations to students with learning disabilities or to even exclude such students from standardized testing based on uninformed assumptions regarding the appropriateness of such testing for children with learning problems. The recent IDEA authorization has opened the door for Congress to limit certain protections children with handicaps formerly had from expulsion and has made it more difficult for parents to pursue their disagreements regarding their children's special education and related services by allowing school districts to sue for recovery of legal fees if parents lose such actions.

Carol Turkington and I bring somewhat different but complementary perspectives to this book. Turkington is a journalist who specializes in medical and psychological topics. I am a licensed and certified school psychologist, former school district special education director, and college instructor, and I have extensive predoctoral and postdoctoral training in neuropsychology, special education law, and diagnostic testing. As chief psychologist for the South Carolina Department of Juvenile Justice, I have discovered that our latest information shows that 37 percent of the juveniles coming through my door receive some sort of special education or related services. I was a second-year graduate student in school psychology when President Ford signed Public Law 94-142 into law, so I have been involved with the implementation of federal special education law from the beginning. I have helped school districts and families advocate for children with handicaps: I have sat on both sides of the negotiating table, representing variously school districts, families, and state agencies. As a special education director who has built special education programs in three school districts and helped write some of the policies and procedures with which school districts must comply in my home state, I am familiar with the challenges that school districts face in implementing unfunded and underfunded mandates. As a school psychologist formerly employed both by school districts and in private practice, I am very familiar with the challenges experienced by people with handicaps and the people who love them. I have worked with attorneys to help many individuals with disabilities obtain Social Security Disability benefits and have worked with college counselors who have invariably been eager to help them obtain appropriate educational accommodations in higher education. I have tried very hard to lend those perspectives to providing helpful information gained from more than 30 years' experience in special education.

This book provides entries on a wide variety of terms and concepts related to learning disabilities that Carol Turkington and I hope parents, teachers, physicians, students, and others will find useful. We have tried to present terms ranging from the basic to the highly technical, from the matter-of-fact to the controversial, in a thorough but straightforward manner that allows readers to decide their positions on those issues for themselves. We have explained much of the "alphabet soup," such as LRE, IEP, PL 94-142, ADA, and IDEA, that so often confuses parents. We hope that we have provided information that readers will find helpful and informative in their attempts to navigate their way through this frequently confusing and controversial field.

—Joseph Harris, Ph.D.

INTRODUCTION

One in five children in the United States struggles with learning disabilities, a broad category that includes a wide range of problems with speech, language, reading, mathematics, concentration, and reasoning. But not all learning *problems* are necessarily learning *disabilities*. Some children are simply slower than others in developing certain skills. How do you tell the difference? This is why early identification and treatment are vital in treating symptoms of learning difficulties. Although learning disabilities themselves have always been a part of the human condition, they have only recently been identified. Many of the symptoms experts consider to be learning disabilities were observed and described more than a century ago, but the term itself was coined by Samuel Kirk in 1963—less than 40 years ago. The discipline continues to evolve.

For much of this century, for example, conditions such as dyslexia have been called many different names, such as strephosymbolia and minimal brain dysfunction. But in the United States, it was really only with the advent of special education legislation and services in the 1970s that this label for a broad, complex, and often poorly understood range of learning problems came into common usage. Likewise, while less than a decade ago attention disorders were viewed primarily as a problem of hyperactive male children, today experts understand that attention deficit and hyperactivity disorder (ADHD) is far more complex, affects many more girls, and extends into adulthood.

As recently as a generation ago, learning disabilities were poorly understood and often ignored. Even when parents were able to obtain special education services for their child, these services were often ineffective. With the advent of educational legislation, the quality of educational services has dramatically improved. The past two decades have also seen a dramatic increase in the scope and depth of research into the underlying issues involved in various learning disorders. Methods of investigation such as brain imaging and genetic research have begun to produce concrete support for scientific theories of the origin and nature of learning disorders. Within the past 10 years, the role of medications in treating some disorders and the development of assistive technology have revolutionized the treatment of learning disabilities.

Even the terminology used in the area of special education has undergone dramatic change. The ways that experts describe individuals and their learning have become far more diagnostically accurate and, at the same time, far more humane. Likewise, with the ongoing refinement of legislation to protect the rights of those with learning disabilities over the last 30 years, the terminology used in the field of special education has taken on legal as well as educational connotations.

In this revised edition, we have tried to present the latest information in the field. There are many new topics, including

- auditory processing disorder
- autism spectrum disorder
- childhood disintegrative disorder
- discrete trial training

- environmental toxins such as dioxins, mercury, and toxic black mold
- Feingold diet
- Landau-Kleffner syndrome
- pervasive developmental disorders
- Scholastic Aptitude Test (with information on updates and accommodations)
- spasmodic dysphonia
- speech disorders
- tardive dyskinesia
- tests, including the Vineland Adaptive Behavior Scales, Stanford Achievement Test, Metropolitan Achievement Test, and Millon Clinical
- Williams syndrome

In addition, almost every entry has been revised, many with extensive updates, including the newest information on the revisions to the IDEA law, passed in 2004. We have updated entries on a variety of conditions, adding details and fresh information on auditory processing; the cause, incidence, and treatment of ADHD; diagnosis and treatment of dyslexia; conduct disorder; bipolar disorder; dysphasia; dysnomia; epilepsy; verbal apraxia; traumatic brain injury; stuttering; tactile defensiveness; nonverbal learning disabilities; and new research into the genetic causes of Angelman syndrome.

The latest information on medication has also been added, including new information on Adderall, a new entry on nonstimulant Strattera (atomoxetine), and the latest information on the manufacturer's decision to stop producing Cylert (pemoline) because of dropping sales. (Cylert is banned in Canada and England because of links to liver disease.) The encyclopedia also includes the latest information on antidepressants and teenage suicide risk, along with updates on other side effects of medications.

Because treatments are very important in this field and are constantly being updated, based on new research, there are expanded entries on diet and ADHD, special education, early childhood assessment, EEGs and ADHD, neurofeedback, and other key topics.

The appendixes in the back have been updated, with many new organizations added and the latest addresses, phone numbers, and Internet Web sites checked for accuracy.

This book has been designed as a guide and reference to a wide range of terms related to learning disabilities and to additional information and addresses of organizations that deal with these issues. It is not a substitute for prompt assessment and treatment by experts trained in the diagnosis of learning problems. Information in this book comes from the most up-to-date sources available and includes some of the most recent research in learning disabilities. Readers should keep in mind, however, that changes occur very rapidly in this field. References have been provided for readers who seek additional sources of information. All entries are cross-referenced, and appendixes provide additional information.

—Carol Turkington
Cumru, Pennsylvania

ENTRIES A–Z

ability grouping   Placing children of similar ability in one group; also called "tracking" or "whole class ability grouping." Some experts believe such grouping harms children with lower ability, who tend to perform more poorly in lower-track classes than in mixed-ability classes. At the same time, studies suggest that children of higher ability do not achieve more in tracked classes than in mixed-ability classes. Moreover, placing students with lower ability in tracked classrooms reduces self-esteem, with a particularly negative effect on students' sense of their own academic competence. Critics of tracking also maintain that the process reduces opportunities to develop relationships among students from different racial, ethnic, and socioeconomic groups, and has a negative effect on race relations.

Placement decisions about ability grouping are often made very early in a student's school career, and are often based on questionable data.

According to the National Association of School Psychologists, mixed-ability grouping can give all students equal access to an enriched curriculum and the highest quality instruction that schools have to offer, and avoids labeling and stigmatizing students with lower ability. It also promotes higher expectations for student achievement and reduces school segregation based on socioeconomic status, race, gender, ethnicity, or disability. Ideally, mixed-ability classes should not "teach to the middle" but should accommodate individual differences in learning styles, abilities, and interests. This type of grouping should include cooperative learning groups, peer tutors, flexible grouping practices, team teaching, multi-age groupings, and instruction in higher order thinking and problem-solving skills.

ability test   Tests (such as INTELLIGENCE TESTS) that measure an individual's ability to perform a task, manipulate information, or solve problems. Typically, tests of ability are used to assess specific performance abilities or potential for future learning, rather than stored information. Among the most commonly used ability tests are the WECHSLER INTELLIGENCE SCALE FOR CHILDREN, either revised or third edition, the SCHOLASTIC APTITUDE TEST (SAT) and AMERICAN COLLEGE TEST, which are widely used in college admissions processes, and the WOOD-COCK-JOHNSON, THIRD EDITION cognitive battery, which is commonly used in public school settings to define a baseline of aptitude against which achievement can be measured in determining the existence of a LEARNING DISABILITY.

Ability tests can be physical or mental. They can test verbal or nonverbal areas, and are also frequently used to assess potential employees for specific tasks.

Depending on the nature of the test, a wide spectrum of individuals may be involved in administration. Specific clinical training in psychology is required in order to administer the Wechsler or other intelligence tests, while the Woodcock-Johnson may be administered by school guidance counselors with appropriate training. Standardized tests such as the SAT must be administered in specific contexts and according to specific testing procedures, but overseeing such tests requires no formal professional training.

Ability tests have particular importance in relation to the AMERICANS WITH DISABILITIES ACT, which protects individuals with disabilities from discrimination, especially in the workplace. Ability tests designed to assess mechanical abilities, clerical abilities, and other job-related abilities can prevent equal access. Individuals can request alternative assessment of their abilities if they can provide documentation of a disability and they are otherwise qualified for a position.

academic classes The core classes in a student's program, such as reading, English, history, and mathematics. Children are generally moved into subject-area classes in elementary school, with different teachers for each subject. As students enter middle school, content areas take on more significance. Often, considerable reading, writing, and critical thinking are required in academic classes that may not be required of such electives as music, art, or physical education.

Typically, students with learning disabilities will perform significantly worse in academic classes involving reading and writing skills. This can be the result of problems with decoding, reading comprehension, or basic study skills. It is generally in academic classes where students with learning disabilities (LD) require accommodations or extra support. In fact, learning disabilities are usually first evaluated as a result of poor academic performance. For LD classification, federal law requires discrepancy between *potential* (usually measured by IQ tests) and *achievement* (usually measured by *individual* achievement tests, never group standardized tests), as supported by anecdotal evidence of academic difficulties in the classroom.

academic skills disorders Problems with reading, writing, or arithmetic skills that can be divided into DEVELOPMENTAL READING DISORDER, DEVELOPMENTAL WRITING DISORDER, and developmental arithmetic disorder (DYSCALCULIA).

Developmental reading disorder (also known as DYSLEXIA) is quite widespread, affecting between 2 percent and 8 percent of elementary school children. The ability to read requires a rich, intact network of nerve cells that connect the brain's centers of vision, language, and memory. While a person can have problems in any of the tasks involved in reading, scientists have found that a significant number of people with dyslexia share an inability to distinguish or separate the sounds in spoken words. For example, a child might not be able to identify the word *cat* by sounding out the individual letters, c-a-t, or to play rhyming games.

Fortunately, remedial reading specialists have developed techniques that can help many children with dyslexia acquire these skills. However, there is more to reading than recognizing words. If the brain cannot form images or relate new ideas to those stored in memory, the reader will not be able to understand or remember the new concepts. This is why other types of reading disabilities can appear in the upper grades when the focus of reading shifts from word identification to comprehension.

Writing, too, involves several brain areas and functions. The brain networks for vocabulary, grammar, hand movement, and memory must all work well if the child is to be able to write well. A developmental writing disorder may be caused by problems in any of these areas. A child with a writing disability, particularly an expressive language disorder, might be unable to compose complete, grammatical sentences.

Arithmetic involves recognizing numbers and symbols, memorizing facts such as the multiplication table, aligning numbers, and understanding abstract concepts like place value and fractions. Any of these may be difficult for children with *developmental arithmetic disorders*. Problems with numbers or basic concepts are likely to show up early, whereas problems that appear in the later grades are more often tied to problems in reasoning.

Many aspects of speaking, listening, reading, writing, and arithmetic overlap and build on the same brain capabilities, so it is not surprising that people can be diagnosed as having more than one type of learning disability. For example, the ability to understand language underlies the ability to learn to speak. Therefore, any disorder that interferes with the ability to understand language will also interfere with the development of speech, which in turn hinders learning to read and write. A single problem in the brain's operation can disrupt many types of learning activity.

acalculia Also known as anarithmia, this is an acquired inability to do simple mathematics that does not involve normal difficulties with mathematics. Both oral and written calculations are commonly affected. The problem is caused by lesions usually caused by brain damage to the left parietal lobe.

Primary acalculia is an acquired problem in calculation that cannot be explained by problems in writing numbers (AGRAPHIA), or by spatial disorganization for numbers. *Spatial acalculia* is the impaired ability to perform written calculations because of the failure to process spatial aspects of written problems properly. Spatial acalculia is more often associated with right brain-hemisphere lesions.

accommodations Any modifications to an educational program to meet the needs of students with disabilities, or to provide access to individuals in the workplace. The AMERICANS WITH DISABILITIES ACT (ADA), INDIVIDUALS WITH DISABILITIES EDUCATION IMPROVEMENT ACT (IDEIA), and Section 504 of the REHABILITATION ACT OF 1973 (PL 93-112) and 1990, all require accommodations in one way or another so that qualified individuals with disabilities have access to educational and employment opportunities.

Although children with disabilities are protected under IDEIA and provided with SPECIAL EDUCATION SERVICES, college students are not protected under IDEIA. They must request accommodations under ADA or the Rehabilitation Act.

Under the ADA, the term *reasonable accommodation* may include

- making existing facilities readily accessible to people with disabilities
- job restructuring, part-time or modified work schedules, reassignment to a vacant position
- modifying equipment, examinations, training materials
- providing qualified readers or interpreter

For example, the ADA requires that someone with a physical disability who needs a wheelchair must be given a desk of the right width and height. However, that person must be "otherwise qualified" for the position. This means that a person who is blind cannot be hired as an air traffic controller; antidiscriminatory legislation is designed to ensure that access is reasonable but not automatic.

However, employers and schools also have legal protection as to whether they are required to provide accommodations. For example, under the ADA an institution or employer may claim that modifications would impose a hardship under certain conditions. Those conditions include

- the nature and cost of the accommodation
- the overall financial resources of the facility involved
- the number of employees
- the impact of the accommodation on the operation of the facility
- the overall size of the business
- the type of operation

Compliance with the ADA has been slow, especially because of the cost of removing physical barriers. Nonetheless, it is this legislation that provides the guidelines for accessibility as a UNIVERSAL ACCESS/DESIGN. For people with LEARNING DISABILITIES (especially for students enrolled in college), accommodations can be provided if a specific request is made to an institution's disability support office. Typical accommodations might include

- academic modifications: note-taking services, course requirement waiver or substitution, reduced course load
- exam accommodations: extended time, alternative test formats, computer availability
- auxiliary aids or services: taped tests, taped books, tutoring, writing or academic center support; remedial skills development courses or workshops; priority registration and course selection

In order to receive services or accommodations, students must have a recommendation from a psychologist based on a specific diagnosis. Program modifications may include waivers or course substitutions. The law states that accommodations should be made on a case-by-case basis, without compromising the academic standards of a program of study.

University faculty members vary in their willingness to provide accommodations to students with learning disabilities. Teachers should not question the need for accommodation nor are they legally allowed to ask for information about the specific disability, but they can decide if the accommodation is reasonable and how it will be implemented. Some studies have suggested that faculty are more willing to provide "teaching accommodations" such as allowing students to record lectures. They tend to be less eager to provide alternative exam formats because they are concerned with keeping academic standards high.

The U.S. Supreme Court has ruled on only one case pertaining to college access for students with disabilities. In *Southeastern Community College v. Davis* (1979), the Court upheld that a student with a hearing problem could be denied admission to a nursing program because the essential program requirements could not be modified. In this and subsequent case law, the courts have repeatedly deferred to faculty expertise regarding what constitutes the essential requirements of a program and whether these requirements can be waived.

See also AUXILIARY AIDS.

accuracy   The correctness or precision in test performance. In general, the term *accuracy* is used with tests that measure different types of performance. For example, some reading tests measure both reading accuracy and reading rate; it is possible that a student might have markedly different scores for reading accuracy and reading rate.

Students with DYSLEXIA or a specific reading disability who have had some reading help could have a relatively high accuracy score compared to their reading rate, showing that they are capable of decoding accurately but that they require more time to do so effectively. On the other hand, a student with an ATTENTION DEFICIT HYPERACTIVITY DISORDER might score very high in terms of reading rate, but have a relatively lower level of accuracy, reflecting careless mistakes and inattention.

achievement   What an individual has learned; achievement generally refers to the kind of knowledge and skills that are taught in school. It may be measured by actual school performance or by STANDARDIZED TESTS of achievement. ACHIEVEMENT TESTS often focus on specific content areas such as grammatical structures or American history, or on general areas such as writing or READING COMPREHENSION.

Because the classification of LEARNING DISABILITY may depend on a discrepancy between achievement on standardized tests and intellectual potential, the concept of achievement can be extremely important. Within most states, whether a person is recognized as having a learning disability and thus qualifies for SPECIAL EDUCATION services depend on a discrepancy between performance on standardized achievement and aptitude tests. Depending on which tests are used, the same student may score very differently, which may affect whether the student qualifies for services.

achievement test   A standardized measure of knowledge, information, or procedural learning (such as how to do something). This type of assessment is used to measure student learning in comparison to a norm.

Achievement tests may assess general academic skill areas such as reading, writing, or mathematics, or they may test for content knowledge in a specific academic subject, such as biology or American history. Achievement tests are used by school systems to provide a standard measure of individual student performance, and to provide an aggregated measure of performance that enables school systems to evaluate their effectiveness. Achievement tests are also used as part of the diagnostic assessment of individuals to determine whether they have a LEARNING DISABILITY and qualify for SPECIAL EDUCATION services.

ACID profile   A pattern of lower scores on specific subtests of the WECHSLER INTELLIGENCE SCALE FOR CHILDREN—THIRD EDITION or the WECHSLER ADULT INTELLIGENCE SCALE—THIRD EDITION that is associated with one subtype of LEARNING DISABILITY. This pattern of significantly low scores on the Arithmetic, Coding, Information, and Digit Span subtests has been associated with learning disabilities in reading, spelling, and arithmetic.

acoustic cortex   A part of the temporal region of the brain that receives all auditory stimuli.

active reading   A term that refers to the process of reading in which students actively engage with the text by applying a variety of strategies. These might include

- previewing the essay or chapter in order to get a sense of the whole
- underlining and/or highlighting main ideas, key terminology, and unfamiliar vocabulary
- margin-noting with main ideas or questions about the material
- outlining a chapter or essay after reading it, in order to show the relationship between ideas and sections
- paraphrasing the information
- summarizing main ideas

For individuals with a LEARNING DISABILITY, READING COMPREHENSION is often an area of weakness because of problems with vocabulary and background knowledge.

Using active reading skills can increase comprehension by exercising critical thinking skills and improving memorization. Research suggests that new information that is manipulated and rehearsed is more likely to be stored in long-term memory. The use of active reading skills helps individuals to understand the relationships between ideas, and to learn the information more efficiently and effectively. Teaching specific cognitive strategies, also known as STRATEGY INSTRUCTION, has been studied since 1960. Since then, other approaches have been developed for helping students with learning disabilities to more efficiently process information.

Studies also support the idea that children with learning disabilities do not have or cannot apply the strategies for reading that more efficient learners do automatically. This emphasizes the need for explicit instruction in active reading, as well as many other skills.

ADA   The acronym for the AMERICANS WITH DISABILITIES ACT.

adaptive behavior   The ability of an individual to adapt to the expectations of society and a particular environment (such as the workplace or the classroom). Initially, the term was applied to those with DEVELOPMENTAL DISABILITIES.

Adaptive behavior is based on how well the person has already mastered basic living skills. Rather than completing a series of tasks or test items, individuals are rated based on interviews with care providers, family, and teachers. The assessment of adaptive behavior is now considered important in the field of LEARNING DISABILITIES.

Some research has indicated that children with learning disabilities often have problems with classroom adaptive behavior, involving difficulties with extroversion, creativity, curiosity, and completing tasks. Research suggests that these difficulties are not simply the result of academic failure, but relate to problems in adapting behavior to the classroom environment. Although this research is not conclusive, it does pose significant implications for MAINSTREAMING students with learning disabilities.

A person's functional intelligence is not the same thing as a person's IQ. Rather, functional intelligence is a combination of skills, IQ, and adaptive behavior—how well the person can function in the community. Most federal and state educational assistance programs require that a person's IQ be below a standard (usually 70) *and* that the level of adaptive behavior be consistent or below with expected levels for the IQ in order for the person to be classified as mentally handicapped.

adaptive behavior rating scale   A standardized scale that measures a person's ADAPTIVE BEHAVIOR. The scale is determined after an interview that typically requires either teachers or parents to rate an individual on a wide variety of specific behavior, such as coping skills, use of language, development of peer relationships, the ability to stay focused, and so on. For example, questions in the "daily living" component might ask whether the person understands that hot things are dangerous, or whether the person can drink from a cup or glass without help.

Adaptive behavior scales are typically used in conjunction with INTELLIGENCE TESTS, and are rarely used alone. These standardized behavior scales can provide important objective information about development and are considered to be more consistent than informal observations by a mental health professional. Although several scales for measuring adaptive behavior have been developed since the 1940s, among the most widely accepted scales are the VINELAND ADAPTIVE BEHAVIOR RATING SCALES (VABS). The VABS are used primarily with children and adolescents from birth to age 18 years but may be used on adults suspected of having a mental handicap based on obtained IQ. The scales measure adaptive behavior in four major areas: communication, daily living skills, socialization, and GROSS MOTOR SKILLS. Also in common use are the AMERICAN ASSOCIATION ON MENTAL RETARDATION ADAPTIVE BEHAVIOR SCALES. Both tests have different forms for children and adults.

adaptive skills   Daily living skills that a person needs to be able to live, work, and play independently. There are 10 skills that are included in this area: communication, self-care, home living, social skills, leisure, health and safety, self-direction, functional academics, community use, and work.

Adaptive skills are assessed in the person's typical environment, in all aspects of an individual's life. A person with limited intellectual functioning but who does *not* have limits in adaptive skill areas may not be diagnosed as having MENTAL RETARDATION. By law, such a person is not retarded.

ADD   See ATTENTION DEFICIT HYPERACTIVITY DISORDER.

Adderall   See DEXTROAMPHETAMINE/AMPHETAMINE.

ADHD   The abbreviation for ATTENTION DEFICIT HYPERACTIVITY DISORDER.

ADHD rating scale—IV   An instrument used to diagnose ATTENTION DEFICIT HYPERACTIVITY DISORDER (ADHD) in children and adolescents and for assessing treatment response. Containing 18 items, the scale is linked directly to *DSM-IV-TR* diagnostic criteria for ADHD and provides three versions of the scale: a parent questionnaire on home behaviors in English or Spanish and a teacher questionnaire on classroom behaviors.

Administration on Developmental Disabilities (ADD)   The principal agency providing funding for services to people with DEVELOPMENTAL DISABILITIES.

The administration implements the provisions of the DEVELOPMENTAL DISABILITIES ASSISTANCE BILL OF RIGHTS ACT of 1990, which calls for more independence, productivity, community integration, and inclusion for those with developmental disabilities.

The ADD administers numerous grant programs for planning, administration, and advocating services for those with developmental disabilities, and to protect their legal and human rights. Activities under these programs include job promotion, community living arrangements, child development, case management, and support for services to help families of those with developmental disabilities.

affect   A visual representation of a person's feelings that conveys emotions through body language and facial expression, rather than through words. The affective component in LEARNING DISABILITIES is sometimes overlooked, but this may play a major role in helping to understand the nature of a person's learning needs.

For example, some individuals with learning disabilities or ATTENTION DEFICIT DISORDERS may display what psychologists call a "flat affect," which means they do not reveal their underlying feelings. This may be interpreted by a teacher or parent as boredom or a lack of emotional engagement, when in fact it may be caused by delayed processing of verbal information or internal distractibility. Such a person may seem to be indifferent to discipline, when in fact the person really feels overwhelmed—and responds by shutting down. On the other hand, an individual may show a highly animated or inappropriate affect because of external stimuli, or because of internal problems with self control.

Affect can be described as

- blunted: significant reduction in the intensity of emotional expression
- flat: absence of any sign of emotional expression
- labile: repeated, rapid, abrupt shifts in expression
- restricted or constricted: mild reduction in the range and intensity of emotional expression

agnosia   A defect in the ability to recognize and interpret complex objects or experiences; the stimuli are received, but their meaning is absent or distorted. Individuals with various forms of agnosia may be unable to recognize people or objects, despite the fact that their basic senses are normal. It is often caused by a lesion in a part of the brain called the angular gyrus.

Agnosia bears some similarities to APHASIA, a condition characterized by problems in naming and describing objects. However, aphasia involves a disorder of language—individuals with aphasia do not improve their ability to name objects when information is presented in another way.

For example, a person with visual agnosia may be able to describe what an object looks like, but still not recognize it; although the person's perceptual system may be intact, the individual has no meaningful associations with the perceived object.

Some types of agnosia are far more common than others. Visual agnosia (especially agnosia for faces, called prosopagnosia) is the most commonly encountered form of recognition disturbance, a disorder of recognition confined to the visual realm despite normal visual perception and alertness, attention, intelligence, and language. Most patients with visual agnosia cannot recognize new visual stimuli that would normally have been learned after adequate exposure.

The condition of auditory agnosia is more rare, and tactile agnosia is even less common.

agraphia The inability to write resulting from brain disease. Agraphia is a type of APHASIA, which is an absent or impaired language ability. The problem may include difficulty with language function, or it may be restricted to problems with written expression. This term is used to describe writing impairment *after* a person has learned to write. Agraphia may involve problems with the formation of letters, spelling, word selection, grammar, or arrangement of letters on the page.

Symptoms and Diagnostic Path

People with *spatial agraphia* cannot place writing on the page; this most often occurs as a progressive upward slant from the left to right side of the page and is associated with lesions of the dominant hemisphere. Someone with *micrographia* will write smaller and smaller letters over the course of a sentence; this problem is associated with Parkinsonism or Alzheimer's disease.

Most patients with aphasia also have agraphia. In ALEXIA with agraphia, a patient distorts letters and has problems with spelling, in addition to reading impairment; this is associated with brain lesions in the left angular or supramarginal gyrus. In *Gerstmann syndrome,* loosely associated with brain damage in the parietal lobe, agraphia occurs with a number of other problems, including the inability to do simple arithmetic (ACALCULIA) and left-right disorientation. *Callosal agraphia* affecting the left hand only can follow brain lesions in the front half of the corpus callosum. *Phonological agraphia* involves a specific defect resulting in the inability to write pronounceable pseudowords.

Agraphia may be caused by almost any brain disease, but stroke, injury, tumor, and Alzheimer's disease are the most common. Agraphia also is often one of the early behavioral signs of confusion due to metabolic problems or poisoning.

The condition can be diagnosed with a simple writing test in which a patient copies a sentence, takes dictation, and spontaneously creates a sentence or two. Although persons with agraphia may still be able to write something learned extremely well (such as a patient's own name), this should not be used to infer normal writing ability. Treatment of the underlying condition may help improve the basic problems with agraphia. Conditions that cannot be treated effectively will typically indicate that agraphia does not improve.

alcohol A substance found in several forms but which is most commonly consumed as ethyl alcohol in the form of beer, wine, and liquor. It is a naturally occurring by-product of the chemical breakdown of sugars. Alcohol exposure to the fetus can cause devastating, lifelong damage, including brain damage, MENTAL RETARDATION, HYPERACTIVITY, and behavioral disorders. FETAL ALCOHOL SYNDROME is a pattern of facial abnormalities, growth retardation, and brain damage that only occurs in babies whose mothers drank during pregnancy and is the leading known cause of preventable mental retardation. Milder exposure to alcohol in the womb can cause FETAL ALCOHOL EFFECT, a less severe, but still very debilitating, lifelong condition resulting in lowered intelligence, hyperactivity, and behavioral disorders.

Because alcohol is present in breast milk shortly after ingestion, and there is no known safe level of alcohol consumption during pregnancy, experts typically advise pregnant or breast-feeding women, and women likely to become pregnant, to abstain from alcohol altogether.

alexia The loss of the ability to read caused by lesions on the brain or from other brain injury. Alexia is a separate condition from DYSLEXIA, and generally does not respond to treatment the way that dyslexia does.

The most common cause of acquired alexia is stroke. Other forms of brain problems, including tumors, inflammation, and head injury, also can cause alexia. In addition, there are some cases of degenerative disease (such as Alzheimer's) in which a reading problem occurs early.

Symptoms and Diagnostic Path

While relatively pure cases of alexia occur, they usually are associated with APHASIA or problems in writing (AGRAPHIA). There are a number of different subtypes, but all types cause reading problems so that reading is slow or impossible, and comprehension of reading material is impaired. In the United States, alexia almost always describes acquired defects in reading that occur as the result of a brain condition in a person who was previously literate.

Treatment Options and Outlook

Some patients respond to repeated reading-aloud practice with familiar text passages, eventually moving to new text passages.

American Association on Mental Retardation Adaptive Behavior Scales—Second Edition (AAMR ABS) An assessment of behavior developed by the American Association on Mental Retardation, the oldest professional organization devoted to MENTAL RETARDATION in the United States. The ADAPTIVE BEHAVIOR RATING SCALE is available in two forms—one for school, the other for residential and community settings. Both versions assess the manner in which an individual copes with the natural and social demands of the environment.

American College Test (ACT) A college entrance and placement exam that assesses high school stu-

dents' general educational development and their ability to complete college-level work. The multiple choice tests include four skill areas: English, mathematics, reading, and science. The optional writing test measures a student's skill in planning and writing a short essay; it was available for the first time in February 2005.

Some colleges require that student applicants submit writing test scores, while others will not. Both versions of the exam—the traditional ACT Assessment and the ACT Assessment Plus Writing—are available to students who want to take them.

The ACT is curriculum-based and is not an aptitude or an IQ test. Instead, the questions on the ACT are directly related to what students have learned in high school, sometimes called "competency-based tests" by testing experts.

In addition to testing the four skill areas, the ACT also provides test takers with an interest inventory that provides information for career and educational planning and a student profile section that provides a comprehensive profile of a student's work in high school and his or her future plans.

The test takes more than four hours for the ACT without the writing test, including administration instructions and a break after the first two tests. Actual testing time is two hours and 55 minutes, broken down as follows

- English: 45 minutes
- math: 60 minutes
- reading: 35 minutes
- science: 35 minutes
- writing test: 30 minutes

The highest possible ACT score is 36; the national average composite score for 2004 was 20.9. Only one in 5,000 students who took the ACT scored a perfect 36. There are a total of 215 questions: 75 English questions, 60 math questions, and 40 questions each in reading and science.

The ACT was first administered in 1959; in 2003–2004, more than 2 million tests were given.

Students may take the ACT as often as they wish, but only once per national test date. Many students take the test twice, once as a junior and again as a senior. ACT research shows that of the students who took the ACT more than once, 55 percent increased their composite score, 22 percent had no change in their composite score, and 23 percent decreased their composite score on the retest.

Americans with Disabilities Act (ADA) Legislation enacted in July 1990 that prohibits discrimination against individuals with disabilities. It guarantees equal opportunity for people with disabilities in jobs, public accommodations, transportation, and telecommunications, as well as other state services.

The ADA represents a significant addition to the scope of protections defined by the Civil Rights Act of 1964, which was not intended to protect the rights of individuals with disabilities. It also augments other laws that address issues of disability and access to education and employment opportunities, such as the INDIVIDUALS WITH DISABILITIES EDUCATION IMPROVEMENT ACT (IDEIA) and the REHABILITATION ACT OF 1973.

While the ADA covers many areas of possible discrimination (including schools), it is used primarily to protect individuals with disabilities on the job. The IDEIA and CRA offer more specific protections and regulations in regard to schools and colleges.

On the job, employers are required to provide fair opportunities to individuals with disabilities if they are "otherwise qualified" for a position. For example, a person who is partly blind cannot perform the essential functions of airline pilot. A person in a wheelchair, however, may be able to perform the essential functions of a bookkeeper, and therefore should not be discriminated against based on physical limitations.

Employers and schools may also be required to provide accessibility to buildings for those who have physical disabilities. Employers with more than 15 employees also may be required to provide accommodations for employees with specific needs based on their disability, such as equipment or more frequent breaks. "Disability" is an important term from a legal perspective, as it distinguishes those with temporary limitations or less severe limitations from those for whom a physical or mental impairment limits major life activities.

For people with LEARNING DISABILITIES, the ADA provides legislative support for accommodations within both educational and workplace settings. Unlike the federal legislation governing public education for children with learning disabilities, the ADA places a much greater burden of responsibility on the person seeking services or accommodations. The ADA also clearly protects educational institutions and employers from being required to provide accommodations that place unreasonable burdens or that represent significant lowering of educational standards. At the same time, the ADA also provides broad protection for individuals with learning disabilities in a wide variety of contexts.

analogy A comparison between two different but related things. The ability to comprehend and create analogies is an important component of critical reasoning abilities. For example, an analogy might compare the biological process of a tree growing from small seed to tall oak, to the human process of development from infancy to adulthood. This analogy would be written:

SEED : OAK AS INFANT : ADULT

Another type of analogy is the visual analogy. For example, in a 2 × 2 cell grid, the two cells on the left might contain blue stars, and the top cell on the right might contain a green square. The person taking the test must then select which of several presented figures (including the correct green square) must go in the empty cell.

For some students with LEARNING DISABILITIES, understanding analogies may be very difficult. They may process information in fairly concrete ways, and miss more subtle connections between dissimilar things.

Often, however, the ability to reason analogically is a relative strength for students with learning disabilities.

anarithmia See ACALCULIA.

Angelman syndrome A childhood disorder characterized by HYPERACTIVITY, seizures, inappropriate laughter, and developmental delays. Initially presumed to be rare, it is now believed that thousands of children with Angelman syndrome have gone undiagnosed or misdiagnosed as having CEREBRAL PALSY, AUTISM, or other childhood disorders.

In 1965, English physician Harry Angelman, M.D., first described three children with characteristics now known as Angelman syndrome (AS), including stiff, jerky gait; lack of speech; excessive laughter; and seizures. Other cases were eventually published, but the condition was considered to be extremely rare. Since the first reports in the 1980s, many new cases have been diagnosed.

In the United States and Canada, there are about 1,000 diagnosed individuals, but it has been reported throughout the world among divergent racial groups. In North America, most patients seem to be of Caucasian origin.

Recent research has discovered that several different types of genetic abnormalities are implicated in AS. Scientists have discovered a very small missing area on chromosome 15 in about 70 percent of people with AS. The deleted area, although extremely small, is actually quite large when viewed at the molecular level. The deleted region is known to contain genes that are turned on or off depending on the chromosome's origin. This gene is turned on when inherited from the mother but off when inherited from the father. Because the AS deletions occur only on the chromosome 15 inherited from the mother, the gene or genes responsible for AS are believed to be found only on the mother's chromosome 15.

In 1997, a gene within the AS deletion region called UBE3A was found to be mutated in approximately 5 percent of AS individuals. All mutations known to cause AS appear to cause inactivation or absence of this gene. In some families, AS caused by a UBE3A mutation can recur in more than one family member. Inheritance of a UBE3A mutation from the mother causes AS; inheritance of a UBE3A mutation from the father has no detectable effect on the child. In 2–3 percent of AS cases, the child inherits both copies of chromosome 15 from the father, with no copy inherited from the mother. In this case, there is no deletion or mutation, but the child is missing an active UBE3A gene because the paternal-derived chromosomes have only inactivated UBE3A genes. (Only the mother's chromosome 15 contain the activated type of this gene).

Symptoms and Diagnostic Path

Hyperactivity and a short attention span are probably the most typical behaviors, which affect boys and girls about equally. Infants and toddlers may be continually active, constantly keeping their hands or toys in their mouth, moving from object to object. In extreme cases, the constant movement can cause accidental bruises. There may be grabbing, pinching, and biting in older children. A child's attention span can be so short that it interferes with social interaction, since the child cannot pay attention to facial and other social cues.

Laughter is also quite common, which seems to be a reaction to physical or mental stimuli. Although AS children experience a variety of emotions, apparent happiness is most common. Parents may first notice this laughter at the age of one to three months. Giggling, chortling, and constant smiling soon develop and appear to represent normal reflexive laughter, but cooing and babbling are delayed.

Other symptoms include

- developmental delay
- severe speech impairment with almost no use of words
- movement or balance disorder
- easily excitable personality, often with hand-flapping movements
- abnormally small head
- seizures

Angelman syndrome is usually not recognized at birth or in infancy, since the developmental problems are hard to spot at that time. Children are typically not diagnosed until ages three to seven, when the characteristic behaviors and features become evident.

Treatment Options and Outlook

A complete range of enrichment programs should be provided. Persistent and consistent behavior modification helps decrease or eliminate unwanted behavior. In milder cases, the child's attention may be good enough to learn sign language and other communication techniques. For these children, educational and developmental training programs are much easier to structure and are generally more effective.

Physical therapy can help improve motor skills; OCCUPATIONAL THERAPY may help improve fine motor and oral-motor control. Speech and communication therapy is essential and should focus on nonverbal methods of communication, including sign language, picture cards, or communication boards.

Extremely hyperactive children may need special help to be included in a regular classroom. AS children with attention deficits and hyperactivity need room to express themselves. Individualization, effective behavior management, and flexibility are important.

Consistent behavior modification at school and at home can help the AS child learn to perform most self-help skills related to eating, dressing, toileting, and performing general activities.

As these patients enter adolescence, they can continue to learn since they do not have significant mental deterioration. Their physical health appears to be remarkably good, and some patients may be able to stop their seizure medications by early adolescence.

AS individuals with severe ATAXIA may lose their ability to walk if they are not encouraged to move around. Scoliosis can develop in adolescence and is a particular problem in those children who cannot walk. Scoliosis can be treated with early bracing to prevent worsening of the condition; surgery or stabilization may be necessary for severe cases. People with AS usually live a normal life span.

Most children do not receive drug therapy for hyperactivity, although some may benefit from use of medications such as METHYLPHENIDATE (Ritalin).

angular gyrus A part of the brain that plays an important role in language processing. It is involved in recoding visual information for interpretation as auditory code. Some research suggests that during reading tasks, the brains of individuals with DYSLEXIA may be less active than nondyslexics in the angular gyrus, as well as in a part of the brain called WERNICKE'S AREA.

anomia The inability to find the correct word. Anomia is Latin-derived and means "without a name" or "unnamed." It is a type of APHASIA that involves the loss of ability to recall words, such as the names of objects, persons, activities, and so on.

anoxia The total deprivation of oxygen. In general, it refers to the ways in which oxygen deprivation damages the brain. Brain damage caused by anoxia can range from subtle LEARNING DISABILITIES to profound MENTAL RETARDATION, depending on severity.

Anoxia during birth may cause brain damage that affects the ability to learn. Brain damage resulting from anoxia also may occur in any situation in which a person is deprived of oxygen for a significant period of time.

antecedent event A stimulus that results in a response, one of the three key elements of the BEHAVIORAL UNIT, a model at the core of behavioral psychology. The other two elements are behavior (response) and consequence (reinforcement). For example, a teacher's cue to sit quietly at a desk and take out paper and pencil might be viewed as an antecedent event designed to stimulate the students to take out paper and pencil (response).

antisocial personality disorder A type of personality disorder characterized by disregard for the feelings and rights of others. Patterns of irresponsibility, aggression toward others, and impulsive "acting out" in social situations recur and interfere with a person's ability to function in society. Antisocial personality disorder exists in 2 percent to 3 percent of the general population, and is three to four times more common in men than in women. The popular term *sociopath* has replaced the older term *psychopath* to describe a person with this disorder.

People with this disorder may be in trouble with the law and have trouble maintaining interpersonal relationships. Antisocial personality disorder is an adult diagnosis that is often given to individuals (typically male) who were diagnosed with CONDUCT DISORDER as children. Research suggests that antisocial personality disorder can coexist with ATTENTION DEFICIT HYPERACTIVITY DISORDER (ADHD).

Research suggests that the condition may be caused by an interaction between a genetic predisposition and environment, since other risk factors include regular exposure to substance abuse and criminal behavior, as well as a childhood characterized by chaotic, neglectful, harsh, or abusive parenting. A combination of ADHD and conduct disorder in childhood can herald the subsequent development of antisocial personality disorders in adulthood.

Symptoms and Diagnostic Path

Although the diagnosis is limited to people over age 18, there is always a history of antisocial behavior since at least age 15, including repetitive lying, truancy, delinquency, and substance abuse. As an adult, there is a pattern of unlawful behavior, failure of job and family responsibility, reckless personal behavior, promiscuity, failure to sustain long-term relationships, and aggressive behavior. Superficial charm and wit can be highly developed and skillfully used. Symptoms of antisocial personality disorder include

- impulsiveness and a lack of concern for consequences
- pattern of criminal behavior
- lying and deceit for personal profit or pleasure
- lack of empathy
- irritability, aggressiveness, and violent behavior
- disregard for safety or responsibility
- lack of remorse

Treatment Options and Outlook

Drug treatment has not proven to be helpful. The fact that antisocial personality disorder develops early and is the natural way these patients define themselves makes treatment more difficult. Effective treatment must address a person's basic behavioral patterns, attitudes, relationship styles, and function. In most cases, antisocial personality disorder can respond to therapy, but changing habits of thought, feeling, and behavior requires extensive and repetitive examination, evaluation, and relearning. Definitive inpatient treatment must be provided in a specialized hospital unit so that a patient's problems with the inability to trust, to fantasize, to feel, and to learn can be addressed.

Some experts believe that the single most effective factor in helping individuals with antisocial personality turn their behavior around is a close, personal relationship with a significant older mentor, to whom the antisocial person looks as a role model.

Typically, most antisocial people do not actively seek therapy; instead, they usually come to treatment as a result of court orders. However, outlook for successful treatment is poor.

anxiety   A feeling of apprehension, fear, or worry not connected to a specific threat. Many experts believe that anxiety is a learned response to stress. For example, a child who has been stung by a bee will run away crying on the next appearance of a flying buzzing insect. Should the avoidance continue to be reinforced, the anxiety continues.

Cognitive psychologists believe that anxiety is the result of inappropriate thinking about circumstances. For someone who has an irrational fear of snakes, a picture of a snake can cause anxiety even though it is not possible to be hurt by a two-dimensional picture.

People with LEARNING DISABILITIES may often have accompanying problems with anxiety, especially in connection to schoolwork. Reading aloud, taking timed tests, or trying to start a writing assignment all may trigger anxiety and cause even further problems with the required task. Someone experiencing a high level of anxiety may "freeze up" and find it impossible to perform at all, or may show signs of restlessness and agitation, leading to erratic and inconsistent performance.

There is also a significant link between attention deficits and anxiety. To some degree, it can be hard to tell the difference between the two. An inability to focus and sustain attention may often lead to anxiety, and anxiety itself can make it very difficult for a person to pay attention to a task. In some cases, attention deficit disorders coexist with anxiety disorders.

It is also possible for someone with an anxiety disorder to be misdiagnosed as having ATTENTION DEFICIT HYPERACTIVITY DISORDER (ADHD). In evaluating ADHD, a differential diagnosis for anxiety may be important. It is equally important that those who work with individuals with ADHD take into account the possibility that anxiety may underlie some expressions of learning, communication, and social difficulties.

aphasia A language disorder characterized by profound difficulties with both expressing and understanding language. Individuals with aphasia experience problems understanding language; there are problems with word-finding ability, and speech may be incoherent. There is often a combination of naming, fluency, comprehension, and repetition deficits that are accompanied by reading and writing impairments (AGRAPHIA). However, aphasia does not include SPEECH DISORDERS. Most patients have disturbed language function rather than complete loss of language.

Caused by damage to the temporal or FRONTAL LOBE in the brain, aphasia may be the result of a stroke, brain injury, or infection. Its severity can vary; some people cannot communicate at all, while others may have problems with just one aspect of language (such as word retrieval).

Types of Aphasia

There are a number of types of aphasia that are characterized by different symptoms, including

- amnesic: word-finding difficulties that imply words have been "forgotten"
- anomic: problems with naming ability sometimes called nominal aphasia or amnesic aphasia
- conduction: fluent aphasia with severely impaired repetition but relatively preserved language comprehension, with word-finding difficulties. Patients with conduction aphasia have difficulty reading aloud but they may have relatively good comprehension
- global: involves loss of nearly all fluency, comprehension, repetition, reading, and writing. Large brain lesions in both Broca's and WERNICKE'S AREA (and nearby tissue) are usually involved
- jargon: characterized by fluent speech that may be incomprehensible. Speech contains numerous incorrect word selections with significant repetition. Jargon aphasia is an acute expression of Wernicke's aphasia
- mixed transcortical: a rare subtype in which patients are unable to name, read, and write
- nonfluent: effortful speech production and lack of normal emotional tone or quality in speech. Nonfluent aphasia includes Broca's aphasia,

global aphasia, transcortical motor aphasia, and mixed transcortical aphasia

- posterior: fluent aphasia, also known as Wernicke's aphasia. The term is no longer widely used
- pure motor: nonfluent speech with largely preserved language functioning demonstrated by the ability to write. It is also called apraxia of speech
- transcortical motor: nonfluent aphasia characterized by preserved repetition and relatively preserved language comprehension
- transcortical sensory: fluent aphasia in which language comprehension is severely impaired. It may occur in the later stages of Alzheimer's disease

aphasia, developmental A term used to describe an individual whose difficulties in learning to speak are severe and pervasive. Developmental APHASIA is generally linked to a problem in the central nervous system present since birth, as opposed to acquired aphasia, which describes the loss of the ability to speak due to brain damage.

aphasoid A mild or moderate retardation in the development of language competence, associated with mild problems in expressing language (APHASIA).

aphemia Loss of the ability to speak. In this condition, written communication is possible, but spoken communication is impossible. Both speech and written words are understood, however. Some experts use the term interchangeably with motor APHASIA.

apraxia A general term describing impairment of the ability to carry out physical movements involved in communication. Children with this problem have trouble transmitting the speech message from their brain to their mouths, and have problems translating their thoughts into a correct sequence of movements using their mouth, tongue, and lips. A child with apraxia of speech can have speech that is very limited and unclear, making it difficult for others to understand the child. This is not something a child will outgrow, but with early speech therapy by a trained SPEECH-LANGUAGE PATHOLOGIST, many children with apraxia are capable of learning to speak clearly and communicate effectively. However, without the necessary and appropriate therapy, children with apraxia may never speak clearly and experience a lifetime of frustration.

Some forms of apraxia involve impairments in the ability to use gestures or movement in nonverbal communication, such as waving or pointing.

aptitude   An individual's ability to learn, without reference to specific instruction or prior knowledge. Aptitude is most often measured by STANDARDIZED TESTS such as INTELLIGENCE TESTS (for example, the WECHSLER INTELLIGENCE SCALE FOR CHILDREN [WISC]) or cognitive batteries of tests that also include achievement components (such as the WOODCOCK-JOHNSON). Other important aptitude tests include the SCHOLASTIC APTITUDE TEST and the AMERICAN COLLEGE TEST, each of which plays a prominent role in college admissions.

Determining whether someone has a learning disability is generally based on a discrepancy between achievement and aptitude, as measured by standardized tests. Consequently, tests of aptitude such as the WISC and the Woodcock-Johnson play a central role in determining who is eligible to receive special education services.

aptitude test   A measurement of a person's ability to learn, typically using tests for specific abilities in order to predict achievement in these areas. For example, the SCHOLASTIC APTITUDE TEST is commonly used to assess potential ability to succeed in college.

See also APTITUDE.

arcuate fasciculus   A pathway of fibers in the parietal lobe of the brain that connects WERNICKE'S AREA with BROCA'S AREA. When this connection first develops at about age two, children become able to form words into sentences. If it is damaged, the child will be able to understand words that are heard or read but will not be able to repeat them. This condition is called conduction APHASIA.

arithmetic disability   A subtype of a specific LEARNING DISABILITY that relates to computational arithmetic skills, rote learning or memorizing, writing, or difficulties with fine motor coordination. Federal law differentiates two subareas of arithmetic disability: mathematics calculation and mathematics reasoning.

There can be a variety of reasons for problems with arithmetic. The more severe subtypes (such as DYSCALCULIA) are based in the brain and relate to visual spatial ability. For others, mathematics ability is impaired by cognitive difficulties or poor information processing.

Those affected with arithmetic disability have a particular cognitive and neuropsychological profile that is different from those with primarily reading deficits, although the two disabilities may coexist in a single individual.

arousal regulation   The regulation of arousal and alertness is associated with the frontal lobe and the BASAL GANGLIA in the brain. Difficulties in regulating arousal have been connected to ATTENTION DEFICIT HYPERACTIVITY DISORDER (ADHD), and in some theories are seen as the central deficiency in attention disorders. There is some evidence that the way in which Ritalin and other stimulants help a person with ADHD is by stimulating the basal ganglia.

A person who has problems with arousal regulation may have difficulty staying alert and focused, and may also have problems with over-arousal and difficulty falling asleep at an appropriate time. For some individuals, difficulty with arousal regulation may be so severe that they may be classified as having a sleep disorder.

articulation   The production of speech sounds. In the human body, speech is produced through the combined work of several organs, including the larynx (voice box), tongue, lips, and pharynx. The respiratory system is also involved in producing basic speech sounds.

Articulation also involves other aspects of speech production, including intonation and enunciation of specific sounds. Difficulties with articulation are sometimes associated with language-based learning disorders, or with speech-language disabilities.

A person who has difficulty pronouncing certain sounds may have a speech disorder, rather than a specific language disorder. In order to produce speech, a person must coordinate muscle movement, including the respiratory system and larynx. Articulation skills and remediation of speech disorders are addressed by a SPEECH/LANGUAGE SPECIALIST.

articulatory phonetics The study and classification of speech sounds based on the way they are produced by the vocal cords.

Asperger's syndrome (Asperger disorder) A condition characterized by sustained problems with social interactions and social relatedness, and the development of restricted, repetitive patterns of interests, activities, and behaviors. The disorder was named after Hans Asperger, a Viennese pediatrician who first documented this cluster of characteristics in the 1940s.

It is believed to be a milder variant of AUTISM, but without the delays in cognitive or language development. In 1994, Asperger's was first classified as a PERVASIVE DEVELOPMENTAL DISORDER (a designation that includes AUTISTIC DISORDER).

Many children with pervasive developmental disorders such as Asperger's syndrome also meet the diagnostic criteria for ATTENTION DEFICIT HYPERACTIVITY DISORDER (ADHD). However, ADHD should not be diagnosed when there is Asperger's, since all the ADHD symptoms can be attributed to the other condition. Clinicians who overlook other symptoms of Asperger's tend to diagnose these children as having ADHD.

As with many LEARNING DISORDERS, Asperger's is believed to be more common in males, although more research needs to be done to understand its genetic origins. According to the National Institutes of Health, Asperger's syndrome occurs in one out of every 500 Americans—more often than multiple sclerosis, DOWN SYNDROME, or cystic fibrosis. It is estimated that more than 400,000 families are affected by this condition.

While biological factors are of crucial importance in the etiology of autism, so far brain imaging studies with Asperger's cases have found no consistent pattern or evidence of any type of lesion.

Associated medical conditions such as FRAGILE-X SYNDROME, tuberous sclerosis, neurofibromatosis, and hypothyroidism (sluggish thyroid) are less common in Asperger's disorder than in classical autism. Therefore, scientists suspect there may be fewer major physical brain problems associated with Asperger's than with autism.

Symptoms and Diagnostic Path

Children have normal IQ (many are highly intelligent), and often there are no obvious delays in language or cognitive development, or in age-appropriate self-help skills. While these individuals possess attention deficits, problems with organization, and an uneven profile of skills, they usually have average and sometimes gifted intelligence.

Individuals with Asperger's syndrome typically have problems with social situations and in developing peer relationships. They may have noticeable difficulty with nonverbal communication and an impaired use of social gestures, facial expressions, and eye contact. There may be certain repetitive behaviors or rituals. Although grammatical, speech is peculiar due to abnormal inflection and repetition. Clumsiness is prominent both in speech and physical movements.

Individuals with this disorder also usually have a limited area of interest that usually excludes more age-appropriate, common interests. Some examples of these single-minded obsessions may include cars, trains, Russian literature, door knobs, hinges, astronomy, or history.

Asperger's vs. Autism When compared to autism, Asperger's syndrome usually appears later in life, with less severe social and communication problems. Clumsiness and single-minded interests are more common, and verbal IQ is usually higher than performance IQ (in autism, the reverse is usually true). The prognosis is usually more positive than for autism.

Treatment Options and Outlook

While there is no cure, early intervention has been proven to be effective. The need for academic and social supports increases through the school years, and by adolescence many children develop symptoms of DEPRESSION and ANXIETY. It is important to continue supports into adulthood to make sure that affected adults can lead productive lives.

Symptoms can be managed using individual psychotherapy to help the individual process the feelings aroused by being socially handicapped. Other treatments may include parent education and training, BEHAVIORAL MODIFICATION, social skills training, educational interventions, and medication. Drug therapy may include

- hyperactivity, inattention, and impulsivity: stimulants such as METHYLPHENIDATE, DEXTROAMPHETAMINE, methamphetamine, pemoline, clonidine, and tricyclic antidepressants (desipramine, nortriptyline)
- irritability and aggression: mood stabilizers (valproate, carbamazepine, lithium), beta blockers (nadolol, propranolol), neuroleptics (risperidone, haloperidol)
- preoccupations, rituals, and compulsions: antidepressants (fluvoxamine, fluoxetine, clomipramine)
- anxiety: antidepressants (sertraline, fluoxetine, imipramine, clomipramine, nortriptyline)

assessment A general term that covers a wide range of activities, instruments, and approaches involved in evaluating prior performance, describing present abilities and behaviors, and predicting future performance and behaviors. "Assessment" differs from "testing," which reflects performance on particular tasks at a specific time. Instead, assessment interprets overall patterns and relationships among testing results and other observations.

In the areas of LEARNING DISABILITIES and SPECIAL EDUCATION, assessment generally has two purposes. The first is to classify the nature of the problems an individual is experiencing and to provide a diagnosis. The second involves planning treatment, including instruction, social and behavioral interventions, and medications (in the case of ATTENTION DEFICIT HYPERACTIVITY DISORDER [ADHD]).

Traditional assessment procedures tend to focus on STANDARDIZED TESTS including tests of ability and tests of achievement. A typical school assessment might include an intelligence test (such as the WECHSLER INTELLIGENCE SCALE FOR CHILDREN—III or STANFORD-BINET INTELLIGENCE SCALE) and ACHIEVEMENT TESTS (such as the WOODCOCK-JOHNSON battery).

The typical assessment in special education includes individual tests measuring intelligence, achievement, behavior and adaptive behavior. Other assessments may be added depending on the nature of the child's disability.

A neuropsychological assessment might include a more comprehensive group of tests designed to identify functioning in specific areas such as memory or visual processing. In most cases, such standardized testing is used together with case histories, interviews, and details on actual performance at school, among friends, and at home. In some cases, assessment may also incorporate testing in specific areas of brain function. Assessment may also include testing designed to identify emotional, psychological, and personality factors that may be involved in learning difficulties.

The field of assessment is in a state of continuous development in order to discover more accurate methods of evaluating performance and behavior. Portfolios may be used as an alternative to assessing a student's academic achievement. Evaluators may assess an individual's ability to learn—rather than test for what the person already knows. Finally, contemporary assessment may also focus on an individual's abilities in the areas of strategy development and problem solving.

Types of Assessment

"Authentic assessment" is usually done at school, and places demands on the individual linked to the actual academic program, such as reading from a passage assigned in class and answering questions about it, giving a short speech about an experience or a topic assigned in class, or solving mathematics problems that have a real-life component.

"Performance assessment" is similar to authentic assessment; it is intended to evaluate how well a student performs in relationship to the actual school curriculum. This sort of assessment is typically part of a teacher's effort in evaluating students' performances on assigned tasks. Portfolio assessment is an increasingly common form of performance assessment, used to measure student progress in reading, writing, and mathematics over time. Portfolio assessment involves collected multiple samples of a student's work over time, keyed to the specific objectives of the curriculum and derived from a wide range of different activities.

"Dynamic assessment" evaluates what students already know plus their ability to learn new skills, strategies, and information. For this, a student might be given, as a baseline, a set of problems to assess initial performance, followed by a similar set of problems after instruction. Assessment of this sort may help to more accurately predict a student's potential to learn and to be successful.

Assessment of problem-solving and strategy development is related to dynamic assessment in that it attempts to evaluate a student's ability to learn, rather than to create a static picture of what a student already knows. Assessment of this sort attempts to identify student's ability to reflect on their own knowledge and strategies, and to develop new strategies and problem-solving procedures based on this. Students who performs well on an assessment of this sort, but performs poorly on more standard or traditional assessment measures, may be demonstrating a gap between the quality of their school experience and their actual potential to learn and succeed. Likewise, a student who has significant problems in assessment of this sort may require much more extensive and focused school interventions.

In general, assessment is an area in which the field of learning disabilities is continuing to change and develop. New developments in this area are likely to include continued questioning of the usefulness of intelligence testing and the discrepancy formula for defining learning disabilities. There will be greater focus on both traditional testing and on more performance-based approaches to measuring a student's actual academic capabilities.

assistive technology Any technology that enables an individual with a LEARNING DISABILITY to compensate for specific deficits. This includes a broad scope of learning tools ranging from the use of tape recorders to voice-activated software programs. Since the onset of the age of computers, assistive technology often refers to computer technology.

Computers are extremely useful to everyone, but they are especially important to people with learning disabilities because they offer powerful and flexible tools for reading and writing. For example, computers allow individuals to find ways to become independent learners. At any point in the writing process, computer software programs can provide the help that once was provided by a teacher, tutor, or parent.

However, not all uses of technology are helpful for everyone. With a wide range of ever-changing products in the market, one of the hardest tasks is to link the most effective technology with an individual's learning profile.

Many people see assistive technology as a way of circumventing deficits; for example, a student with writing problems that make taking notes in class virtually impossible may be allowed to tape the lecture as a way of bypassing this area of weakness. After all, the goal is to learn the information from the lecture—not to improve note-taking skills. This is what is referred to as a *compensatory approach.*

In a *remedial approach,* technology is used to directly address skill deficits. For example, in this approach the same person who relied on taped lectures could use a keyboarding program to improve note-taking skills.

Furthermore, the two approaches are not necessarily mutually exclusive. In many cases, the use of assistive technology to bypass a problem also improves the area of weakness at the same time. For example, students who tape a lecture may be sketching written notes (by pencil or keyboard) at the same time. Later, students may revisit the tape to supplement written notes, while improving writing skills in class.

The chart on page 18 outlines some of the most commonly used assistive technologies.

Because computers allow users to control, customize, and manipulate the learning environment, more so than static text environments, assistive technology offers flexibility and options to individuals with learning disabilities. While it is not the only answer, the explosion in modern technology has made an enormous impact on the lives of individuals with learning disabilities who have access to such tools.

FORMS OF ASSISTIVE TECHNOLOGY AND USES FOR INDIVIDUALS WITH LEARNING DISABILITIES

Technology	Strengths	Limitations	LD Characteristic
Word processing	• circumvents handwriting and spelling difficulties • easily allows deleting, inserting, moving, and copying text • allows information to be arranged graphically into charts and tables • can customize text by size, color, style	• does not directly improve spelling • spell check and grammar check can be confusing or distracting • spell/grammar check can give a false sense of accuracy	• writing aversion • handwriting difficulties • visual weakness • short-term memory weakness
Spell checker	• identify misspelled words • suggest correct spellings	• proper nouns are flagged as spelling errors • does not catch errors that are real words/homonyms • suggestions for severe mis-spellings are unhelpful	• poor spellers • some phonological awareness • strong visual discrimination
Word prediction	• limits the amount of keyboarding • used in conjunction with synthesized speech can be very useful in spelling • assist spelling/word choice during writing rather than during revisions	• can interrupt the flow of writing • visually similar words are displayed • severe spelling problems • eye-hand/keyboarding difficulties	• poor spellers • writing aversion
Voice recognition	• transcribes spoken language into text	• does not work with 100% accuracy	• oral language skills exceed written language
Outlining/Semantic webbing	• provides visual-graphic structures to show relationships among ideas • allows ideas to be "dumped" into the program and then organized later	• weak in terms of spelling/word processing functions	• visual learner • "big picture"learners • difficulties generating ideas • difficulties moving from generating ideas to starting papers
Screen reader/ Synthesized speech	• enables user to hear text on computer screen spoken aloud • uses a computer (synthe-sized) voice • scan or import text • improves decoding and fluency • some versions provide study skills and active reading support • allows users to hear what they have written • helps identify errors in syntax and spelling	• unnatural speech voices can be distracting • uses significant computer memory when used with other programs	• poor spellers • oral language skills exceed written language

Assistive Technology Act of 2004   This law replaced the Assistive Technology Act of 1998, which had replaced the Technology-Related Assistance for Individuals with Disabilities Act of 1988. Signed into law by President George W. Bush on October 25, 2004, it ensures the continued existence of a major source of funding for ASSISTIVE TECHNOLOGY. The goal of the act is to provide assistive technology to allow people with disabilities to more fully participate in education, jobs, and daily activities equally with other members of their communities.

Under the law, each U.S. state and territory receives a grant to fund an Assistive Technology Act Project (ATAP). These projects provide services to persons with disabilities for their entire life span, as well as to their families or guardians, service providers, and agencies and other entities that are involved in providing services such as education and employment to persons with disabilities.

Although the program has been on the books for some time, the new legislation makes significant strides toward providing appropriate assistive technology to every person with a disability who needs it. Up until now, the law expired each year unless its authorization was renewed, which constantly put its existence into jeopardy. This new law eliminates these so-called sunset provisions, representing the federal government's commitment to people with disabilities. In the past, projects were created on a state-by-state basis, which meant that services and organization varied greatly. The new law is more consistent.

The law created 56 ATAPs to provide a place where consumers can go for demonstrations of products they may be interested in buying, along with low-cost loans for the purchase, information, and referral on these products. For example, the state ATAP is the place to go to compare prices before buying a screen magnifier, adapted personal digital assistant, or braille printer. If traveling to the location of the ATAP is a problem, arrangements can be made to ship equipment to the person's home for a trial period. States also must provide alternative financing for the purchase or lease of equipment, training and technical support for equipment, short-term loans of equipment, referrals for repairs and servicing of equipment, demonstration of equipment, and referrals for evaluation and assessment of assistive technology. Although various states were providing some of these services already, under the new legislation, all states need to provide all of them in some manner.

astereognosis   Deficient ability to recognize objects by touch alone, including the inability to discriminate shape, texture, weight, and size of objects. Astereognosis often occurs with lesions in the PARIETAL LOBE of the brain.

ataxia   The complete or partial inability to control or coordinate body movements; this may include an unsteady gait and poor coordination of speech. Ataxia is caused by a group of rare, hereditary diseases known as the hereditary ataxias, which vary in age of onset and severity of symptoms. They are generally characterized by breakdown of the CEREBELLUM, brain stem, and spinal cord.

Another type of ataxia (nongenetic ataxia) can be acquired as a result of multiple sclerosis, alcoholism, or other diseases.

There is no direct relationship between ataxia and LEARNING DISABILITIES, although DEVELOPMENTAL DISABILITIES are common with the problem. Ongoing evaluation, diagnosis, and educational assessment are necessary. In acquired ataxia, there may be specific treatments for the underlying diseases.

atomoxetine (Strattera)   The first and only nonstimulant medication approved by the U.S. Food and Drug Administration (FDA) for the treatment of ATTENTION DEFICIT HYPERACTIVITY DISORDER (ADHD) in children, adolescents, and adults. Strattera is a norepinephrine reuptake inhibitor, a class of ADHD treatment that works differently from other ADHD medications currently available.

Scientists suspect Strattera reduces ADHD symptoms by blocking or slowing the reabsorption of norepinephrine, a chemical in the brain considered important in regulating attention, impulsivity, and activity levels. Blocking the reabsorption of norepinephrine keeps more of this substance at work in the spaces between neurons in the brain. Improved efficiency in the norepinephrine system is associated with improvement in symptoms of ADHD.

Strattera provides full-day relief of ADHD symptoms from school or work through family time, when taken as directed once or twice a day. It takes up to a month before the effects of this medication become effective. It is important to understand this delay will occur so parents do not stop the drug when there is no effect after one or two doses.

In each of six clinical trials, Strattera worked better than placebo in reducing the symptoms of ADHD—including hyperactivity, impulsivity, and inattention—in children, adolescents, and adults. Both Strattera and older treatments, such as METHYLPHENIDATE (the active ingredient in Ritalin and Concerta), are effective in treating ADHD. However, Strattera is the first FDA-approved treatment for ADHD that is not a stimulant nor a controlled substance under the Controlled Substance Act. Research has shown that Strattera does not have abuse potential because it does not have stimulant effects on the brain. To date, there is no known black-market demand for Strattera. As a noncontrolled substance, Strattera can be given as a free physician samples and can be refilled over the phone.

Side Effects

The most common side effects in children and adolescents are temporary weight loss, upset stomach, decreased appetite, nausea and vomiting, dizziness, fatigue, and mood swings. In adults, the most common side effects are constipation, dry mouth, nausea, decreased appetite, dizziness, problems sleeping, sexual side effects, problems urinating, and menstrual cramps.

Because of two reports of severe liver injury after taking Strattera among several million patients, in December 2004 manufacturer Eli Lilly added a warning in bold type to Strattera's product label indicating that the drug should be discontinued in patients with jaundice (yellowing of the skin or whites of the eyes) or laboratory evidence of liver injury. Both patients recovered with normal liver function after discontinuing the medication. The 6,000 patients taking Strattera in clinical trials experienced no evidence of liver injury.

Strattera should not be taken at the same time as, or within two weeks of taking a monoamine oxidase inhibitor (MAOI); it should not be taken by patients with narrow angle glaucoma or who abuse ALCOHOL. Patients with a history of high or low blood pressure, increased heart rate, or any heart or blood vessel disease should tell their doctor before taking Strattera.

This medication has not been tested in children less than six years of age or in geriatric patients.

attention   The focus of consciousness on something in the environment, or on a sensation or an idea. Attention includes a number of elements that are essential to all activities, including

- arousal: being ready to receive stimuli
- vigilance: being able to select stimuli from those presented over a period of time
- persistence or continuity: being able to sustain a mental effort and select stimuli that are presented often
- monitoring: checking for and correcting errors

The length of time in which a child can pay attention to something (the attention span) increases with age, interest, and intelligence level.

Breakdowns in these different elements can cause a variety of problems. A breakdown in vigilance, for example, might cause someone to select or focus on the wrong details. A breakdown in monitoring might lead to repeated careless errors. Persistence or continuity is necessary for a complex task to be completed.

attention deficit disorder with or without hyperactivity   The former term used to define ATTENTION DEFICIT HYPERACTIVITY DISORDER, used in the *Diagnostic and Statistical Manual of Mental Disorders—Third Edition, Revised (DSM-III-R)*. It was replaced by the term *ADHD*, used in the current *DSM-IV-TR*.

attention deficit hyperactivity disorder (ADHD)   A condition that may occur in both children and adults who consistently display INATTENTION, HYPERACTIVITY, and IMPULSIVITY. ADHD is a disorder featuring problems in two major areas: impulse control and ability to focus attention on tasks.

People who are inattentive may have trouble keeping their mind focused, and may get bored with a task after just a few minutes. Those who are hyperactive seem to feel restless and are constantly in motion, finding it hard to sit still. People who are impulsive have a problem curbing their immediate reactions and tend to act before they think. Other symptoms may include problems in school, with friends, and with behavior.

ADHD and LEARNING DISABILITIES frequently occur together, but they are not the same. Learning disabilities include difficulty with receiving, organizing, understanding, remembering, and offering information. ADHD involves difficulty with paying attention to information. Between 10 percent and 20 percent of all school-age children have learning disabilities. Between 3 percent and 5 percent of all school-age children have ADHD, (one out of 20) making it the most common childhood neurobehavioral disorder.

Once thought to be a disorder primarily affecting young hyperactive boys, ADHD is both more complicated and more pervasive. In particular, experts now know that children do not typically "outgrow" the condition, nor does it affect only males. In the past, gender ratio were given at 3 to 1 males to females, but recent research suggests the ratio is nearly equal.

ADHD is presumed to be a problem with brain function. Since the early 1990s, scientists have worked to pinpoint the differences found in brain scans between the normal brain and the ADHD brain.

Most experts believe that there may be several causes of ADHD, including genetic problems, abnormal brain structure, or low levels of certain brain chemicals. Stress in parenting or life situations can make ADHD worse, but they do not cause the disorder.

Structural differences Computer imaging of the brain structure of people with ADHD sometimes reveals areas of shrunken size (especially in the part of the brain called the BASAL GANGLIA) and in slowed brain activity in the frontal lobes. The basal ganglia are involved in routine behaviors, and the frontal lobes are involved in planning and organizing, attention, impulse control, and inhibition of responses to sensory stimulation. In some studies, scientists have identified differences in brain scans between normal students and those

with ADHD, specifically located in the frontal lobe and the basal ganglia, which are about 10 percent smaller and less active in children with ADHD. Over the past few years, studies have suggested that boys with ADHD tend to have more symmetrical brains than boys without the condition in three areas—the prefrontal cortex, caudate nucleus, and the globus pallidus. The prefrontal cortex is believed to be the part of the brain that acts as a command center, and the other two sections help translate those commands into actions.

Other research suggests that there is an abnormal increase of activity in the front lobe and nearby areas that help to control voluntary action. In one study, boys with ADHD worked harder to control their impulses than boys without ADHD. When the boys with ADHD were given Ritalin (a drug often used to treat ADHD), this abnormal activity quieted down. Ritalin did not have any effect in the boys without ADHD, which also suggests that Ritalin may act differently on the brains of ADHD children compared to unaffected students.

Experts also suspect that the tendency toward ADHD may be inherited in many cases.

Heredity More than 20 genetic studies have shown evidence that this disorder is a neurological condition caused by a combination of genetic and environmental factors. At least three separate yet interactive brain regions appear to be associated with the condition.

Research also clearly indicates that ADHD tends to run in families. ADHD is a complex condition that is probably the result of multiple interacting genes. Recently published data indicate that the child of an adult with ADHD has approximately a 25 percent chance of also having ADHD. There are also indications that the type of ADHD that persists into adulthood is more highly genetic than the type that diminishes in childhood. A family history of alcoholism and other mood disorders also seems to be associated with an increased risk of ADHD. This may imply some type of genetic link between these disorders.

Brain chemicals Chemical imbalances (especially with the chemical neurotransmitter DOPAMINE) also may play a role in the development of ADHD. Dopamine is involved in controlling emotions and reactions, concentrating, reasoning, and coordinating movement. An abnormally low level of dopamine can cause inattention, impulsiveness, and hyperactivity—the three primary symptoms of ADHD.

Moreover, the fact that stimulants (such as Ritalin) increase the levels of dopamine and other brain chemicals and also ease ADHD symptoms suggests that complex interactions between these chemicals are involved in ADHD.

Fetal damage   A pregnant woman who abuses ALCOHOL or drugs can cause poor motor and muscular development and sensory impairment; problems with learning, memory, attention, and problem solving; and problems with mental health and social interactions in her unborn baby.

Environmental toxins   Lead poisoning has been implicated in the development of ADHD, causing irritability, poor concentration, and distractedness. In particular, children raised in older homes with flaking lead-based paint have a high incidence of ADHD.

Coexisting conditions   Several other medical problems are associated with ADHD, although ADHD is not necessarily caused by them. Generally, children who experience brain damage during pregnancy, delivery, or immediately after birth are at a greater risk for ADHD. About half of children with pediatric autoimmune neuropsychiatric disorder associated with streptococcal infections (PANDAS) have ADHD.

Between 20 to 30 percent of the 4 million children in the United States with learning disabilities also suffer from ADHD, according to the National Institute of Mental Health. Twenty percent to 40 percent of children with learning disabilities may be prone to recurrent defiance or malicious conduct and may be diagnosed with ADHD and either OPPOSITIONAL DEFIANT DISORDER (ODD) or CONDUCT DISORDER (CD). About 70 percent of people who suffer from involuntary twitching or spasms (tics) caused by TOURETTE'S SYNDROME also have ADHD, although Tourette's is not common among people with ADHD.

Symptoms and Diagnostic Path

The American Academy of Pediatricians recommends an ADHD evaluation if a child shows signs of school problems, underachievement, problems with family members or friends, or other behavioral problems. The assessment should include information obtained directly from parents, caregivers, teachers, or other school professionals about symptoms, when they began, and how much they affect the child's life. It also should include assessments of cognitive development, memory, and behavior.

Typically, ADHD is diagnosed between ages four and 10, but although it is a common childhood behavioral disorder, it can be difficult to diagnose and even harder to understand. Once viewed as a disorder of childhood primarily involving hyperactivity and the inability to pay attention, ADHD is now seen as a lifelong condition that may not include physical restlessness or hyperactive behavior at all. It also may be a source of unusual talents or giftedness in specific areas.

In recent years, there has been growing interest in ADHD as well as concern about possible overdiagnosis. In surveys among pediatricians and family physicians across the country, wide variations were found in diagnostic criteria and treatment methods for ADHD. Indeed, the definition and treatments of ADHD continue to evolve; over the past decade, there has been an extraordinary surge in the level of focus on ADHD and in the incidence of diagnosis among children and adults. It is likely that the present level of understanding of the disorder, as well as current methods of diagnosis and treatment, will continue to develop rapidly in the coming years.

ADHD is primarily diagnosed by a combination of individual and family history, individual behavioral assessments, and information about behavior from parents, teachers, and others. Some tests also contain factors for inattention, distractibility, and memory that can be affected by ADHD, and may contribute to a diagnosis.

Although ADHD is a common childhood behavioral disorder, it can be difficult to diagnose and even harder to understand. Many of the symptoms of ADHD are common in other conditions, and all of the symptoms occur at times in normal children. It is important to obtain a comprehensive evaluation from a qualified professional or team with experience in ADHD. This team may include a pediatrician, behavioral neurologist or psychiatrist, a clinical psychologist or school psychologist, and other less-specialized professionals such as a classroom teacher.

Unfortunately, some physicians "diagnose by prescription." That is, some physicians, when confronted by parents of children with objectionable behavior, will administer ADHD medication as a first step, without obtaining the other assessments discussed above, to see if it helps. Such practice has, in the opinion of many professionals, led to gross overdiagnosis of ADHD with undersocialized, aggressive, conduct-disordered children.

In addition, certain medical conditions such as hypothyroidism, juvenile diabetes, and seizure disorders must be ruled out as causes for the child's inability to pay attention. Increasingly, psychologists and physicians are reluctant to make the diagnosis alone, favoring a joint diagnosis after they have gathered all necessary medical, psychological, and behavioral information.

Formerly called "attention deficit disorder with or without hyperactivity," this disorder was renamed attention deficit hyperactivity disorder (ADHD) and includes three subtypes:

- *inattentive subtype* (formerly known as ATTENTION DEFICIT DISORDER, or ADD); easy distraction; an inability to pay attention to details; not following directions; losing or forgetting things like toys, notebooks, or homework
- *hyperactive-impulsive subtype* (formerly known as attention deficit hyperactivity disorder, or ADHD): fidgeting, squirming, blurting out answers before hearing the full question, difficulty waiting, running or jumping out of a seat when quiet behavior is expected
- *combined subtype* (the most common of the subtypes): signs from both of the subtypes above; also seen with or without hyperactivity

To be considered for a diagnosis of ADHD, a child must display maladaptive behaviors before age seven and the behaviors must last for at least six months. The behavior also must negatively affect at least two areas of a child's life (such as school, home, or friendships).

ADHD is diagnosed using the criteria in the *Diagnostic and Statistical Manual of Mental Disorders,* *Fourth Edition, Text Revision (DSM-IV-TR)*. Diagnostic criteria include

Inattention

- often fails to give close attention to details or makes careless mistakes in schoolwork, work, or other activities
- often has difficulty sustaining attention in tasks or play activities
- often does not seem to listen when spoken to directly
- often does not follow through on instructions and fails to finish schoolwork, chores, or duties in the workplace (not due to oppositional behavior or failure to understand instructions)
- often has difficulty organizing tasks and activities
- often avoids, dislikes, or is reluctant to engage in tasks that require sustained mental effort (such as schoolwork or homework)
- often loses things necessary for tasks or activities (such as toys, school assignments, pencils, books, or tools)
- is often easily distracted by extraneous stimuli
- is often forgetful in daily activities

Hyperactivity-Impulsivity

- often fidgets with hands or feet or squirms in seat
- often leaves seat in classroom or in other situations in which remaining seated is expected
- often runs about or climbs excessively in situations in which it is inappropriate (in adolescents or adults, may be limited to subjective feelings of restlessness)
- often has trouble playing or engaging in leisure activities quietly
- is often on the go
- talks excessively
- often blurts out answers before questions have been completed
- often has difficulty awaiting turn
- often interrupts or intrudes on others

Unfortunately, there are no reliable medical or psychological tests that can specifically reveal

ADHD at this time. Typically, tests for ADHD include measures to evaluate inattention, distractibility, and memory, along with tests to identify coexisting conditions (learning and language problems, aggression, disruptive behavior, DEPRESSION, or ANXIETY). This type of assessment should take at least one or two hours or more if the picture is complicated or unclear. The interview should include input from several people, including at least one parent.

It is also necessary to rule out other medical conditions, such as juvenile diabetes, thyroid disorder, and various neurological disorders that can cause ADHD-like symptoms.

The American Academy of Pediatrics developed guidelines for the diagnosis of ADHD designed for primary care physicians diagnosing ADHD in children aged six to 12 years. The guidelines include the following recommendations

- ADHD evaluations should be performed by the primary care clinician for children who show signs of school difficulties, academic underachievement, troublesome relationships with teachers, family members, and peers, and other behavioral problems.

- Questions to parents, either directly or through a previsit questionnaire, regarding school and behavioral issues may help alert physicians to possible ADHD.

- In diagnosing ADHD, physicians should use *DSM-IV-R* criteria, which require symptoms to be present in two or more of a child's settings, and that the symptoms interfere with the child's academic or social functioning for at least six months.

- The assessment of ADHD should include information obtained directly from parents or caregivers, as well as from a classroom teacher or other school professional, regarding the core symptoms of ADHD in various settings, the age of onset, duration of symptoms, and degree of functional impairment.

- Evaluation of a child with ADHD should also include assessment for coexisting conditions: learning and language problems, aggression, disruptive behavior, depression, or anxiety.

- Because as many as one-third of children diagnosed with ADHD also have a coexisting condition, other diagnostic tests (sometimes considered positive indicators for ADHD) have been reviewed and considered not effective. These tests include lead screening, tests for generalized resistance to thyroid hormone, and brain image studies.

Of course, all children sometimes have trouble paying attention, following directions, or being quiet, but for children with ADHD, these behaviors occur more frequently and are more disturbing.

Although the primary symptoms associated with ADHD are inattention, distractibility, and hyperactivity, some current researchers now recognize ADHD as a condition that primarily affects impulse controls that delay response to external or internal stimuli. The inability of impulse controls to delay response has a significant effect on memory and executive functions that involve holding verbal or visual information in mind in order to process it, reflecting on previous experience and learning to change behavior based on it, and reconstituting prior emotional states as a means to self-understanding and development.

Symptoms of ADHD may include failing to sustain attention while playing or performing tasks, difficulty completing tasks, difficulty with organization and planning, difficulty with impulsive behavior, such as blurting out answers, acting inappropriately, and/or fidgeting and restlessness. There may also be an inability to self-monitor or self-regulate behavior, and an impaired sense of the passage of time. Individuals with ADHD frequently have difficulty getting started, lose focus, and do not finish projects. Short- and long-term planning abilities may be greatly diminished, and disorganization can result from an inability to mindfully plan, act, and complete even the most basic tasks, such as cleaning a room. Individuals with ADHD often display risk-taking or conflict-seeking behaviors, and may exhibit poor judgment in social or interpersonal contexts.

At the same time, individuals with ADHD may also display paradoxical behaviors, such as the ability to focus intensively on a task over a period of time; very strong intellectual, verbal, and problem-solving skills; and extraordinary creativity. Characteristically, both types of behavior may occur within a single place, such as a class or work environment. Because the performance of individuals with ADHD can be strong, especially when they are very interested, subsequent failure to perform at the same level is often perceived as a lack of self-discipline or effort.

The symptoms for ADHD must be pervasive and long-lasting, usually appearing before age seven. Adults who are diagnosed late in life often report severe and lifelong problems in school, job, or with personal relationships. They may feel misunderstood and are frequently misdiagnosed, given the range of varying symptoms that can develop as a result of an attention disorder.

ADHD and Other Disorders As discussed previously, ADHD can coexist with a number of psychological conditions, including conduct disorders, mood disorders (such as depression), anxiety disorders, and IMPULSE CONTROL disorders (such as eating disorders and ALCOHOL abuse). Some children may be depressed as a result of having ADHD, whereas others may have a mood disorder that exists independently of ADHD. Nearly half of all children with ADHD also have OPPOSITIONAL DEFIANT DISORDER, characterized by stubbornness, outbursts of temper, and defiance.

Many children with ADHD also have a specific learning disability, which means that they might have trouble mastering language or other skills, such as math, reading, or handwriting. Although ADHD is not categorized as a learning disability, its interference with concentration and attention can make it even more difficult for a child to perform well in school. The issue of coexisting conditions makes diagnosis, treatment, and understanding of ADHD particularly complex.

Overdiagnosis Many experts believe that in some situations ADHD probably is overdiagnosed. On the other hand, many diagnoses of ADHD may be missed in situations where adequate medical services and evaluation are not available for a family. Approximately one out of 20 children in the United States would receive a diagnosis of ADHD using accepted, established diagnostic criteria.

Treatment Options and Outlook

There is no cure for ADHD, but a combined program of medication and behavioral therapy can help and is often prescribed to treat ADHD. With the advice and cooperation of a child's pediatrician, teachers, counselors, and family members, the child can have a normal life in spite of this disorder.

Medication For most children and adults with ADHD, medication is an important part of treatment that is not used to "control" behavior but to ease the symptoms of ADHD. The newest medication used to treat children with ADHD is ATOMOXETINE (Strattera), the first and only nonstimulant medication approved by the U.S. Food and Drug Administration (FDA) for the treatment of ADHD in children, adolescents, and adults. Strattera is a norepinephrine reuptake inhibitor, a class of ADHD treatment that works differently from other ADHD medications currently available. Because Strattera does not have stimulant effects on the brain, it does not have abuse potential, as other stimulant ADHD drugs do. More than 2 million prescriptions for Strattera have been filled since the FDA approved it in 2002. Strattera provides full-day relief of ADHD symptoms when taken as directed once or twice a day; typically, it takes about a month before it effectively manages ADHD symptoms.

Stimulants also appear to work by altering the levels of transmitters in the brain by which the different nerve cells communicate.

Between 70 and 80 percent of children with ADHD respond positively to these medications, with improvements in attention span, impulsivity, and behavior, especially in structured environments. Some children also demonstrate improvements in frustration tolerance, compliance, and even handwriting. Relationships with parents, peers, and teachers may also improve.

This type of medication also may be effective in adults who have ADHD. The reaction to these medications can be similar to that experienced by children with ADHD—a decrease in impulsivity and an increase in attention. Many ADHD adults treated with medication report that they are able to bring more control and organization to their lives. Other medications, such as antidepressants, can be helpful when depression and phobic, panic, anxiety and/or OBSESSIVE-COMPULSIVE DISORDERS are present.

The drugs usually include regular, fairly small doses of stimulants such as METHYLPHENIDATE

(Ritalin) DEXTROAMPHETAMINE, (Dexedrine, Dextrostat) (Adderall), or CYLERT (pemoline). While these drugs can be addictive in teenagers and adults, they do not seem to be addictive in children. Nine out of 10 children improve on one of these stimulants; so if one does not work, others are tried. It may seem strange to give stimulants to children with hyperactivity and attention deficit problems, but instead of making the child act out more, these drugs reduce the hyperactivity and increase the attention span. The drugs also help children with ADHD control their behavior. A child using these drugs actually becomes quieter and more attentive.

Sometimes, however, none of these medications work. In this case, some children may respond well to antihistamines usually prescribed for allergies, or to antidepressants such as Elavil, Prozac, Tofranil, or Norpramin. Clonidine, a drug normally used to treat high blood pressure, may ease some symptoms of ADHD. With any of these medications, adjusting the dosage for each child is vital for treating the symptoms of ADHD.

Side Effects

All ADHD drugs cause side effects, and most doctors believe the potential side effects should be carefully weighed against the benefits before prescribing drugs to children with ADHD.

While taking stimulant medications, some children may lose weight, have stomachaches or have less appetite, and temporarily grow more slowly. Others may have trouble falling asleep and become irritable. Some doctors worry that stimulants may worsen the symptoms of Tourette's syndrome, although recent research suggests this is not true. Many doctors believe if they carefully monitor a child's height, weight, and overall development, the benefits of medication far outweigh the potential side effects. Side effects that do occur can often be handled by reducing the dosage.

Unfortunately, the long-term effects of taking these drugs are not known. Cylert may cause more serious side effects and is therefore not considered to be a first-line medication for ADHD. Otherwise, side effects are usually dose related.

Drug Controversy In particular, the use of stimulants for children with ADHD (especially Ritalin) is not without controversy, which is why

Strattera became popular so quickly. Critics worry that Ritalin and other stimulant drugs are prescribed unnecessarily for too many children, since many things—including anxiety, depression, allergies, seizures, problems at home or school—can make children seem overactive, impulsive, or inattentive. They argue that many children who do not have ADHD are drugged anyway as a way to control disruptive behaviors.

Critics also worry that so many of the nation's children are given these drugs without any real understanding of the future side effects. Although Ritalin is one of the most commonly prescribed drugs for children, there are concerns about its long-term effects.

There are no studies on children who have taken Ritalin for more than 14 months. Ritalin affects the brain in a way very similar to cocaine, one of the most addictive substances known. Critics worry that the child who takes Ritalin may be more likely to use illegal drugs in the future, or that he or she might be more likely to smoke as an adult. These concerns are fueled by research showing that rats who were exposed to stimulants were more likely to choose cocaine, suggesting that early exposure to some drugs may make a person more likely to abuse drugs in the future. However, the data on whether there is a link between Ritalin and later substance abuse are controversial, and some researchers insist that ADHD children are not more likely to use drugs of any type later in life.

Behavioral Treatment Many experts believe that the best way to manage the symptoms of ADHD is to combine drug treatment with BEHAVIORAL MODIFICATION. Although medication can help to control some of the behavior problems that may have led to family turmoil, more often there are other aspects of a child's problem that medication will not affect.

Even though ADHD primarily affects a person's behavior, the simple fact of having ADHD can trigger serious emotional problems as well. Some of these children have very few experiences that build their sense of worth and competence. If they are hyperactive, they are often punished for being disruptive. If they are too disorganized and unfocused to complete tasks, they may be branded "lazy." If they are impulsive, shove classmates, and interrupt, they may lose friends. If they are unlucky enough to have a related conduct disorder, they may get in trouble at school or with the police.

The daily frustrations that are a part of having ADHD can make people feel abnormal or stupid. In many cases, the cycle of frustration and anger has persisted for so long that it may take years to alleviate.

For this reason, parents and children may need special help to develop techniques to manage behavior patterns that have become ingrained. In such cases, mental health professionals can help the child and family develop new attitudes and ways of relating to each other.

Behavior treatments include coaching, a process of individual support that focuses on understanding maladaptive patterns of behavior, identifying goals and strategies for change, and providing consistent reinforcement and feedback. For younger children, such an approach may involve behavioral rating scales, consistent feedback, and reinforcement for positive behavioral change. For adults, the approach may focus on identifying and describing goals and strategies. In either case, focusing on the role of individual responsibility and choice is a vital component, as is developing a consistent pattern of feedback and reinforcement.

In individual counseling, the therapist helps children or adults with ADHD learn to feel better about themselves. The therapist can also help people with ADHD identify and build on their strengths, cope with daily problems, and control their attention and aggression.

In group counseling, people learn that they are not alone in their frustration and that others want to help. Sometimes only the child with ADHD needs counseling, but often the entire family can benefit from support. If the child is young, parents can learn techniques for coping with and improving their child's behavior.

Several intervention approaches are available and different therapists tend to prefer one approach or another. Knowing something about the various types of interventions makes it easier for families to choose the best therapist for their own situation.

In psychotherapy, patients talk with the therapist about their thoughts and feelings, explore problem behaviors, and learn different ways to handle their emotions. If someone who has ADHD wants to gain control of symptoms more directly, more direct kinds of intervention are available.

Cognitive-behavioral therapy helps people directly change their behavior instead of concentrating only on understanding their feelings and actions. The therapist may help an individual learn to think through tasks and to organize work, or may encourage new behavior by giving praise each time the person acts in the desired way. A cognitive-behavioral therapist can use these techniques to help an ADHD child learn to control his fighting, or an impulsive teenager to think before speaking.

Social skills training can help children learn new behaviors by watching the therapist model appropriate behavior, like waiting for a turn, sharing toys, or responding to a bully.

Support groups can also be helpful, linking people who have common concerns. Many adults with ADHD and parents of children with ADHD find it useful to join a local or national support group. Many groups deal with issues of children's disorders. Members of support groups share frustrations and success, and provide referrals.

Because ADHD affects all aspects of a child's home and school life, experts recommend parent education and support groups to help family members learn how to help the child cope with frustrations, organize environments, and develop problem-solving skills. Special parenting skills are often needed because children with ADHD may not respond as well to typical parenting practices, especially punishment. Instead, children with ADHD should learn how to reinforce their positive behaviors themselves, and learn how to solve problems. Children who take medications and practice these behavior techniques do better than those who rely on medication alone.

Parenting skills training, offered by therapists or in special classes, gives parents tools and techniques for managing their child's behavior. One such technique is the use of "time out" when the child becomes too unruly or out of control. During time outs, the child is removed from the agitating situation and sits alone quietly for a short time to calm down. Parents may also be taught to give the child quality time each day, in which they share a relaxed activity. During this time together, the parent looks for opportunities to point out what the child is doing right and to praise strengths and abilities. An effective way to modify a child's behavior is through a system of rewards and penalties. The parents (or teacher) identify a few desirable behaviors that they want to encourage in the child, such as asking for a toy politely. The child is told exactly what is expected in order to earn a small reward, which is given when he or she performs the desired behavior. The goal is to help children learn to control their own behavior and to choose the more desired behavior. The technique works well with all children, although children with ADHD may need more frequent rewards.

Parents also may learn to structure situations in ways that will allow their child to succeed. If a child is easily overstimulated, parents may try allowing only one or two playmates at a time. If the child has trouble completing tasks, parents may help the child divide a large task into small steps, then praise the child as each step is completed.

Stress management methods such as meditation, relaxation techniques, and exercise can increase the parents' tolerance for frustration, enabling them to respond more calmly to their child's behavior.

Other behavioral treatments that may be helpful in treating children with ADHD include play therapy and special physical exercise.

Although play therapy may help a child who has fears and anxieties, these are not the key problems among most ADHD children. Special physical exercises usually try to boost coordination and increase a child's ability to handle activities that can be overstimulating. Most ADHD children do have problems in these areas, but this is not the cause of ADHD. While these exercises may help, they seem to work mostly because they get parents to pay more attention to the child, which boosts self-esteem.

Controversial Treatments   In addition to more traditional treatments, there are a range of controversial therapies that may sound reasonable. Some come with glowing reports, and a few are outright quackery. Some are developed by reputable doctors or specialists but, when tested scientifically, results cannot be proven.

One of the most widely used controversial treatments is a special diet based on the unproven idea that certain foods cause ADHD. These diets look at specific groups of foods, such as additives, sugar, and foods to which children are commonly allergic, such as corn, nuts, chocolate, shellfish, or wheat. While there is scientific evidence that these diets do not work, many parents strongly believe they help. Some of these diets are healthy and will not hurt, but most experts agree that no special diet alone can solve the problems of ADHD and should not be used as the only treatment for a child's behavior.

Other types of treatment that have not been shown scientifically to be effective in treating the majority of children or adults with ADHD include

- biofeedback
- allergy treatments
- drug treatments for inner-ear problems
- megadoses of vitamins
- chiropractic treatments
- yeast infection treatment
- eye training or special colored glasses

Education

ADHD occurs in children with all levels of intelligence, yet even bright or gifted children with ADHD may experience school failure. Despite their natural ability, problems with inattentiveness, impulsivity, and hyperactivity often lead to poor grades, retention, suspension, and expulsion. Without proper diagnosis, accommodations, and intervention, children with ADHD are more likely to experience negative consequences.

Children suspected of having ADHD must be evaluated at the school's expense and, if found to be eligible, provided services under either of two federal laws, the INDIVIDUALS WITH DISABILITIES EDUCATION IMPROVEMENT ACT (IDEIA) Part B, and Section 504 of the REHABILITATION ACT OF 1973. These two laws guarantee children with ADHD a free and appropriate public education. Both laws also require that children with disabilities be educated, to the maximum extent appropriate, with children who do not have disabilities. Because there are different criteria for eligibility, different services available, different procedures for implementing the laws, and different procedural safeguards, it is important for parents, educators, clinicians, and advocates to be well aware of the variations among these laws and to be fully informed about their respective advantages and disadvantages.

The most substantial difference between these two laws is that eligibility for IDEIA mandates that a child have a disability requiring special education services, while eligibility for Section 504 may occur when the child needs special education or related services. Because of this distinction, children covered under Section 504 include those who typically either have less severe disabilities than those covered under IDEIA, or have disabilities that do not neatly fit within the categories of eligibility under IDEIA. Most students classified as ADHD are served under the Rehabilitation Act.

Some of the services that could be provided to eligible children include modified instructions, assignments, and testing; help from a classroom aide or a special education teacher; ASSISTIVE TECHNOLOGY; behavior management; and the development of a behavioral intervention plan.

Adjustments may be necessary for a child with ADHD in the classroom, such as having the child sit in front of the room so as to help him pay better attention. The teacher can try to limit open spaces in the classroom, which may encourage hyperactive behaviors. Teachers should provide clear instructions and have the child write down homework assignments in a notebook. Both parent and teacher should keep oral instructions brief and provide written instructions for tasks that involve many steps.

Formal feedback (such as a star chart) can be used to reinforce positive behaviors and progress even if it falls a little short of the goal. The child should work hard on organization, establishing daily checklists.

Parents and teachers also can help the child with ADHD

- control impulses: urge the child to slow down when answering questions and to check homework before turning it in
- foster self-esteem: the child should be encouraged and not be asked to perform a task in public that is too difficult

- design a specific behavior program: focus it on a few unacceptable behaviors with clear and consistent consequences. These consequences should not be publicly humiliating (hand signals can warn a child that his or her behavior is inappropriate)
- encourage active learning: have the child underline important passages in his or her school books as he or she reads and to take notes in class

Even when suspended or expelled, children covered by IDEIA are still entitled to education services that meet the standards of a free appropriate education. Parents can request an impartial due-process hearing when they disagree with a school's decision.

Under a separate provision, a child can remain in the then-current educational placement until all administrative proceedings are concluded (unless the child has brought a weapon or drugs to school, or is proven to be substantially likely to harm himself, herself, or others).

If a child's behavior interferes with learning, IDEIA requires that a functional behavior analysis be conducted and a positive behavior plan be developed. IDEIA prohibits schools from suspending such a child for more than 10 days or expelling students whose behavior results from their disability, unless drugs or weapons are involved or the child is a danger to himself, herself, or others.

attention deficit hyperactivity disorder in adults

ADHD has been recognized and treated in children for almost a century, but only in the last few decades have experts realized that the condition often persists into adulthood. In fact, up to 4 percent of children diagnosed with ADHD will continue to have symptoms that significantly interfere with school, work, or social functioning throughout their adult lives.

ADHD in adults is sometimes viewed as a "hidden disorder" because the symptoms are often concealed by problems with relationships, organization, mood, substance abuse, or employment.

Symptoms and Diagnostic Path

Symptoms in adult may be different from those in children. Childhood symptoms of hyperactivity may turn into feelings of being overwhelmed or talking too much in adulthood. Lack of attention may evolve into an inability to focus on everyday tasks. Impulsive children may grow into adults who are quick to anger, who have rude thoughts, and who are often irritable.

To be diagnosed with ADHD as an adult, an individual may

- fail to pay close attention to details
- make careless mistakes at work
- fidget or squirm
- have trouble paying attention in tasks or fun activities
- feel restless
- not follow through on instructions and fail to finish work
- have problems engaging in leisure activities quietly
- have trouble organizing activities
- feel "on the go" or "driven by a motor"
- avoid, dislike, or be reluctant to perform work that requires sustained mental effort
- talk excessively
- lose things
- blurt out answers before questions have been completed
- be easily distracted
- be impatient
- be forgetful in daily duties
- interrupt others

Since these symptoms are common to many other psychiatric and medical conditions, adults should never try to diagnose themselves but should seek a comprehensive evaluation from a qualified professional or a team with experience in ADHD. This team may include a behavioral neurologist or psychiatrist, a clinical psychologist or an educational psychologist. Evaluation for ADHD should include a comprehensive clinical interview surveying ADHD symptoms, and a comprehensive history of health, school, work, and mental problems, including any medications, social adjustment, and general day-to-day function. This should not simply be a brief, sur-

face-level exam, but an in-depth survey that should require at least one or two hours. Ideally, the interview should rely on several people, including a parent or significant other, if possible. It is also imperative that the clinician rule out other psychiatric diagnoses that may better explain symptoms.

A proper diagnosis can help adults better understand their problems and the reasons for lifelong symptoms. Proper diagnosis and effective treatment can improve self-esteem, job performance, and social relationships. Many adults with ADHD are offered protection under the AMERICANS WITH DISABILITIES ACT of 1990, which prohibits job discrimination for anyone with a physical or mental impairment that substantially limits one or more major life activities, such as school and job.

Treatment Options and Outlook

Although there is no cure, treatment can help an adult manage symptoms. The best treatment plan combines medication, education, and psychotherapy. Several studies suggest that counseling can be effective in treating adults with ADHD, helping the patient identify how the disability might be linked to a history of below-average performance and trouble in personal relationships. Therapy also can help control mood swings, stabilize relationships, and alleviate guilt and discouragement. This long-term combined treatment approach can help affected adults lead more satisfactory and productive lives.

attention disorders   See ATTENTION DEFICIT HYPERACTIVITY DISORDER.

attention span   A phrase commonly used to refer to a person's ability to sustain attention, maintaining focus and alertness over a period of time. It is also referred to as sustained attention. Individuals with ADHD are often seen as having a "short attention span," although in reality such individuals may be capable of sustained attention when presented with information that engages them. The breakdown in attention lies in the ability to distinguish between essential and nonessential information.

For example, Mary (who does not have ADHD) pays attention to the teacher's lesson, while Jim, who has ADHD, is noticing that the car driving by the school is making a strange sound and there is a grasshopper sitting on a rock outside the classroom window.

attribution The ways in which an individual understands the sources of success, difficulty, or failure. Often, people with LEARNING DISABILITIES attribute their successes and failures to factors they do not control, such as luck, the nature of the task, or their own inadequacies. By contrast, successful learners tend to attribute failure or success to their own level of effort and perseverance, and see themselves as having control over the outcomes of their work.

Attribution theory provides an approach to understanding the difficulties with motivation experienced by some people with learning problems, and also suggests that direct guidance in changing attribution styles may be helpful to those with learning disorders.

atypical learner A general term for a child who is different from the typical student in physical, intellectual, social, or emotional development, and who differs in mental characteristics, sensory abilities, communication abilities, or social behavior to the extent that SPECIAL EDUCATION services are required for the child to develop.

audiologist A licensed or certified specialist trained to identify and measure hearing loss and rehabilitate those with hearing and speech problems. Audiologists also can fit hearing aids. A child who is experiencing learning problems, especially in early grades, may see an audiologist in order to identify or rule out physiological factors.

Audiologists are trained to determine where hearing loss occurs, and to assess the effect of the loss on the ability to communicate. They also offer hearing aid evaluation and orientation, auditory training, training in speechreading techniques, and speech counseling. Audiologists are not physicians, and thus cannot treat infections or other ear diseases.

Audiologists work in a wide variety of settings, including universities, hospitals, schools, medical offices, and private practice. Since most school districts require some type of hearing screening tests for their students, audiologists serve as directors of these programs and work with teachers to help with special educational needs of students with hearing problems. In schools with special classes for students with hearing problems, audiologists equip and maintain classroom amplification systems.

audiology The study of hearing and hearing disorders. It involves identification and assessment of hearing, including the nature and degree of hearing loss and the rehabilitation of individuals with hearing disorders, with an emphasis on the communication skills.

auditory discrimination The ability to distinguish one speech sound from another, and to identify whether words are the same or different. People with problems in auditory discrimination have difficulty distinguishing between words that sound alike or differ in a single phoneme, such as between the words *bake* and *make* or *lick* and *like*. In order to read efficiently, a child must be able to distinguish one sound from another, especially those sounds that match letters in the alphabet.

Children with problems in this area may find it difficult to learn to read or understand spoken language, follow directions, and remember details. Problems with auditory discrimination may be part of a group of problems in the area of AUDITORY PERCEPTION that can have a significant effect on learning, especially in the area of reading development, and on academic and social performance.

In addition, a serious weakness in auditory discrimination in the classroom setting can be confused with inattention, as the child appears not to have listened closely.

See also PHONEMIC AWARENESS; INFORMATION PROCESSING DISORDERS.

auditory figure-ground discrimination The ability to pick out important sounds from background noise. Some disorders of attention are associated with auditory figure-ground discrimination difficulties. Children with problems in this area may find it harder to separate meaningful sounds from background noise. For example, a child may not be able to easily isolate the words spoken by a teacher standing at the front of the classroom in the presence of sounds made by children playing in the next room or the traffic outside.

Problems in this area may be physiological or may have to do with selective attention and filtering problems.

In order to be successful, a child with this condition will need to stay focused on auditory information in order to complete tasks.

See also FIGURE-GROUND DISCRIMINATION; FIGURE-GROUND DEFICITS.

auditory integration training (AIT) A somewhat controversial treatment method used to help people with auditory processing problems by reducing sensitivity to specific sound frequencies. The treatment is used to help people with AUTISM, DYSLEXIA, ATTENTION DEFICIT HYPERACTIVITY DISORDER (ADHD), vestibular processing problems, and reading problems. The training was developed by French otolaryngologist Guy Berard, who believes that abnormal auditory processing occurs when there is a discrepancy between how well someone hears different sound frequencies. For example, a person with auditory processing problems may be hypersensitive to the frequencies 2,000 and 8,000 hertz but hear all the other frequencies normally. Auditory processing problems seem to be linked to a defect in the brain stem's reticular activating system, responsible for regulating information from the auditory and vestibular systems and focusing on certain types of sensory input.

Researchers who believe that AIT is effective suspect that many children diagnosed with ADHD and other problems really have an AUDITORY PROCESSING DISORDER. This condition is particularly common if the child has SENSORY INTEGRATION DISORDER, such as touch sensitivity. AIT seems to help improve ATTENTION SPAN deficits, correct poor auditory discrimination skills, and improve the ability to follow directions, all of which are common problems in ADHD children.

Other experts believe that dyslexia may also affect the auditory processing system. Brain scans of dyslexic people show fewer neurons on the left side of the medial geniculate nucleus, one of the most important parts of the auditory system and an area that processes fast-changing sounds. AIT focuses on training the child to improve discrimination of this type of sound.

Other experts believe AIT helps poor readers by enhancing listening skills and the ability to perceive sounds more accurately, which may help the child hear the spoken sounds more clearly. In order to read an unfamiliar word, a child must understand that letter combinations represent spoken sounds. For example, he or she must understand the "it" sound in order to read "sit" or "hit" correctly. A child who has an auditory perceptual problem may not be able to read because he or she is not able to hear the "it" sound properly.

The Training Process
The first step in AIT is to schedule an audiogram to determine whether the person has auditory sensitivity. After the first five hours of treatment, the child will get a second audiogram to determine if the sensitivities are still present and whether new sensitivities have developed. A final audiogram is given after the completion of the listening sessions. The goal of the training is that all frequencies should be perceived equally well, and the sensitivities should be eliminated.

The training begins with twice-a-day, 30-minute sessions for 10 days. During the first five hours of training, each ear receives the same sound-level input. For children with a speech or hearing impairment, the sound level is reduced in the left ear during the second five hours of training.

The left hemisphere is largely responsible for processing speech and language; since the right ear is connected more directly to the left hemisphere, proponents believe that a higher sound level in the right ear will stimulate the left hemisphere. Using a cassette or CD player, the child listens to unpredictable, modulated music that has been specially processed to stimulate the reticular activating system. If the child is sensitive to certain frequencies, these frequencies are filtered out. The special music can train the child to filter out unimportant sounds in order to focus on certain frequencies. It works by allowing a sound-sensitive child to adapt to sounds. Adaptation is a built-in mechanism, which after continued exposure to a stimulus reduces the perception of that stimulus. This results in better sound discrimination. Because the vestibular system is also integrated in this part of the brain, the unique sounds used in AIT also may produce better posture, balance, and spatial orientation.

To be effective, the music used for AIT should cover a wide range of frequencies and have a good tempo or beat. Most music does not meet these criteria. AIT experts have reviewed more than 1,000 CDs and created a list of 70 CDs—mostly jazz, pop, reggae, and contemporary rock—that can be used in AIT training. Very few classical pieces fit the requirements.

Effectiveness

Current research has not supported the benefits of this treatment. Studies into the effectiveness of the training have been inconclusive; some researchers have found benefits and others have not. However, since the training is not invasive, some experts believe there is little to be lost by trying the approach. Although the treatment period is short (only two weeks), it is expensive (on average, about $2,000).

However, treatment is not without problems. Some patients report behavior changes, including agitation, hyperactivity, and rapid mood swings. Experts do not know why, but this type of reaction occurs with other forms of sensory integration training as well. Many children become less compliant, perhaps as a result of an improved attention span. A child with a short attention span is easy to redirect; as the attention span lengthens, the child may become more focused and hence, more reluctant to change tasks.

auditory memory The ability to store and retrieve information presented as sounds, most important in the acquisition of language. An individual who has problems with auditory memory might not be able to follow a sequence of oral directions, or to remember and discuss information presented in a class. In general, difficulties in the area of auditory memory are common among those with diagnosed LEARNING DISABILITIES, especially in the area of reading.

There are two kinds of auditory memory, long- and short-term. Long-term auditory memory is the ability to recall something heard long ago. Short-term auditory memory is the ability to remember something heard very recently. Children with problems in this area may find it difficult to remember people's names, memorize and recall telephone numbers, follow multistep spoken directions, or recall stories or remember words from songs.

auditory perception The ability to process and make sense of information that is received as sound. Involving recognition and interpretation, rather than hearing itself, auditory perception is related to the ways in which the brain recognizes and discriminates sounds in order to make sense of them.

Problems with auditory perception are frequently associated with LANGUAGE DISORDERS and may have a significant effect on an individual's language development in areas such as reading, EXPRESSIVE LANGUAGE, and receptive vocabulary. These problems are a major factor in language learning disabilities.

auditory processing The full range of mental activity involved in reacting to sounds (especially speech sounds) and in considering their meanings in relation to past experience and to their future use. Auditory processing is what happens when the brain recognizes and interprets the sounds in the environment. Humans hear when energy recognized as sound travels through the ear and is changed into electrical information that can be interpreted by the brain. Anything that adversely affects the processing or interpretation of the information can result in an AUDITORY PROCESSING DISORDER.

auditory processing disorder (APD) A complex problem that leads to difficulty recognizing subtle differences between sounds in words, even though the sounds themselves are loud and clear. For example, the request "Are a chair and a couch alike?" may sound to a child with APD like: "Are a hair and a cow alike?" These kinds of problems are more likely to occur when a person with APD is in a noisy environment or when he or she is listening to complex information. APD goes by many other names. Sometimes it is referred to as central auditory processing disorder, an auditory perception problem, auditory comprehension deficit, central auditory dysfunction, central deafness, or word deafness.

There are three types of auditory processing deficits: that involve problems with AUDITORY DISCRIMINATION, AUDITORY FIGURE-GROUND DISCRIMINATION, and AUDITORY SEQUENCING.

Auditory discrimination problems are characterized by difficulty in discriminating between similar sounds such as "t" and "b" or "m" and "n." People with an auditory discrimination problem may have trouble distinguishing between tones of voice, such as knowing how to tell the difference between when someone is making a joke or being serious.

Someone with an auditory figure-ground problem would have trouble hearing sound in the presence of background noise, such as hearing someone speak in a noisy restaurant.

A person with an auditory sequencing problem would have difficulty hearing sounds in the correct order, so that "ten-four" becomes "four-ten."

Human communication relies on taking in complicated perceptual information from the outside world through the ears and other sensory organs and interpreting that information in a meaningful way. Human communication also requires certain mental abilities, such as attention and memory. WERNICKE'S AREA of the brain directs the comprehension of language. Scientists still do not understand exactly how all of these processes work and interact or how they malfunction in cases of communication disorders. Even though a child seems to hear normally, he or she may have trouble using those sounds for speech and language.

The cause of APD is often unknown. In children, auditory processing difficulty may be associated with conditions such as DYSLEXIA, ATTENTION DEFICIT HYPERACTIVITY DISORDER, AUTISM, autism spectrum disorder, specific language impairment, PERVASIVE DEVELOPMENTAL DISORDER, or developmental delay. Sometimes this term has been misapplied to children who have no hearing or language disorder but have challenges in learning.

Symptoms and Diagnostic Path
Children with auditory processing difficulty can have normal hearing and intelligence, but they may have trouble paying attention to and remembering information presented orally. They also may

- have poor listening skills
- need more time to process information
- have low academic performance
- have behavior problems
- confuse syllable sequences and have problems developing vocabulary and understanding language
- have difficulty with reading, comprehension, spelling, and vocabulary

Parents, teachers, or day-care providers may notice symptoms of auditory processing difficulty. A pediatrician or a family doctor can help rule out possible diseases that can cause some of these same symptoms, measuring growth and development. If there is a disease or disorder related to hearing, an otolaryngologist (a physician who specializes in diseases and disorders of the head and neck) may then try to determine whether the child has a hearing function problem. An audiologist will give tests that can determine the softest sounds and words a person can hear and other tests to see how well people can recognize sounds in words and sentences. For example, the audiologist might have a child listen to different numbers or words in the right and the left ear at the same time. Another common audiologic task involves giving the child two sentences, one louder than the other, at the same time in order to identify the processing problem.

A speech/language pathologist is extremely important in this diagnostic process and can find out how well a person understands and uses language, while a mental health professional can provide information about cognitive and behavioral challenges that may contribute to problems in some cases. Because the audiologist can help with the functional problems of hearing and processing, and the speech-language pathologist is focused on language, they may work as a team.

Treatment Options and Outlook
Much research is still needed to understand APD problems, related disorders, and the best intervention for each child or adult. Several strategies are available to help children with auditory processing difficulties, some of which are now available and others of which have not been fully studied. Researchers are currently studying a variety of treatment approaches, including auditory trainers, electronic devices that allow a person to focus attention on a speaker and reduce the interference of background noise. They are often used in classrooms, where the teacher wears a microphone to transmit sound and the child wears a headset to receive the sound. Children who wear hearing aids can use them in addition to the auditory trainer.

Environmental modifications such as classroom acoustics, placement, and seating may help. An audiologist may suggest ways to improve the listening environment, and he or she will be able to monitor any changes in hearing status. Exercises to improve language building skills can increase the ability to learn new words and increase a child's language base.

Auditory memory enhancement, a procedure that reduces detailed information to a more basic representation, may help, as well as informal auditory training techniques, used by teachers and therapists to address specific difficulties.

AUDITORY INTEGRATION TRAINING may be promoted by practitioners as a way to retrain the auditory system and decrease hearing distortion, but current research has not supported the benefits of this treatment.

In recent years, scientists have developed new ways to study the human brain by using brain scans that can monitor brain activity without surgery. Imaging studies are already giving scientists new insights into auditory processing, and some of these studies are directed at understanding auditory processing disorders. One of the values of imaging is that it provides an objective, measurable view of a process, since many symptoms related to APD are described differently by different people. Imaging can help identify the source of these symptoms.

Other scientists are studying the central auditory nervous system. Cognitive neuroscientists are helping to describe how the processes that mediate sound recognition and comprehension work in both normal and disordered systems.

auditory sequencing Also called auditory sequential memory, this is the ability to remember verbal items presented orally in the sequence in which they were presented.

Children with auditory sequencing problems may have trouble learning the alphabet or the months of the year. Difficulties with such basic auditory sequencing tasks may persist into later childhood or adulthood if not recognized and treated. In addition, subtle difficulties with auditory sequencing may persist throughout life.

Auditory sequencing is measured by tests such as digit span and memory for sentences and nonsense syllables. People with auditory sequential memory problems may also have difficulty following a series of instructions. However, such a problem may be confused with or coexist with ATTENTION problems. Such an attention problem may also be marked by an inability to respond correctly to a series of verbal directions.

autism This complex DEVELOPMENTAL DISABILITY (known correctly as AUTISTIC DISORDER) typically appears during the first three years of life. The result of a neurological disorder that affects the functioning of the brain, autism and its associated behaviors have been estimated to occur in as many as one in 500 people. This means that more than a half-million Americans have autism or some other form of PERVASIVE DEVELOPMENTAL DISORDER. Its prevalence rate makes autism one of the most common developmental disabilities. The condition is four times more common in boys than in girls and is not related to race, ethnic origin, family income, lifestyle, or education.

Autism significantly impairs a child's ability to communicate and socialize with others. While severity and symptoms vary according to age, the disorder is significant and sustained. Children with autistic disorder demonstrate little interest in friends or social interactions, often failing to develop verbal and nonverbal communication skills. Typically, these children function at a low intellectual level; most experience mild to severe mental retardation. However, this is by no means true for all individuals with autistic disorder; the condition may be accompanied by average or strong abilities in an isolated area such as reading or computation.

During the course of childhood and adolescence, children with this condition nevertheless usually make some developmental gains. Those who show improvement in language and intellectual ability have the best overall outlook. Although some individuals with autism are able to live with some measure of partial independence in adulthood, very few are able to live entirely on their own.

Autism impacts the normal development of the brain in the areas of social interaction and communication skills. Although a single specific cause of autism is not known, current research links autism to biological or neurological differences in the brain. In many families there appears to be a pattern of autism or related disabilities—suggesting a genetic basis to the disorder—although at this time no gene has been directly linked to autism. Scientists think that the genetic basis is complex and probably involves several combinations of genes.

Autism is not a mental illness or a behavior problem, and it is not caused by bad parenting. No known psychological factors in the development of children have been shown to cause autism.

Symptoms and Diagnostic Path

Autism is a spectrum disorder, which means that the symptoms and characteristics of autism can appear in a wide variety of combinations, from mild to severe. Although autism is defined by a certain set of behavior, children and adults can exhibit any combination of behavior in any degree of severity. Two children with the same diagnosis can act very differently from one another and have varying skills.

Children and adults with autism typically have problems in verbal and nonverbal communication, social interactions, and leisure or play activities in many of the following ways:

- communication: language develops slowly or not at all; uses words without attaching the usual meaning; communicates with gestures instead of words; short ATTENTION SPAN

- social interaction: spends time alone rather than with others; shows little interest in making friends; less responsive to social cues such as eye contact or smiles

- sensory impairment: may have overly sensitive sight, hearing, touch, smell, and taste

- play: lack of spontaneous or imaginative play; does not imitate others or initiate pretend games

- behavior: may be overactive or very passive; throw tantrums for no apparent reason; show an obsessive interest in a single item, idea, activity, or person; lack common sense, show aggression, often has difficulty with changes in routine

The disorder makes it hard for children to communicate with others and relate to the outside world. There may be repeated body movements (hand flapping, rocking), unusual responses to people, or attachments to objects and resistance to changes in routines.

In some cases, there may be aggressive or self-injurious behavior. Autism may affect a child's range of responses and make it more difficult to control how body and mind react. Sometimes visual, motor, or processing problems make it hard for these children to maintain eye contact, and some use peripheral vision rather than looking directly at others. Sometimes touching or being close to others may be painful to a person with autism. Because they cannot make sense of the world in a normal way, people with autism may experience ANXIETY, fear, and confusion.

In addition, people with autism may have other disorders that affect brain function, such as epilepsy, MENTAL RETARDATION, DOWN SYNDROME, or genetic disorders such as FRAGILE X SYNDROME or TOURETTE'S SYNDROME. Many people diagnosed with autism will also be mentally retarded, and between 25 and 30 percent may develop a seizure pattern.

Although there is no standard type of person with autism, these children can learn and function productively and show gains from appropriate education and treatment.

Diagnostic categories have changed over the years as research progresses and as new editions of the DIAGNOSTIC AND STATISTICAL MANUAL OF MENTAL DISORDERS have been issued.

Because there are no medical tests for autism, an accurate diagnosis must be based on observing the person's communication, behavior, and developmental levels. However, because many of the behaviors associated with autism are similar to other disorders, various medical tests may also be ordered to rule out or identify other possible causes of symptoms.

Because the characteristics of the disorder vary, a child should be evaluated by a team including a neurologist, psychologist, developmental pediatrician, speech/language therapist, learning consultant, or other professionals experienced in autism. Problems in recognizing autism often lead to a lack of services to meet the complex needs of these individuals.

It is important to include a history from parents and caregivers in coming to an accurate diagnosis. Some people with autism may seem to have developmental disabilities, a behavior disorder, problems with hearing, or eccentric behavior. It is important to distinguish autism from other conditions, since early identification is required for an effective treatment program. While there is no "cure" for the brain abnormalities that cause autism, patients can learn coping mechanisms and strategies to ease various symptoms. Some of these symptoms may lessen as the child ages and others may disappear altogether.

Treatment Options and Outlook

Early intervention is crucial and can provide dramatic improvements for young children with autism. While various preschool models may differ, all emphasize early, appropriate, and intensive educational interventions for young children, including

- some degree of inclusion, mostly behaviorally based interventions
- programs that build on the interests of the child
- extensive use of visuals to accompany instruction
- structured activities
- parent and staff training
- transition planning
- follow-up

Because of the nature of autism, no single approach can ease symptoms in all cases. Therapies include applied behavior analysis, AUDITORY INTEGRATION TRAINING, special diets, DISCRETE TRIAL TEACHING, medications, MUSIC THERAPY, OCCUPATIONAL THERAPY, physical therapy, SENSORY INTEGRATION, SPEECH/LANGUAGE THERAPY, and VISION TRAINING.

Studies show that individuals with autism respond well to a highly structured, specialized education program tailored to individual needs. A well-designed treatment approach may include work on communication and social skills, sensory integration therapy, and applied behavior analysis by autism experts.

More severely ill children may require a structured, intensive education and behavior program with a one-on-one teacher-to-student ratio. However, many other children with autism may do well in a normal education environment with appropriate support.

In addition to an academic program, children with autism should be trained in functional living skills at the earliest possible age. Learning to cross a street, to buy something in a store or ask for help are critical skills, and may be hard even for those with average intelligence. Training is aimed at boosting a person's independence and providing opportunity for personal choice and freedom.

With appropriate treatment, many problem behaviors can be changed so that the person may appear to no longer have autism. However, most patients continue to show some faint symptoms to some degree throughout their entire lives. Contrary to popular belief, many children and adults with autism can make eye contact, and can show affection and demonstrate a variety of other emotions in varying degrees. Like other children, they respond to their environment in both positive and negative ways.

With appropriate treatment, some behaviors associated with autism may lessen over time. Although communication and social problems will continue in some form throughout life, difficulties in other areas may improve with age, education, or stress level. Many individuals with autism enjoy their lives and contribute to their community in a meaningful way, as they learn to compensate for and cope with their disability.

Some adults with autism live and work independently in the community, and can drive a car, earn a college degree, and even get married. Some may need some support only for daily pressure, while others require a great deal of support from family and professionals.

Adults with autism may live in a variety of residential settings ranging from an independent home or apartment, to group homes or supervised apartment settings with other family members, or more structured residential care. More and more support groups for adults with autism are appearing, and many patients are forming their own networks to share information, support each other, and speak for themselves. Individuals with autism are providing valuable insight into the challenges of this disability by publishing articles and books and appearing on TV to discuss their lives and disabilities.

See also GRANDIN, TEMPLE; AUTISM SPECTRUM DISORDER.

autistic disorder   The medical term for AUTISM.

autistic spectrum disorders (ASD) A group of related problems that are all present from birth or very early in development and affect three primary areas of a child's life: social interaction, the ability to communicate ideas and feelings, and flexibility in adapting to the environment. The disorders on the autistic spectrum include ASPERGER'S SYNDROME (sometimes considered "mild autism" or "high functioning autism"), AUTISM (also called "autistic disorder"), PERVASIVE DEVELOPMENTAL DISORDER—NOT OTHERWISE SPECIFIED (PDD-NOS), and two much more rare conditions, RETT SYNDROME and CHILDHOOD DISINTEGRATIVE DISORDER (CCD). Many of these terms for different problems on the autistic spectrum overlap, although different professionals try to create distinctions among them.

Most children occasionally behave in an odd or eccentric way, or may sometimes be shy, without having a diagnosable disorder. What differentiates children with ASD is the consistency and severity of the unusual behavior. This typically includes a lack of social interaction and problems with nonverbal behavior.

The three main conditions found along the autism spectrum—autism, Asperger's, and PDD-NOS—overlap to such a degree that they are often considered as different measures of severity along the same disorder spectrum.

Autism (autistic disorder) seriously affects verbal and nonverbal communication, as well as the ability to relate to others, and presents as various restricted, repetitive, or stereotyped behavior patterns.

Asperger's syndrome is a milder condition featuring social deficits and certain unusual behavior patterns, without significantly affecting overall intelligence or basic language skills. Asperger's syndrome is sometimes called "high-functioning autism" (autism with minimal deficits in language, IQ, or adaptive skills), but experts disagree about whether these are the same or separate disorders.

PDD-NOS includes children with enough autistic symptoms to receive a diagnosis on the spectrum, but who do not fit completely into either of the other two categories.

In the past, experts guessed that one out of every 500 children had an autistic spectrum disorder, including autism itself, which experts thought occurred once in 2,000 to 5,000 children. More recent estimates of the prevalence of autism is one in 1,000; estimates for having any of the autistic spectrum disorders is about one in 167. Some experts suggest that Asperger's disorder may occur less often than autism (2.5 per 10,000). Rett syndrome and CDD are clearly much more rare, occurring less often than one child in 10,000.

Experts agree that there has been a dramatic increase in reported cases of autism in the past decade, especially in California. Most experts believe that there are not that many more cases of autism now than in the past; rather that the increase can be attributed to a better ability to identify these conditions and more widespread availability of health care for young children. Since more people are now aware of autism, there has been more research into the disorder, and more services (such as intensive behavior modification) are now available only when a child has a formal diagnosis of autism. At the same time, the diagnostic criteria are loosening to include milder forms of autism. Most experts believe there is little sound evidence for either genetic or environmental exposure reasons for an increase in actual number of cases.

Experts do not know what triggers the onset of the autistic spectrum disorders, although it is clear that they reflect a problem in the developing brain linked to subtle abnormal changes in brain structure or differences in brain chemicals (serotonin, DOPAMINE, and epinephrine). In most cases, the onset of these problems is probably influenced by genetics and is much less likely to be primarily caused by the environment or various toxins. Postmortem and brain scan studies have suggested many different major brain structures implicated in autism, including the cerebellum, cerebral cortex, limbic system, CORPUS CALLOSUM, BASAL GANGLIA, and brain stem.

These disorders may be caused by a combination of abnormal genes that affect brain development, since families who have one child with an autistic spectrum disorder have a higher risk of having another child with a similar disorder. Evidence clearly points to these genetic factors, bolstered by twin and family studies that have suggested an underlying genetic vulnerability to ASD.

Although many parents and some researchers have suggested there might be a link between autism and the use of thimerosal, a mercury-based preservative in the measles-mumps-rubella (MMR) vaccine, a growing collection of well-designed, large-scale studies have failed to show a link between thimerosal and autism. Thimerosol is no longer used in childhood vaccines in the United States in response to this concern.

Symptoms and Diagnostic Path

To be considered as having one of the autistic spectrum disorders, a child must have problems with social relationship and communication skills and have stereotyped behavior, interests, and activities. (For example, HYPERSENSITIVITY is one type of stereotyped behavior, in which sounds seem louder, lights brighter, or smells stronger.) Although many people with autism also are mentally retarded, some are of average or high intelligence.

Symptoms of unusual behavior typically begin during infancy or very early childhood, with the child avoiding touch and direct eye contact or exhibiting persistent odd behaviors. Autistic disorders are unique in their pattern of symptoms and sometimes in their areas of relative strength, and they typically have lifelong effects on how children interact, care for themselves, and participate in the community.

Symptoms typically vary from one person to the next, depending on where in the autistic spectrum the person falls. In addition, coexisting conditions often include DEPRESSION, ANXIETY, ATTENTION DEFICIT HYPERACTIVITY DISORDER, and BIPOLAR DISORDER. A disorder on the autism spectrum often occurs together with MENTAL RETARDATION or language disorders.

Social skills Autistic children often prefer to be alone and have trouble using nonverbal communication such as facial expressions, body posture, or eye contact. Children often have trouble making friends and may lack empathy, so that they have trouble understanding someone else's feelings.

Communication skills Children along the autistic spectrum typically have problems with both the spoken and written word, making it hard for them to participate in conversation. Many have language problems and either learn to speak later than average or never learn to speak at all. Some

repeat words or sentences (echolalia) or use only single words. Language problems may contribute to behavioral problems, so that a child who is frustrated by not being able to use language to communicate may resort to screaming or lashing out.

Behavioral problems Problem behaviors are typical and may include inappropriate, annoying, repetitive, aggressive, or even dangerous behavior. This may include self-stimulatory behavior such as hand-flapping, finger-snapping, rocking, or head-banging. Children with autism may try to hurt themselves, smashing their head against the wall or biting their arms. They may show little or no sensitivity to pain and may physically lash out for no reason. Changes in routine may be difficult.

Extreme behavioral problems may involve property destruction and constant devastating tantrums, which can severely limit the child's function in the world. These behaviors can be triggered by a variety of situations, such as the child's inability to understand demands, communication problems, social problems, changes in routine, or confusion about the effects and consequences of actions.

The earlier the diagnosis is made, the earlier treatment can begin, which is important since evidence indicates that intensive early intervention and the best possible educational settings for at least two years during preschool and kindergarten time can improve the outlook for most young children with ASD. A doctor should check for certain behavioral characteristics, even in children as early as one year of age. In addition to general behavioral characteristics discussed above, several screening instruments have been developed to quickly gather information about a child's social and communicative development. These include the Checklist of Autism in Toddlers (CHAT), the modified Checklist for Autism in Toddlers (M-CHAT), the Screening Tool for Autism in Two Year Olds (STAT), the Social Communication Questionnaire (SCQ) for children four years of age and older, the Autism Spectrum Screening Questionnaire (ASSQ), the Australian Scale for Asperger's Syndrome, and the Childhood Asperger Syndrome Test (CAST).

If the doctor suspects ASD, the parent may be referred for a comprehensive evaluation by a multidisciplinary team. To reach a diagnosis of ASD, the child must have significant problems in social skills, communication, and stereotyped behaviors before age three.

Because ASDs may involve other neurological or genetic problems, the most comprehensive evaluations sometimes entail neurologic and genetic assessment, along with intelligence testing.

Treatment Options and Outlook

The basic problems that children face with ASD typically cannot be treated with medications (although some people may take medicine to improve certain symptoms, such as aggressive behavior).

Instead, children with ASD are taught how to do the things that are difficult for them and coaxed into greater participation with the outside world. The best results are usually seen with children who begin treatment when they are very young, as soon as they are diagnosed. As soon as a child's disability has been identified, intervention should begin. Effective programs can teach early communication and social interaction skills.

In children younger than age three, appropriate interventions may involve the home or a child-care center targeting deficits in learning, language, imitation, attention, motivation, compliance, and initiative of interaction.

Any effective treatment program will be designed around a schedule and focus on the child's interests, teaching tasks in a series of simple steps that actively engage the child's attention in highly structured activities. Reinforcing positive behavior is an important part of this treatment. Parental involvement is considered a major factor in treatment success, and parents are asked to work with teachers and therapists to identify problem behaviors that need to be changed. Often parents are trained how to continue therapy at home.

Specially designed education programs are very effective, especially if they involve intensive behavior modification. These programs teach the child to communicate (sometimes by pointing or using pictures or sign language) and to interact with others. Basic living skills, such as how to buy something in a store or ask for directions, are also emphasized in SPECIAL EDUCATION programs. A good treatment program might include speech therapy, physical therapy, and/or occupational therapy.

Most interventions are based on the theory of applied behavior analysis (ABA), in which desired

behavior is rewarded so as to be more likely repeated. Undesired behavior is ignored. Although ABA is a theory, many people use the term to describe a specific treatment approach, and it has become widely accepted as an effective treatment. The basic research done by Ivar Lovaas at UCLA recommends an intensive, one-on-one child-teacher interaction for 40 hours a week.

ABA typically involves DISCRETE TRIAL TRAINING, an intensive approach in which the therapist breaks tasks into short simple tasks (or "trials"), asking the child to do something, getting a response from the child, and then earning subsequent reaction from the therapist. This approach is designed to teach skills ranging from basic daily living, such as dressing and eating, to more complicated skills such as social interaction. Intensive in-home behavioral modification programs using ABA and discrete trials learning programs are available for up to 30 or 40 hours a week. These programs are particularly effective in teaching the very basic skills children need, such as paying attention to adults, maintaining eye contact, and following directions.

Learning how to communicate is also important for children with ASD. Although some children with ASD speak, others never learn to talk. In these cases, a communication program such as Picture Exchange Communication Systems (PECS) can help provide a way of communicating for children who do not speak. PECS, which was developed in 1985 at the Delaware Austistic Program, uses behavioral-based methods to teach children to exchange a picture for something they want, such as an item or activity.

In this method, a child hands the teacher or parent a picture of a desired item, which is immediately granted. Verbal prompts are not used, and eventually the pictures can be put together in simple sentences. As PECS training proceeds, the child is taught to comment and answer direct questions. Many preschoolers using PECS also begin developing speech.

Because children with ASD often have oversensitive nervous systems, they either underreact or overreact to sounds, taste, touch, or bright lights. SENSORY INTEGRATION THERAPY by occupational, physical, or speech therapists desensitizes the child, helping to reorganize sensory information.

Medication If other methods do not success-fully manage all of a child's problems associated with ASD, medications can sometimes be used to treat certain symptoms. This is particularly impor-tant if the child's symptoms are severe and involve aggression, self-injurious behavior, or tantrums. Medications that are typically used with children who have ASD are those that have been developed to treat similar symptoms in other disorders. How-ever, many available medications are prescribed "off-label," which means they have not been offi-cially approved for use in children but are widely believed by doctors to be effective in children.

Antidepressants, such as the newest SSRIs, are the medications most often prescribed for symp-toms of anxiety, depression, or OBSESSIVE-COMPUL-SIVE DISORDER (OCD) that may appear in children with ASD. Treatment with these drugs may lessen repetitive, ritualistic behavior and improve eye con-tact and social interactions. Only one of the SSRIs, fluoxetine (Prozac), has been approved for both OCD and depression in children age seven and older. Three approved for OCD include fluvoxam-ine (Luvox), age eight and older; sertraline (Zoloft), age six and older; and clomipramine (Anafranil), age 10 and older.

Some "atypical" antipsychotics, such as risperi-done (Risperdal), appear to be effective and well tolerated by autistic children with severe behav-ioral problems. The most common side effects were increased appetite, weight gain, and sedation. Fur-ther long-term studies are needed to determine any long-term side effects. Other atypical antipsy-chotics that have seemed to be effective in recent studies include olanzapine (Zyprexa) and ziprasi-done (Geodon). Ziprasidone has not been associ-ated with significant weight gain.

Antipsychotics that have been used to treat severe behavioral problems in children with ASD work by interfering with the neurotransmitter dopamine. Among the older antipsychotics, haloperidol has been found to be more effective than other drugs in this class. Although haloperidol can reduce symp-toms of aggression, it also can have adverse side effects, such as sedation, muscle stiffness, and abnor-mal movements.

Because seizures occur in one out of every four people with ASD, these children are often treated with an anticonvulsant drug, such as carbamazepine (Tegretol), lamotrigine (Lamictal), topiramate (Topa-max), or valproic acid (Depakote). The level of the medication in the blood should be carefully moni-tored so that the smallest effective amount is used. Although medication usually reduces the number of seizures, it cannot always eliminate them.

Stimulant medications such as METHYLPHENIDATE (Ritalin), more typically used to treat children with attention deficit hyperactivity disorder, also have been prescribed for children with autism to decrease impulsivity and hyperactivity, especially in higher-functioning children.

Although several other medications have been used to treat ASD symptoms, their safety and use-fulness have not been supported. These other drugs include antidepressants, naltrexone, lithium, and some of the benzodiazepines such as diazepam (Valium) and lorazepam (Ativan).

Dietary interventions based on the idea that ASD may be linked to allergies or a lack of certain vitamins or minerals are unsupported, although some parents swear by their usefulness. A gluten-free, casein-free diet has helped some ASD chil-dren, according to their parents. Casein is the primary protein in milk, and gluten is a casein-like substance in wheat, oat, rye, and barley seeds. However, since gluten and milk are found in many common foods, following a gluten-free, casein-free diet can be challenging.

In the search for autism treatment, there has been discussion in the last few years about the use of secretin, a substance approved by the U.S. Food and Drug Administration (FDA) to help diagnose of a gastrointestinal problem. Anecdotal reports have shown improvement in autism symptoms, including better sleep patterns, eye contact, lan-guage skills, and alertness. However, several recent studies have found no significant improvements in symptoms in patients who received secretin com-pared to those who received a placebo.

Education

Children older than three years usually can enroll in individualized SPECIAL EDUCATION programs in their public school districts. High-functioning autistic children may be enrolled in mainstream classrooms and child-care facilities, which can help them pattern their behavior after the behavior of other normally developing children. However, a child who is overstimulated in a regular classroom may work better in a smaller, more structured environment.

The EDUCATION FOR ALL HANDICAPPED CHILDREN ACT OF 1975 (P.L. 94-142), which has been updated during the ensuing 30 years, mandates the education of children with ASD. However, the goals, methods, and resources available vary from one school to the next.

Each state is required to provide special education and related services for every eligible child. The INDIVIDUALS WITH DISABILITIES EDUCATION IMPROVEMENT ACT (IDEA; now reauthorized as IDEIA 2004) is a federally mandated program that assures a free and appropriate public education for children with diagnosed educational deficits; ASD is included in this category. Usually, children with autism are placed in public schools and the school district pays for all necessary services, including a speech therapist, occupational therapist, school psychologist, social worker, school nurse, and often a classroom aide.

By law, public schools must prepare an INDIVIDUALIZED EDUCATION PROGRAM for every child in a special education program, which is a plan about what the child's goals are and how they will be met.

A child under age three with special needs should be eligible for an early intervention program available in every state, provided by qualified workers in the child's home or a place familiar to the child. This might include a physical activity to help develop coordination and body awareness, such as stringing beads or working on a puzzle. Social interaction is encouraged, and children learn by doing with positive reinforcement. The child may be in a segregated class with other ASD children or in an integrated class with children without disabilities for at least part of the day.

In elementary school, the child should receive help in any delayed skill area. Many schools include the child in a regular classroom for most of the day, with special instruction in social skills for part of the day. During middle and high school, instruction may address practical matters such as independent living, work, and recreation. This might include work experience and using public transportation.

automatization   A form of learning in which a skill or procedure becomes automatic and virtually unconscious. Most people experience some degree of automatic skills, such as driving a car, forming letters, spelling common words accurately, and performing simple arithmetic equations.

Individuals with LEARNING DISABILITIES may have difficulty with automatic skills, taking longer to develop automaticity with such basic skills as spelling, decoding, and handwriting, and requiring more repetition, practice, and reinforcement.

This means that people who experience inadequate automatization may take longer to complete academic tasks, and expend an enormous amount of mental energy on relatively low-order elements of an assignment, leaving little capacity to work on more complex components such as problem-solving or coming up with new ideas.

auxiliary aids   ACCOMMODATIONS made to help students with disabilities, such as taped books, voice recognition software, and note-takers. Under Section 12102 [Section 3] of the AMERICANS WITH DISABILITIES ACT, the term *auxiliary aids and services* includes

- qualified interpreters or other effective methods of making aurally delivered material available to people with hearing problems
- qualified readers, taped texts, or other effective methods of making visually delivered materials available to people with visual impairments
- acquisition or modification of equipment or devices
- other similar services

Determining what auxiliary aids may be necessary to provide access is primarily the role of the individual seeking such accommodations, working with human resources personnel, compliance officers, or college disability support services. Providing specific auxiliary aids must be based on documented disabilities.

background knowledge Information an individual has acquired through previous learning and experiences that creates a familiar context in which to learn new ideas. Activating background knowledge before introducing a new concept is a learning strategy that improves comprehension by connecting new information to existing information.

Many individuals with LEARNING DISABILITIES do not have good background knowledge due to poor reading, memory, or COMPREHENSION skills. Children who have not developed age-appropriate decoding skills will not have the reading rate and fluency they need to understand what they read. For these children, the energy and focus needed to decode words makes reading inefficient and interferes with reading comprehension. In addition, children who spend significant time in resource rooms learning basic skills miss out on practicing the use of background information in areas such as history, geography, and literature.

Through remediation of basic skills, many individuals with learning disabilities are able to develop the skills required to perform high school and college-level academic work. However, many find that they are not successful in higher level courses because they do not have solid background knowledge in certain areas.

back-to-basics movement An educational movement emphasizing explicit instruction in basic academic skills. This movement represents the preferences of some parents in public school districts, although it is often at odds with contemporary teacher-instruction practices in colleges and universities.

"Back to basics" includes such elements as a phonics approach to teaching reading and attention to rote memorization of math facts.

basal ganglia A group of small nerve structures inside the brain located under the center of the CEREBRAL CORTEX and above the THALAMUS that play an important role in movement, routine behavior, and sensory information. The basal ganglia includes the caudate nucleus, globus pallidus, putamen, subthalamus, substantia nigra, and red nucleus.

Computer imaging of the brain structure of people with ADHD sometimes reveals smaller basal ganglia. Researchers at Stanford University have shown that these specific areas of the brain are less active in children with ADHD than in healthy ones. Their studies also show that Ritalin (the drug typically given to ease ADHD symptoms) increases brain activity in the basal ganglia in hyperactive children but decreases basal ganglia activity in healthy children.

basal reader A look-say model of reading instruction designed to teach reading in a structured sequence. Through practice, students memorize key words that are repeated throughout the text. Basal readers often are introduced in first grade, using simple words for simple stories. The words gradually become more difficult until about the sixth or seventh grade. Teachers often use additional materials such as workbooks, activity sheets, and teacher editions to deliver reading instruction and skill development.

basic skill A fundamental ability necessary to function on a daily basis. The mastery of basic skills is necessary to progress to higher levels of achievement. Academically, basic skills include speaking, spelling, reading, writing, and arithmetic.

The basic skills of children with a LEARNING DISABILITY are often not uniformly developed. This makes the achievement of more advanced academic skills like problem solving more difficult to achieve.

For children with learning disabilities, basic skills training may emphasize social skills, study habits, attention training, and other specific tasks that assist in the development of independence and self-esteem.

behavioral rating scales   Major assessment instruments that can help an examiner identify ATTENTION DEFICIT HYPERACTIVITY DISORDER (ADHD) behaviors and other problems.

Rating scales are typically filled out by parents or teachers, and sometimes by the individuals being evaluated. Behavioral rating scales generally contain items intended to assess attention and distractibility, such as "daydreams," "easily distracted," and "does not pay attention."

These scales are generally reliable and easy to use, but they cannot make a precise analysis of the various components of attention. Some commonly-used behavioral scales are the CONNORS PARENT TEACHER RATING SCALES, the CHILD ATTENTION PROFILE, and the ADHD Rating Scale.

behavioral unit   The center of behavioral psychology's theory of behavior management. The behavioral unit consists of three elements: antecedent (stimulus), behavior (response), and consequence (reinforcement).

In behavior management, a person's response is the target behavior of the individual, situated between two sets of environmental influences. Changing a behavior involves carefully and systematically analyzing each of these three components.

This approach is the core of direct instruction techniques: teachers provide specific lessons, assess target behavior (response), and then either reward or repeat the stimulus until the child masters the lesson.

Individuals with LEARNING DISABILITIES often require the structure and objectivity inherent in a behaviorist approach to instruction. Even young children are capable of understanding the fundamental principles underlying this approach, and how to achieve the desired consequence.

Critics of behaviorist approaches typically agree that it is effective, but suggest that other approaches are needed to help develop more complicated thinking and problem-solving skills, since some research suggests that children with learning disabilities are not efficient or organized in their approach to learning. While individuals with learning disabilities require explicit instruction in order to learn basic skills, they also require a range of instructional techniques.

behavior modification   The application of rewards or punishments as a way of reducing or eliminating problem behavior, or to teach people new responses. Behavior modification is based on the idea that since all behavior is learned, with appropriate treatment it also can be *unlearned* by using positive or negative consequences.

Behavior modification is used by psychologists, social workers, teachers, and other professionals to change an individual's reaction to a situation. There are two major approaches to behavior modification, one based on the work of the late psychologist B. F. Skinner, the other based on the work of psychologist Albert Bandura.

Skinner believed that all behavior is learned by interacting with the environment, and that bad behavior is learned the same way normal behavior is learned. Skinner believed that rewarded behavior is likely to be repeated, and punished behavior is likely to be avoided. Therefore, a behavior modification program will set up a program that rewards specific desired behaviors.

Bandura's approach emphasizes learning through imitation, believing that a person can learn to avoid an unpleasant situation without experiencing it. Individuals can also learn new skills by watching and imitating others. Bandura emphasizes the effectiveness of role models who speak and act consistently, and this applies especially to working with young children.

Modeling specific social skills or strategies, communication patterns, and other behaviors is especially important for children with LEARNING DISABILITIES, who require specific direct instruction as well as consistent modeling. Because children with learning disabilities often present behavior issues in the classroom, often a consequence of their frustration with learning, it is important that teachers and parents have consistent approaches to helping these children learn more appropriate and effective behaviors.

Bender Visual-Motor Gestalt Test A test of visual-perceptual and motor development for children aged five to nine-and-a-half years old. This test measures VISUAL-MOTOR SKILLS using nine geometric figures for the child to copy one at a time. The drawings are then scored depending on any distortions of shape, rotations, integration difficulties, and too many dots or extra lines.

The test is useful only for younger children since those over age eight can usually reproduce all the designs perfectly. After age eight, the test is helpful only in distinguishing whether a child's perceptual motor maturity is below that of an eight-year-old.

bias When used to describe a psychometric test, bias denotes "unfairness." Bias can involve any sort of group membership, such as race, social class, gender, age, and so on. Bias in standardized testing can be detected and, when it cannot be eliminated, its effects can be measured so that scores can be fairly interpreted.

Most test makers review items for obvious biases, such as offensive words, but many forms of bias are not superficial. While some test makers also use statistical bias-reduction techniques, these techniques cannot detect underlying bias in the test's form or content. As a result, critics say, biased cultural assumptions built into the test as a whole may not be exposed or removed by test makers.

bilateral motor coordination The ability to use arms and legs in a symmetrical, coordinated manner. An individual needs to have adequate motor coordination to ride a bike, catch a ball, or swim.

See also MOTOR SKILLS; MOTOR PLANNING; MOTOR SEQUENCING.

bilingual approach Teaching in two languages—a person's native language and a second language. The philosophy behind using a bilingual approach in teaching children who do not speak English is to allow students to learn academic courses in their native language while introducing a second language. Gradually, more and more information is taught in the second language. For students with learning disabilities, learning in an environment with two languages may be difficult.

bipolar disorder Popularly known as "manic depression," this condition is characterized by highly energized "manic" episodes alternating with DEPRESSION. Mood swings are often dramatic and unpredictable. Because the manic periods (with impulsive behavior and bursts of energy) can be similar to symptoms of ATTENTION DEFICIT HYPERACTIVITY DISORDER, a good diagnosis is important for anyone experiencing repeated episodes of mania or depression. The feelings of depression, inadequacy, fatigue, and sadness are also similar to emotions experienced by individuals with other disorders.

While everyone experiences normal mood changes during everyday life, bipolar disorder is a medical condition in which people have mood swings totally unrelated to things going on in their lives. These swings affect thoughts, feelings, physical health, behavior, and functioning.

Bipolar disorder affects about 2.3 million American adults (about 1.2 percent of the population), according to the National Institute of Mental Health. It is in the same family of illnesses (called "affective disorders") as clinical depression. Unlike depression alone, which affects more women than men, bipolar disorder seems to affect men and women equally. For a clinical definition of bipolar disorder, symptoms must include one or more manic episodes accompanied by one or more major depressive episodes, which usually occur in cycles.

Bipolar disorder usually begins in the early 20s, although it can sometimes start in early childhood or as late as the 40s or 50s. However, when someone over 50 has a manic episode for the first time, the cause is more likely to be a problem that just mimics bipolar disorder (such as a brain condition or the effects of drugs, ALCOHOL, or some prescription medications).

There is no single, proven cause of bipolar disorder, but research strongly suggests that it is often an inherited problem related to a lack of stability in the transmission of nerve impulses in the brain. This biochemical problem makes people with bipolar disorder more vulnerable to emotional and physical stresses.

This means that if a person experiences stress, substance abuse, lack of sleep, or too much stimulation, the normal brain mechanisms for restoring calm functioning do not always work properly.

Bipolar disorder tends to run in families, and a number of genes have been linked to the condition, suggesting the presence of several different biochemical problems. If one parent has bipolar disorder and the other does not, there is a one in seven chance that the couple's child will develop it. The chance may be greater if one spouse has several relatives with bipolar disorder or depression.

Symptoms and Diagnostic Path

Bipolar disorder can seriously affect a patient's marriage, family, and job. Divorce rates are much higher in patients with bipolar disorder (about two to three times higher than in normal subjects).

A person with bipolar disorder may experience any or all of four different kinds of episodes: mania, low-level mania (hypomania), depression, or a combination ("mixed state").

Mania (manic episode) This episode often begins with a pleasant sense of high energy, creativity, and social confidence, which become more severe until it develops into a full-blown manic episode. People with mania typically lack insight and deny that anything is wrong, angrily blaming anyone who suggests otherwise. A manic episode is characterized by feeling unusually euphoric or irritable for at least a week, plus at least four (and often almost all) of the following symptoms:

- needing little sleep yet having great amounts of energy
- talking fast
- having racing thoughts
- being easily distracted
- having an inflated feeling of power, greatness, or importance
- doing reckless things without concern about possible negative consequences, such as spending too much money, inappropriate sexual activity, or making foolish business investments
- psychotic symptoms in very severe cases, such as hallucinations or delusions

Mild mania (hypomania) This milder form of mania causes similar but less severe symptoms, which often begin with someone feeling better and more productive than usual and then usually build into a full-blown mania or crash into depression.

Depression (major depressive episode) To be considered a full-blown "major" depressive episode, a person will feel sad and lack interest for at least two weeks, in addition to at least four other symptoms:

- trouble sleeping or sleeping too much
- loss of appetite or eating too much
- problems concentrating or making decisions
- feeling slow or agitated
- feeling worthless or guilty
- loss of energy; fatigue
- thoughts of suicide or death
- hallucinations or delusions (in severe cases)

Mixed episode The most disabling episodes are those that include symptoms of both mania and depression at the same time, or that alternate often during the day. A person in this condition will feel excited or agitated but also feel irritable and depressed.

Number of episodes Untreated patients with bipolar disorder may have more than 10 total episodes of mania and depression during their lifetime. Often, five years or more may pass between the first and second episode, but the time periods between subsequent episodes get shorter and shorter. But people do not all experience bipolar dis-order in the same way. Some people have equal numbers of manic and depressive episodes; others have mostly one type or the other.

The average person with bipolar disorder has four episodes during the first 10 years of the illness. Men are more likely to begin with a manic episode, while women tend to experience depression first. While a number of years can elapse between the first two or three episodes of mania or depression, without treatment most people eventually have episodes more often. Sometimes these follow a seasonal pattern, but a few people cycle frequently or even continuously through the year.

Episodes can last days, months, or sometimes even years. On average, without treatment, manic or mild manic episodes last a few months, while depressions often last well over six months. Some individuals recover completely between episodes and may go many years without any symptoms, while others continue to have low-grade but troubling depression or mild swings up and down.

There are two main types of bipolar disorder:

- Bipolar I: the "classic" form of the condition that most often involves widely spaced, long-lasting bouts of mania followed by long-lasting bouts of depression

- Bipolar II: at least one episode of mild mania (hypomania) and one major depressive episode

Although the shifts from one state to another are usually gradual, they can be quite sudden. In this so-called rapid-cycling form of the disorder, a person can experience four or more complete mood cycles within a year's time. Some rapid cyclers can complete a mood cycle in a matter of days (or more rarely, hours). Rapid cycling occurs in between 5 percent and 15 percent of patients.

It is also possible for someone who has bipolar disorder to experience a mixed state, which means their mood includes some characteristics of depression and some of mania or mild mania.

While there are rare documented cases of mania without depression, the *DSM-IV-TR* does not currently include a category for just "mania." Using *DSM-IV-TR* to diagnose the condition, a person with symptoms of mania will almost always be diagnosed as bipolar.

Bipolar disorder cannot yet be identified with a medical test such as a brain scan or blood analysis. Instead, a diagnosis is reached on the basis of symptoms, course of illness, and (when available) family history. The diagnostic criteria for bipolar disorder are described in the *Diagnostic and Statistical Manual for Mental Disorders—Fourth Edition, Text Revision.*

In the opinion of many mental health professionals, bipolar disorder may soon surpass ADHD as the most overdiagnosed mental disorder.

Typically, people with bipolar disorder see three or four doctors over at least eight years before being correctly diagnosed. The earlier the diagnosis and proper treatment, the quicker people can be helped and the more likely they will be able to avoid suicide attempts, alcohol and substance abuse, and other personal problems.

Treatment Options and Outlook

Research suggests that the earlier the treatment the better the outcome; evidence indicates that the more mood episodes a person has, the harder it is to treat each subsequent episode and the more frequent episodes may become. (This is sometimes referred to as "kindling.")

While there is no cure for bipolar disorder, a combination of drug treatment and therapy can lessen the frequency, severity, and consequences of symptoms and improve functioning between episodes. The two most important types of medication used to control the symptoms of bipolar disorder are mood stabilizers and antidepressants; other medications can help ease insomnia, ANXIETY, restlessness, or psychotic symptoms.

Mood stabilizers are used to improve manic symptoms, but they also may sometimes ease depression as well. They are the mainstay of long-term preventive treatment for both mania and depression. Three mood stabilizers are widely used in the United States: lithium, valproate, and carbamazepine. Each of the three affects the body differently, so that if one does not work another may prove to be better. For all three, blood tests determine the correct dose.

Traditionally, lithium has been the primary drug treatment for patients with bipolar disorder. Discovered to be effective in 1949, it has been widely used since the mid-1960s for prevention and treatment. Valproate and carbamazepine are newer drugs used for bipolar disorder since the late 1970s.

Although mood stabilizers (especially lithium) can ease depression, many patients also need a specific antidepressant to treat the depressive episode. However, antidepressants alone can sometimes trigger a manic attack or rapid cycling. For this reason, antidepressants are given together with a mood stabilizer.

Anticonvulsant medications, such as valproate (Depakote) or carbamazepine (Tegretol) also can have mood-stabilizing effects and may be especially useful for difficult-to-treat bipolar episodes. Valproate was FDA-approved in 1995 for treatment of mania. Newer anticonvulsant medications, including lamotrigine (Lamictal), gabapentin (Neurontin), and topiramate (Topamax), are being studied to determine how well they work in stabilizing mood cycles. Anticonvulsant medications may be combined with lithium or with each other.

Children and adolescents with bipolar disorder generally are treated with lithium, but valproate and carbamazepine also are used. Researchers are evaluating the safety and efficacy of these and other psychotropic medications in children and adolescents. However, there is some evidence that valproate may lead to harmful hormone changes in teenage girls and polycystic ovary syndrome in women who began taking the medication before age 20. Therefore, young female patients taking valproate should be monitored carefully by a physician.

Atypical antipsychotic medications, including clozapine (Clozaril), olanzapine (Zyprexa), risperidone (Risperdal), quetiapine (Seroquel), and ziprasidone (Geodon), are being studied as possible treatments for bipolar disorder. Evidence suggests clozapine may be helpful as a mood stabilizer for people who do not respond to lithium or anticonvulsants. Other research has supported the usefulness of olanzapine for acute mania, an indication that has recently received FDA approval. Olanzapine may also help relieve psychotic depression.

If insomnia is a problem, a high-potency benzodiazepine medication such as clonazepam (Klonopin) or lorazepam (Ativan) may help promote better sleep. However, since these medications may be habit-forming, they are prescribed on a short-term basis. Other types of sedative medications, such as zolpidem (Ambien), are sometimes used instead.

Changes to the treatment plan may be needed at various times during the course of bipolar disorder to manage the illness most effectively. To reduce the chance of relapse or of developing a new episode, patients should keep to the treatment plan.

Women with bipolar disorder who wish to conceive, or who become pregnant, face special challenges due to the possible harmful effects of existing mood-stabilizing medications on the developing fetus and the nursing infant. As a result, the benefits and risks of all available treatment options should be discussed with a clinician skilled in this area. New treatments with reduced risks during pregnancy and lactation are under study.

Medication Side Effects   At least half of those who take medication have side effects, especially if high doses and a combination of medicines are needed. Lower doses and fewer medicines help offset symptoms, but some people may have severe enough side effects to require different medicine. Although side effects tend to be worse early in the treatment, some people who have taken lithium for 20 years or more can suddenly develop side effects as they age. Valproate or carbamazepine make excellent alternatives as long as the switch is made gradually. Valproate appears to cause the fewest side effects during long-term treatment.

In an addition to medication, psychotherapy can be helpful in providing support and guidance to people with bipolar disorder and their families. Studies have shown that psychosocial interventions can lead to more stable moods, fewer hospitalizations, and better functioning. A licensed psychologist, social worker, or counselor typically provides these therapies and often works together with a psychiatrist to monitor a patient's progress. Cognitive behavioral therapy, psychoeducation, and family therapy are all helpful in treating bipolar disorder.

Cognitive behavioral therapy helps people with bipolar disorder learn to change inappropriate or negative thought patterns and behaviors associated with the illness. Psychoeducation involves teaching people with bipolar disorder about the illness and its treatment and how to recognize signs of relapse so that early intervention can be sought before a full-blown episode occurs. Psychoeducation also may be helpful for family members. Family therapy uses strategies to reduce the level of distress within the family that may either contribute to or result from the ill person's symptoms. Interpersonal and social rhythm therapy helps people with bipolar disorder to improve interpersonal relationships and regularize their daily routines. Regular daily routines and sleep schedules may help protect against manic episodes.

In situations where medication, psychotherapy, and the combination of these interventions is ineffective (or work too slowly to relieve severe symptoms such as psychosis or suicidal thoughts), electroconvulsive therapy may be considered.

Although ECT has received negative publicity, it can be the safest and most effective treatment for psychotic depression. ECT may also be needed if a patient is severely ill and cannot wait for medicine to work, if there have been several unsuccessful attempts with different antidepressants, or if the patient is pregnant or has a health condition that makes drug therapy less safe.

Hospitalization may be needed but usually lasts only a week or two, and can prevent self-destructive, impulsive, or aggressive behavior. During a depressed phase, hospitalization may be needed if a person becomes suicidal. Hospitalization is also used for people who have medical complications that make it hard to monitor medication or for those who cannot stop using drugs or alcohol. Early recognition and treatment of manic and depressive episodes can lower the chances of hospitalization.

Prognosis   In most cases, proper treatment can help reduce the frequency and severity of episodes and can help people with bipolar disorder maintain a good quality of life. People with bipolar disorder can lead healthy and productive lives when the illness is effectively treated, but without treatment the natural course of bipolar disorder tends to worsen. Over time a person may suffer more frequent and more severe manic and depressive episodes than those experienced when the illness first appeared.

Prevention   Successful management of bipolar disorder can be challenging, especially if a patient wants to stop medication because he or she feels better, does not like the side effects, or misses the "highs." A patient who stops medication probably will not have an acute episode right away, but eventually a relapse will probably occur. And each episode runs the risk of making it harder to manage subsequent flare-ups.

Sometimes a diagnosis of bipolar disorder is not clear after just one episode, and medication can be tapered off after about a year. However, if a patient has had only one episode of mania but has a very strong family history, or if the episode was severe, experts believe the patient should probably take medication for several years—or for life. After two or more manic or depressive episodes, experts strongly recommend taking preventive medication indefinitely.

About one in three people with bipolar disorder will be completely free of symptoms by taking lithium, valproate, or carbamazepine for life, and most people become ill much less often, much less severely, with each episode.

birth weight, low   Low-birth-weight infants are at risk for a wide range of behavior and learning problems, and assessment and intervention are feasible well before the child might be diagnosed as needing SPECIAL EDUCATION services.

Recent research has suggested that extremely low-birth-weight children from age seven through adolescence have poorer reading and math skills; children whose birth weight was less than two pounds lagged behind their peers academically, and displayed other subtle behavioral characteristics that undermined their efforts at school. Poor MOTOR SKILLS and neurological immaturity were defined in many of the children.

This is becoming more of a concern since modern medicine can now save many infants with very low birth weight who would have died 15 years ago. In fact, infants whose birth weight was as low as one pound eight ounces, born after 24 weeks of gestation, have survived in neonatal intensive care units.

Many neonatal intensive care units have follow-up programs to assess the development of children and initiate early intervention strategies, as needed. Unfortunately, physicians traditionally have not received much training in the area of child development and disabilities, although pediatric and family practice training programs today include rotations in child development and rehabilitative services for children. Such assessments are vital since some studies have found that middle-class, low-birth-weight children may not require special education services if they received strong parental support. Early childhood educational partnerships between home and school are essential to help keep low-birth-weight infants on target in their development.

blending   Stringing sounds (PHONEMES) together to create sounds and words.

See also PHONICS.

borderline intellectual functioning   An IQ between 70 and 85, in the absence of functional or adaptive problems; sometimes considered in the "slow learner" educational category. Earlier classifications referred to this IQ range as borderline MENTAL RETARDATION. Neither term has anything to do with BORDERLINE PERSONALITY DISORDER.

borderline personality disorder   A pervasive pattern of instability in interpersonal relationships and self-image, with marked impulsivity, beginning by early adulthood.

Because the impulsivity and inappropriate behavior of this condition may mimic symptoms of ATTENTION DEFICIT HYPERACTIVITY DISORDER, a diagnosis by an experienced clinician is important.

Borderline personality disorder affects about 2 percent of people in the United States. The name "borderline personality disorder" was given because experts once thought the condition fell somewhere between neurosis and psychosis on the mental illness continuum. Professionals who are educated about BPD all agree that the name should be changed as it does not in any way describe the disorder.

Although some experts believe the condition is a true personality disorder acquired from childhood trauma, research does not support this theory. While the exact cause is still unknown, more and more research has discovered that BPD is highly genetic. Mothers who have the condition are five times more likely to give birth to an affected child compared to a mother without BPD.

Symptoms and Diagnostic Path

This type of personality disorder leads to intense feelings of abandonment, poor self-image, and unrealistic expectations of others. Moodiness and angry outbursts may be common, and the individual may seem depressed or suicidal. The hallmark of the disorder is chronic instability, affecting relationships with family members or colleagues, and a lack of close, long-term interpersonal relationships that can add to a sense of isolation and abandonment.

Treatment Options and Outlook

Recent research has shown that medications can significantly relieve the suffering of borderline patients when used in combination with psychotherapy. Treatment may be some combination of antipsychotic or antianxiety drugs, antidepressants, and psychotherapy. Due to their suicide attempts, or brief psychotic episodes, borderline patients frequently are hospitalized.

brain imaging   Imaging technology that offers a way of identifying structural and metabolic differences between the brain functions of individuals with learning and attention disorders and normal subjects. In turn, imaging research offers an increasing potential for clarifying the factors underlying learning problems in terms of brain chemistry and physiology.

These techniques will play an increasingly prominent role in research into learning and attention disorders, and may also become more important in the assessment of individual cases.

For example, research into brain imaging is producing important information about how children learn to read and do arithmetic. Scientists now have a fairly good idea of what areas of the brain are activated in certain skills. These scanning techniques may one day also help teachers objectively decide which are the best methods to help children learn.

In the future, brain scanning may provide ways to understand the effectiveness of various training techniques, although there will probably not be one technique that will be better than another in all children under all circumstances and for all languages.

Brain imaging studies also can reveal specific LEARNING DISABILITY problems. In research at the National Institute of Mental Health (NIMH), brain imaging has revealed dramatic evidence of a deficit in the brain's visual system in people with DYSLEXIA, a disorder that affects the reading ability of millions of American schoolchildren and adults. While it has been commonly believed that only the language related areas of the brain are affected in dyslexia, this study adds to the growing body of research pointing to dysfunction of another portion of the brain as well.

The research confirms that people with dyslexia, hobbled by problems with reading, writing, and spelling, have trouble processing specific visual information. It also confirms that dyslexia is a discrete brain disorder, not a by-product of a poor education. If confirmed by additional research, functional brain imaging could be used as a tool for early and accurate diagnosis of this common and disabling disorder.

According to the research team, the anatomical changes underlying these functional differences may occur during the early stages of development, when regional functional specialization occurs. Future research will provide further insights into the details of visual and language deficits and their effects on reading.

Types of Scans

MRI A technique capable of projecting images of multiple sections of the brain onto a video screen, indicating the shape and location of various structures of the brain.

Functional MRI (fMRI) represents a technological advance over MRI that allows for noninvasive study of the human brain at work. The technique of FMRI is based on the principle that blood flow increases in active areas of the brain at work.

Brain electrical activity mapping (BEAM) An advance over electroencephalogram (EEG) procedures, allowing researchers to convert the electrical brain waves that individuals produce in response to various stimuli into visual form, and map these.

Positron emission tomography (PET) A type of scan that permits researchers to measure metabolic activities and changes within the brain.

brain injury, traumatic Damage to the brain may be caused by a wide range of factors, including injury before birth as a result of maternal illness, substance abuse, or medications; loss of oxygen at birth or because of an accident such as near drowning; stroke or other medical conditions such as tumors; and physical injury. Brain injury may be associated with LEARNING DISABILITIES.

Traumatic brain injury is a federally recognized disabling condition that can change how a student learns and acts in school. The degree of dysfunction varies with the type and location of injury and with the age of the child. School personnel traditionally have had little exposure to this condition, and there is great potential for problems to occur due to lack of knowledge and miscommunication.

Even a mild brain injury such as a concussion or whiplash can cause serious learning and behavioral impairments. Headaches, sleep, concentration, memory, vision, mood, and irritability are but a few of the many continuing problems. The combination of the many thinking and emotional disorders caused by brain injury seriously undermine the ability to learn and fit in.

Children tend to make what appears to be a "good" physical recovery from brain injuries, but parents, teachers, and doctors may be surprised by the behavioral, learning, and emotional problems that soon follow. Due to the nature of the persistent problems that typically follow traumatic brain injury, such as restlessness, disinhibition, and impulsivity, many children with this condition are misdiagnosed as ATTENTION DEFICIT HYPERACTIVITY DISORDER.

Assessment

Assessment procedures, including tests of intelligence, academic achievement, and social/emotional functioning, should be conducted by a multidisciplinary team to determine the special services that may be needed. Appropriate placement should depend upon the specific characteristics of the child. INDIVIDUALIZED EDUCATION PROGRAM objectives should be developed first for achievement over short periods of time.

Modifications in teaching style and methods, testing, behavior management techniques, length of lessons and homework assignments, and student expectations may all be necessary.

Symptoms and Diagnostic Path

Depending on the region of the brain affected, the conditions associated with brain damage or brain injury may vary widely. Physical and mental problems may be severe or highly selective and localized in cases where trauma occurred in a particular brain region. Relatively mild brain injury may express itself more subtly in conditions that have to do with language, behavioral controls, and judgment, or other higher cognitive functions.

Because each injury is unique, some patients may not experience all the symptoms. The impact of the injury really depends on where in the brain the trauma occurred.

Cognitive Symptoms

- problems processing information (decreased speed, accuracy, and consistency)
- shortened attention span

- problems understanding abstract concepts
- impaired decision-making ability
- inability to shift mental tasks or to follow multi-step directions
- memory loss
- problems in expressing thoughts and understanding others, inappropriate word selection

Perceptual Symptoms

- change in vision, hearing, sense of touch, smell, or taste
- loss of sense of time and space
- spatial disorientation
- altered sense of balance
- increased pain sensitivity

Physical Symptoms

- persistent headache
- extreme mental or physical fatigue
- disorders of movement, including spasticity or tremors
- seizures
- sensitivity to light
- sleep disorders
- paralysis
- speech that is not clear due to poor control of the muscles in the lips, tongue, and jaw, or poor breathing patterns

Behavioral/Emotional Symptoms

- irritability and impatience
- reduced tolerance for stress
- lack of initiative, apathy
- dependence
- denial of disability
- aggression, cursing, inappropriate sexual behavior
- inflexibility
- stronger or weaker emotional responses

Broca, Paul Pierre (1824–1880) A brilliant French surgeon and anthropologist who was a superb brain anatomist. Born in Sainte-Foy-la-Grande, France, he was a child prodigy, subsequently earning baccalaureate degrees simultaneously in literature, mathematics, and physics. He entered medical school when he was only 17 years old, graduating three years later. He became a professor of surgical pathology at the University of Paris and a noted medical researcher in many areas, and by age 24 he already had been showered with awards, medals, and important positions. In his early work he studied cartilage and bone, in addition to cancer, the treatment of aneurysms, and infant mortality.

As a brain expert, he made important contributions to the understanding of the limbic system, but he was best known for his discovery of the speech center (now known as BROCA'S AREA) in the third circumvolution of the FRONTAL LOBE. He also studied the brains of patients with APHASIA.

A kind and gentle man with a huge propensity for work, he wrote hundreds of books and papers (53 of them on the brain), and he was also concerned with health care for the poor. Near the end of his life, he was elected a lifetime member of the French Senate, and also was a member of the French Academy, holding honorary degrees from many universities around the world. He died in Paris in 1880, probably of a brain aneurysm.

Broca's aphasia A problem encountered in speaking, although spoken words are understood. Also called expressive APHASIA, the condition occurs with lesions in the motor strip of the FRONTAL LOBE.

See also BROCA'S AREA; BROCA, PAUL PIERRE.

Broca's area A section of the left FRONTAL LOBE involved in the production of language, that also directs speech via the MOTOR CORTEX. Damage to this area results in BROCA'S APHASIA, a speech disorder characterized by the ability to understand language but difficulty in speaking fluently.

Broca's area processes syntax and structural complexity of language. Individuals with neurological damage to this area are unable to understand and make grammatically complex sentences.

See also BROCA, PAUL PIERRE.

Brown v. Board of Education of Topeka The major court ruling on desegregation of public schools in the United States, ending the doctrine of "separate but equal" and requiring integration of schools with "all deliberate speed." It was delivered on May 17, 1954, by the U.S. Supreme Court, which ruled unanimously that racial segregation in public schools violated the Fourteenth Amendment to the Constitution. This amendment states that no state may deny equal protection of the laws to any person within its jurisdiction.

The 1954 decision declared that separate educational facilities were inherently unequal. Based on a series of Supreme Court cases argued between 1938 and 1950, *Brown v. Board of Education of Topeka* completed the reversal of an earlier Supreme Court ruling (*Plessy v. Ferguson,* 1896) that permitted "separate but equal" public facilities. The 1954 decision was limited to the public schools, but it was believed to imply that segregation was not permissible in other public facilities. However, the decision did not actually abolish segregation in other public areas, such as restaurants and restrooms, nor did it require desegregation of public schools by a specific time. It did, however, declare the permissive or mandatory segregation that existed in 21 states to be unconstitutional. While it was a giant step toward complete desegregation of public schools, even partial desegregation of these schools was still very far away.

In the early 1950s, racial segregation in public schools was widespread across America. Although all the schools in a given district were supposed to be equal, most black schools were far inferior to their white counterparts. In Topeka, Kansas, a black third grader named Linda Brown had to walk one mile through a railroad switchyard to get to her elementary school, even though a school for whites was only seven blocks away. When Linda's father, Oliver Brown, tried to enroll her in the white elementary school, the principal of the school refused.

Topeka's branch of the National Association for the Advancement of Colored People (NAACP) was eager to assist the Browns, as it had long wanted to challenge segregation in public schools. Brown was the right plaintiff at the right time, and other black parents joined Brown; in 1951 the NAACP requested an injunction that would forbid the segregation of Topeka's public schools.

The U.S. District Court for the District of Kansas heard Brown's case from June 25 to 26, 1951. At the trial, the NAACP argued that segregated schools sent the message to black children that they were inferior to whites; therefore, the schools were inherently unequal. The board of education's defense was that because segregation in Topeka and elsewhere pervaded many other aspects of life, segregated schools simply prepared black children for the segregation they would face during adulthood. The board also argued that segregated schools were not necessarily harmful to black children; great African Americans such as Frederick Douglass, Booker T. Washington, and George Washington Carver had overcome more than just segregated schools to achieve what they achieved.

Because of the precedent of *Plessy v. Ferguson,* which allowed separate but equal school systems for blacks and whites, the court felt "compelled" to rule in favor of the board of education.

Brown and the NAACP appealed to the Supreme Court on October 1, 1951, and their case was combined with other cases that challenged school segregation in South Carolina, Virginia, and Delaware. The Supreme Court first heard the case on December 9, 1952, but failed to reach a decision. In the reargument, heard from December 7 to 8, 1953, the Court requested that both sides discuss "the circumstances surrounding the adoption of the Fourteenth Amendment in 1868." The reargument shed very little additional light on the issue. The Court had to base its decision not on whether the authors of the Fourteenth Amendment had desegregated schools in mind when they wrote the amendment in 1868, but on whether desegregated schools deprived black children of equal protection of the law when the case was decided, in 1954. On May 17, 1954, Chief Justice Earl Warren read the decision of the unanimous Court:

> We come then to the question presented: Does segregation of children in public schools solely on the basis of race, even though the physical facilities and other "tangible" factors may be equal, deprive the children of the minority group of equal educational opportunities? We believe that it does . . . We conclude that in the field of public education the doctrine of 'separate but equal' has no place.

Separate educational facilities are inherently unequal. Therefore, we hold that the plaintiffs and others similarly situated for whom the actions have been brought are, by reason of the segregation complained of, deprived of the equal protection of the laws guaranteed by the Fourteenth Amendment.

The Supreme Court struck down the "separate but equal" doctrine of *Plessy* for public education, ruled in favor of the plaintiffs, and required the desegregation of schools across America.

Bruininks-Oseretsky Test of Motor Proficiency

An assessment for children aged four and a half through $14^1/_2$ that measures large- and fine-motor development on subtests that assess running speed, balance, coordination, muscle strength, visual tracking, speed of motor response, coordination of eye and hand movements, hand speed, arm speed, and hand and finger dexterity.

cadmium and learning disabilities See ENVIRON-
MENTAL TOXINS.

California Achievement Test (CAT) A national
standardized achievement test that is "norm-referenced" (that is, it compares a person's score against
the scores of a group of people who have already
taken the same exam, called the "norming
group"). A commercial norm-referenced test does
not compare all the students who take the test in a
given year. Instead, test makers select a sample
from a target student population and "norm" the
test on this sample, which is supposed to represent
the entire target population in the nation. Students' scores are then reported in relation to the
scores of this "norming" group.

To make comparing different students easier,
test makers create exams so that most students will
score near the middle and only a few will score low
or high. Versions of the CAT are available from
kindergarten through 12th grade.

case history An essential element of any assessment that represents a record of the person's family,
health, developmental, educational, psychological,
and social experiences. Typically, the creation of a
case history involves the analysis of records as well
as interviews with parents, teachers, and the individual. Case histories are an important component
of assessment in all cases of learning or psychological difficulty.

central auditory dysfunction See AUDITORY PRO-
CESSING DISORDER.

central deafness See AUDITORY PROCESSING DIS-
ORDER.

cerebellum A prominent hindbrain structure
important for coordinating and integrating motor
activity.

cerebral cortex The most complex area of the
brain, the cerebral cortex is the six-layered convo-
luted covering of the two hemispheres (also
known as gray matter). The body's control and
information processing center, it is organized into
four lobes: frontal, parietal, occipital, and temporal, each concerned with different functions.

Microscopic examination of autopsied brains
from people with DYSLEXIA have revealed changes
in the arrangement of nerve cells in the cerebral
cortex. Measurement of nerve cells in visual and
auditory parts of the thalamus revealed smaller
cells. These studies provided the first evidence of a
brain-based cause for developmental dyslexia.

The cerebral cortex is divided into two equal
halves (or spheres) called hemispheres. The left
hemisphere processes information logically; for
example, it helps a person read, speak, and write
language or compute an equation. The right hemisphere is responsible for more processing of spatial
information, such as recognizing a friend's face or
appreciating a piece of artwork. In other words, the
right hemisphere sees the forest (the big picture)
while the left hemisphere sees the trees (details).

Because the brain carries out many different
functions, its cells are also specialized. Different
types of neurons are distributed across different
layers of the cortex in arrangements that characterize the several areas of the hemispheres, each
one with its own functions.

The cerebral cortex represents a highly developed structure concerned with the most familiar
functions associated with the human brain, including intelligence and personality, interpretation of

sensory impulses, movement, and the ability to plan and organize.

Its distinctive shape arose during evolution as the volume of the cortex increased more rapidly than the cranial volume, so that the entire brain structure folded in onto itself.

cerebral palsy (CP) A condition caused by injury to the parts of the brain that control the ability to use muscles. Most often, the injury happens before or during birth, or soon afterward. A child can have mild, moderate, or severe cerebral palsy.

In mild cases, a child simply may be clumsy. With moderate CP, a child might walk with a limp and require a special leg brace or a cane. More severe CP can affect all parts of a child's physical abilities, and the child may need to use a wheelchair and other special equipment.

Sometimes children with CP also can have learning problems, problems with hearing or vision, or MENTAL RETARDATION. Usually, the greater the injury to the brain, the more severe the CP, but the condition does not worsen over time, and most children with CP have a normal life span.

About 500,000 Americans have some form of CP; each year 8,000 infants and nearly 1,500 preschool-age children are diagnosed with the condition.

Symptoms and Diagnostic Path

There are three main types of cerebral palsy: spastic, athetoid, and a combination of these two types known as "mixed."

Spastic CP is the most common form and is characterized by extremely tight muscles, with stiff movements of the legs, arms, or back. Children with this form of CP move their legs awkwardly, turning in or scissoring their legs as they try to walk.

Athetoid CP (also called dyskinetic CP) can affect movements of the entire body. Typically, this involves slow, uncontrolled body movements and low muscle tone that make it hard for the person to sit straight and walk.

Mixed CP is a combination of the symptoms listed above. A child with this form has some muscles that are too tight and others that are too loose, creating a mix of stiffness and involuntary movements.

In some cases of cerebral palsy, only the legs are affected (diplegia) or only half the body (hemiplegia).

Treatment Options and Outlook

With early and ongoing treatment the effects of CP can be reduced. Children younger than age three benefit from early intervention; older children can get SPECIAL EDUCATION services through public schools. Typically, children with CP may need different kinds of therapy, including

- PHYSICAL THERAPY: to help develop stronger muscles, with emphasis on walking, sitting, and keeping his or her balance
- OCCUPATIONAL THERAPY: to help develop FINE MOTOR SKILLS such as dressing, feeding, writing, and other daily living tasks
- SPEECH-LANGUAGE THERAPY: to help develop communication skills

A variety of special equipment may help. This may include braces to hold the foot in place when the child stands or walks, or custom splints to help a child use the hands. A variety of therapy equipment and adapted toys can help children play, and activities such as swimming or horseback riding can help strengthen weaker muscles and relax the tighter ones.

Surgery, Botox injections, or other medications can help lessen the effects of CP, but there is no cure for the condition.

Education

A child with CP can face many challenges in school and is likely to need individualized help. For children up to age three, services are provided through an early intervention system. Schools work with the child's family to develop an INDIVIDUALIZED FAMILY SERVICES PROGRAM (IFSP). The plan describes the child's unique needs as well as the services the child needs. The plan will also emphasize the unique needs of the family, so that parents and other family members will know how to help their young child with CP. Early intervention services may be provided on a sliding-fee basis, meaning that the costs to the family will depend upon their income.

For school-age children (including preschoolers), special education and services will be provided through the school. School staff will work with the child's parents to develop an INDIVIDUAL-

IZED EDUCATION PROGRAM, which is similar to the family services plan in that it describes the child's unique needs and necessary services. Special education and related services, which can include physical and occupational therapy and speech-language pathology, are provided free.

In addition to therapy services and special equipment, children with CP may need ASSISTIVE TECHNOLOGY, like communication devices such as voice synthesizers, or communication boards with pictures, symbols, letters, or words attached. The child communicates by pointing to or gazing at the pictures.

Other types of technology may include electronic toys with special switches or sophisticated computer programs operated by simple switch pads or keyboard adaptations.

The INDIVIDUALS WITH DISABILITIES EDUCATION IMPROVEMENT ACT (IDEIA) guides how early intervention services and special education and related services are provided to children with disabilities. Under IDEIA, cerebral palsy is considered an "orthopedic impairment"—a severe impairment that affects a child's educational performance.

channel   A sensory mode through which information is taken in and processed, as in the "auditory channel" or "visual channel." Individuals often show a preference for a specific sensory channel.

See also LEARNING MODALITIES; MULTIPLE INTELLIGENCES.

Child Attention Profile   A popular BEHAVIOR RATING SCALE used to help diagnose ATTENTION DEFICIT HYPERACTIVITY DISORDER.

Child Behavior Checklist   A type of behavioral questionnaire that contains a list of behavioral problems rated by the parent as "not true," "somewhat true," or "very true." Children are compared with others of the same age on anxiety, depression, hyperactivity, and so on. Because it is helpful on any behavior checklist to obtain input from several teachers and parents, self-report and teacher forms are also available. Because each teacher and parent is likely to see the student from a different perspective, the best overall view of the child's behavior is obtained by comparing many different viewpoints.

childhood disintegrative disorder (CDD)   A fairly rare yet serious condition in which a child older than age three stops developing normally and regresses to a much lower level of functioning, typically after a serious illness, such as an infection of the brain and nervous system. The disorder is associated with seizures and is more common in boys. Patients with the condition usually require lifelong care. CDD was first described in 1908, but it has only recently been officially recognized. The condition resembles AUTISM, and appears only after a relatively prolonged period of clearly normal development (usually two to four years). Although apparently rare, experts believe the condition probably has often been incorrectly diagnosed.

Symptoms and Diagnostic Path

Several different patterns of this condition have been identified. CDD may begin slowly or relentlessly. There may be progressive deterioration, developmental plateaus with little subsequent improvement, or—much less often—marked improvement.

CDD occurs most often in boys, with symptoms typically appearing between ages three and four. Until this time, patients develop appropriate skills in communication and social relationships for their age. Then symptoms appear, beginning with extensive and pronounced losses in motor, language, and social skills, including loss of expressive or receptive language, nonverbal behavior, and play. In addition, the child develops difficulties in social interaction (failing to develop friendships and being unable to start or sustain a conversation) and begins performing repetitive behaviors similar to those that occur in children with autism. Quite often the child gradually deteriorates to a severely retarded level. Once regression begins, the loss of skills, such as vocabulary, are dramatic and are often accompanied by loss of bowel and bladder control, seizures, and a very low IQ.

The condition is diagnosed based on the symptoms and by ruling out both childhood schizophrenia and autism. Generally the diagnosis is made with a loss of functioning in at least two areas in language, motor, or social skills.

Treatment Options and Outlook

Childhood disintegrative disorder cannot be specifically treated or cured, and most children, particularly those who are severely retarded, need lifelong care. Unfortunately, the prognosis for this disorder is limited. The loss of functioning is usually permanent, although to some degree the child's behavior can be modified. The available data suggest that generally the prognosis for this condition is worse than that for autism.

child psychiatrist   A physician who specializes in the diagnosis and treatment of disorders of thinking, feeling, or behavior that affect children and adolescents. Psychiatrists can prescribe medication (as can psychologists in a few states), and often work with psychologists in prescribing drug treatments.

Child psychiatrists must complete four years of medical school, at least three years of residency training in medicine, neurology, and general psychiatry with adults, and two years of training in psychiatric work with children, adolescents, and their families in an accredited residency in child and adolescent psychiatry. After completing medical school, graduates must pass a licensing test given by the board of medical examiners for the state in which they want to work. Psychiatrists must then take and pass the certifying examination given by the Board of Psychiatry and Neurology. (In order to be board-certified in child and adolescent psychiatry, a candidate must first be board-certified in general psychiatry.)

child study committee   A group of school members who review and decide plans of action for students. Typically, a student is referred to the child study committee because of concerns about school performance, either academic or behavioral. The committee usually consists of at least three people, including the school principal or a delegate, the teacher or teachers, and a special educator or school counselor.

See also INDIVIDUALIZED EDUCATION PROGRAM.

chunking   A strategy for enhancing memory by grouping similar information, because smaller "chunks" are easier to remember than larger sequences of information. For example, a telephone number is typically remembered in chunks of three: the area code, the exchange, and the individual four-digit number, which is far easier to remember than a 10-digit number.

classroom management   The array of strategies and techniques a teacher uses to manage the range of learning needs and behaviors that may exist within a given class. Effective classroom management keeps discipline problems to a minimum and addresses them effectively, and provides a safe, secure space for learning that appropriately responds to a variety of learning styles.

clinical observation   The study and analysis of an individual's behavior and performance in a clinical setting. This observation may involve analysis of behaviors during testing, mood and behavior during a clinical interview, or the observations of behavior in more open-ended assessment contexts, such as play in the case of young children. Clinical observation is an important component of assessment.

closure   The idea that information processing and perception typically strives for making things whole. For example, in a CLOZE PROCEDURE TEST (a form of assessment that measures various READING COMPREHENSION skills), individuals read sentences in context; if they understand, they have little difficulty finding correct responses.

cloze procedure test   A form of assessment used to measure various READING COMPREHENSION skills. In a passage of sentences, words are replaced with spaces for the reader to fill in, using contextual cues and the reader's understanding of a variety of language patterns.

Code of Federal Regulations (CFR)   All of the federal regulations that explain, expand on, and are used to implement federal laws. Federal regulations contained in the CFR often define terms that are used in laws but are not clearly defined; the CFR also may specify how a program mandated by law is to be administered. Federal regulations are cited by volume and section number in the CFR.

coding   The ways in which information is represented so it can be placed in and retrieved from long-term memory. When something is seen or heard, it must be associated with existing knowledge or organized if the information to be useful.

Research suggests that some people with a LEARN-ING DISABILITY do not encode information well.

cognition   The process of knowing, thinking, problem solving, remembering, reasoning, planning, and making judgments. It includes the acquisition and manipulation of knowledge, usually by means of symbols.

Cognitive scientists are concerned with this human ability. They are less concerned about the fact that cognition cannot be directly observed; instead, they consider the neurological events that allow the process to occur.

cognitive ability   A general term that refers to the broad cluster of mental skills involved in learning, thinking, and processing information. Examples of cognitive abilities include MEMORY, ATTENTION, LANGUAGE DEVELOPMENT, COMPREHENSION, problem solving, critical analysis, and concept formation.

Although it is possible to generalize about the overall cognitive ability of an individual, it is far more important and valuable to understand the ways in which specific cognitive functions interact and depend on one another, and to assess strengths and difficulties in a more specific fashion.

cognitive style   The preferred way an individual processes information, usually described as a personality dimension that influences attitudes, values, and social interaction. Unlike individual differences in abilities that describe peak performance, styles describe a person's typical mode of thinking, remembering, or problem solving. Having more of an ability is usually considered beneficial, while having a particular cognitive style simply denotes a tendency to behave in a certain manner.

Field Independence/Dependence   A number of cognitive styles have been identified and studied over the years; field independence/field dependence is probably the most well known. Individuals view the world in different ways. Those who are called "field-dependent" perceive the world in terms of larger patterns and relationships, whereas those who are "field-independent" perceive the world in terms of discrete individual elements— they look at the pieces that make up the whole.

Most schools in Western culture favor a field-independent approach, rewarding students who tend to work and organize information on their own. These learners are objective in that they make what is being studied into an object to be analyzed and understood.

Studies have identified a number of connections between this cognitive style and learning. For example, field-independent individuals are likely to learn more effectively by studying by themselves, and are influenced less by social reinforcement.

college admission and learning disabilities   More and more students with LEARNING DISABILITIES are enrolling in two- and four-year colleges and universities, doubling from 15 percent to 32 percent since 1985. Currently, nearly one-third of all freshmen with disabilities report having learning disabilities.

However, universities have different purposes, entrance criteria, programs, and requirements for certifications, associate degrees, and baccalaureate degrees. As a result, students with learning disabilities who want to go to college need to prepare in high school long before their senior year.

First, students with learning disabilities who want to go to college need to learn strategies to help them plan, complete, and evaluate projects, to apply strategies flexibly, and modify or create strategies to fit new learning situations. There are many ways to do this, such as allowing more time to complete tests or projects, listening to audio tapes of textbooks while reading, and so on.

Legal rights   High school students with learning disabilities must understand their rights under Section 504 of the REHABILITATION ACT and the AMERICANS WITH DISABILITIES ACT (ADA), which guarantee the civil rights of people with disabilities, and how these differ from the rights and services they receive under the INDIVIDUALS WITH DISABILITIES EDUCATION IMPROVEMENT ACT (IDEIA).

IDEIA is the legislation that guarantees a free, appropriate public education and governs how SPECIAL EDUCATION services will be provided to students with disabilities in elementary and secondary schools. Under IDEIA, the school is responsible for identifying and testing students with disabilities, and for monitoring services. These special education services, which are described in detail in a student's

INDIVIDUALIZED EDUCATION PROGRAM (IEP) and individualized transition plan (ITP), could significantly change the requirements of the standard high school academic program. Requirements for high school diplomas may be changed under IDEIA as well. For example, depending on the particular disability, some students may not need to take certain language, mathematics, or science courses that are usually required courses for a diploma. However, IDEIA does not apply to higher education; colleges and universities do not offer "special" education.

Under Section 504 and the ADA, universities cannot discriminate against a person because of disability, and must provide reasonable modifications, accommodations, or aids to enable qualified students to participate in college programs. A university, for example, may provide readers, notetakers, extra time to complete exams, or alternate test formats. Decisions about the exact accommodations a college would provide are made on a case-by-case basis. Exactly what they offer is up to the college, as long as it is effective. *Colleges and universities are not required by law to provide aides, services, or devices for personal use or study.*

In addition, colleges are not required to design special academic programs for students with disabilities, but they must provide services so that qualified students with disabilities will have equal access to the regular academic program. After equal access is provided, it is a student's own responsibility to succeed. Section 504 and the ADA do not require colleges to change their requirements for either admission or graduation.

After high school, the level of responsibility about special services changes. Once a student has been admitted to college, it is the student's responsibility to provide documentation of a disability. The college will not provide any ACCOMMODATION until a student

- requests services from the office (or person) on campus responsible for providing services to students with disabilities
- provides documentation of disability. For the student with a learning disability, such documentation is often a copy of the testing report and/or a copy of the IEP or ITP

Confidentiality   To protect the privacy of student records, the Family Educational Rights and Privacy Act (FERPA) was passed in 1974 and later amended several times. FERPA (also known as the Buckley Amendment) gives students the right to access their educational records, consent to release a record to a third party, challenge information in those records, and be notified of their privacy rights. FERPA affects all colleges that receive federal funds. FERPA protects a student's record from being shared (without the student's permission) with "curious" faculty, administrators, other students, the press, or anyone without a legitimate reason for seeing the record. For example, faculty members do not have a right to access information about a student's disability; they need to know only what accommodations are necessary to meet the student's disability-related needs, and then only with permission of the student.

Preparing for college   Under the IDEIA, the IEP for each student receiving special education services must include a statement of the transition services needed. Students with learning disabilities who plan to go to college should participate in the transition planning process.

College options   Hundreds of colleges and universities have comprehensive programs on campus specially designed for students with learning disabilities. Staffed by experts, these programs may offer tutoring or counseling services. Since the services provided in such programs are more than they are required to offer under Section 504 and ADA, many colleges and universities charge for these services. Services required by Section 504 and ADA are provided at no cost.

It is also possible that such programs have their own separate admission requirements. Students who wish to learn more about such programs should either call and ask if such a program exists on campus, or check guidebooks that contain listings of such programs.

IDEIA requires reevaluations to be conducted at least every three years; therefore, high school students with learning disabilities ought to have a comprehensive reevaluation close to graduation to ensure that the documentation they take with them is up to date. Students and parents should discuss the documentation in order to understand what it conveys about the student's strengths, weaknesses, and recommended services.

Many high schools routinely destroy copies of student records after a number of years. Since students with learning disabilities will need copies of some items in their records to show to the college or university as documentation of their disability, they should be sure to have complete copies of all records.

Students with learning disabilities should consider various college options as well as their academic strengths and weaknesses in planning their high school program. Students seeking admission to selective institutions *must* meet the criteria set by the college.

Successful college students with learning disabilities report that high school courses teaching keyboard skills and word processing are especially important. A high school transcript displaying successful completion of a wide array of courses (science, math, history, literature, foreign language, art, music) is attractive to selective college admissions staff. Involvement in school or community sponsored clubs, teams, or performances also enhances a college admission candidate's application.

Students with learning disabilities may benefit from mini-courses in study skills, assertiveness training, and time management. It is very important to list the accommodative services in the ITP, since the types of accommodations students may receive when taking standardized college admission tests or licensing examinations may depend on the evidence of having received them in high school.

Colleges and universities are not required to change admission requirements, nor are they required to alter program requirements for students with learning disabilities once they have been admitted. While colleges and universities need to give consideration to requests of students with learning disabilities for course waivers and substitutions, such waivers and substitutions are not often granted. If the campus academic committee determines that a course is not an essential component of the student's major, a waiver may be granted. Substitution with courses that convey the essential elements of the requirement (such as substituting a course in the culture of another country

for a course in foreign language) are more readily granted than waivers. However, if a course is an essential element to the degree sought, it is unlikely that a waiver or substitution would be granted. Therefore, passing such a course would continue to be a requirement for graduation.

Admission testing With proper documentation, high school students with learning disabilities may take standardized college admission tests such as the PSAT, SAT, and ACT with certain accommodations, including

- individual administration of the test
- audiocassette tape or large-print test editions
- special answer sheets
- extended testing time

However, the procedures for accommodations in each of the standardized tests vary, and students should contact the agency that administers each standardized test for specific information. It is the responsibility of the student to request information and accommodations. Any accommodation given by a testing agency to a student with a learning disability is designed only to give that student equal footing in the testing environment. It is then every student's responsibility to do well. Tests taken by students with disabilities are scored in the same fashion as those taken by students without disabilities. Scores of tests taken with accommodations are so noted when they are reported to the schools.

Disclosure A student will need to decide whether or not to disclose the disability. Colleges may invite applicants for admission to indicate the existence of disabilities on the application form, but may not require this information. Should a student reveal a disability, this information alone cannot be used as a basis for denying admission. On the other hand, colleges do not have to change their admission requirements or standards. This means that having a learning disability does not entitle a student to a place in college.

However, by disclosing the disability, the student may explain possible discrepancies within admission documents, such as a transcript with top grades but low SAT scores. Such discrepancies are typical of a student with a learning disability, but if an admissions committee is not aware of the disability, admission may be denied.

Of course, disclosing a learning disability does not guarantee admission, but it can offer the chance to include additional insights.

communication delay   Speech and language patterns that develop normally but at a slower pace than would be typically expected.

communication disorder   A wide variety of problems in speech, language, or hearing. Students with a communication disorder can quickly fall behind in class and have problems in vocabulary, MEMORY, and PROBLEM SOLVING. Many also encounter trouble in social situations.

Although experts are not sure exactly how many children have communication disorders, estimates suggest it may affect about 5 percent of the school-age population. This figure includes voice disorders (3 percent) and STUTTERING (1 percent). The incidence of elementary school children who experience delayed articulation development is 2 to 3 percent, although the percentage decreases steadily with age. Exact figures on the number of children with hearing problems vary considerably, but many experts use the figure of 5 percent of school-age children with abnormal hearing levels. Of this number, 10 to 20 percent need some type of SPECIAL EDUCATION. About one-third of students who are deaf attend residential schools; two-thirds attend day programs in schools for students who are deaf or day classes in regular schools. The rest are MAINSTREAMED into regular school programs.

According to government estimates, more than 20 percent of students with disabilities (or more than 1 million children ages six to 21) received special services for communication disorders during the 1996–97 school year. A smaller number of students with hearing problems (70,883) received services.

Language-based communication disorders are caused by a difference in brain structure present at birth, which may be inherited or attributed to environmental factors during a woman's pregnancy, including drugs, sexually transmitted diseases such as syphilis, and birthing trauma. Other communication disorders stem from oral-motor problems (such as APRAXIA or DYSARTHRIA of speech), APHASIA (difficulty in using words, usually as a result of a brain injury), traumatic brain injuries, and fluency problems such as stuttering, which is now believed to be a neurological deficit.

The most common conditions that affect children's communication include language-based learning disabilities, attention deficit disorder, ATTENTION DEFICIT HYPERACTIVITY DISORDER, CEREBRAL PALSY, mental disabilities, cleft lip or palate, and AUTISTIC SPECTRUM DISORDERS. The list of conditions in the communication disorders group includes DEVELOPMENTAL ARTICULATION DISORDER, DEVELOPMENTAL EXPRESSIVE LANGUAGE DISORDER, DEVELOPMENTAL RECEPTIVE LANGUAGE DISORDER, and MIXED RECEPTIVE-EXPRESSIVE LANGUAGE DISORDER.

Symptoms and Diagnostic Path

A child with a communication problem may have many different symptoms, such as trouble following directions or paying attention to a conversation; difficulty pronouncing words; slow or incomprehensible speech because of a stutter or a hoarse voice; pronounce difficulties in syntax (the order of words in a sentence) and articulation (the way in which sounds are made); or difficulty understanding what was said. The hallmark of an articulation disorder is the substitution of one sound for another or the omission or distortion of certain sounds. Stuttering (also called dysfluency) is a disorder of speech flow that typically appears between ages three and four and may steadily worsen to be a chronic problem. Stuttering may spontaneously disappear by early adolescence. Voice disorders (hoarseness, breathiness, or sudden breaks in loudness or pitch) are often combined with other speech problems to create a complex communication disorder.

Communication disorders can be grouped into two main categories—hearing disorders and speech/language disorders. A child with a full or partial hearing problem also may have trouble with speech and language development, which is why an assessment of hearing ability is one of the first steps in the investigation of speech and language problems. A child with a physical disability such as a cleft lip and palate, or malformations of the mouth or nose, may have a communication disorder. Other disabilities, such as cerebral palsy, may mean the child cannot speak at all. Some children with a developmental disability, such as DOWN SYNDROME, may be slower to learn to talk.

Hearing disorders A hearing disorder affects the ability to hear sounds clearly. Such disorders may range from hearing speech sounds faintly or in a distorted way to profound deafness. Hearing difficulties also may cause speech problems (such as ARTICULATION or voice) and/or language problems. A child with a hearing problem may strain to hear conversations or have to ask people to repeat things before giving the right answer. These children may have speech inaccuracies, such as dropping the beginnings and endings of words, or seem to be confused during classroom discussions. Detection and diagnosis of hearing impairments have become so sophisticated that it is now possible to detect and evaluate hearing loss in a newborn child.

There are four types of hearing loss: conductive, sensorineural, mixed, and central. Conductive hearing losses are caused by disease or obstructions in the outer or middle ear; these typically can be helped with a hearing aid. Sensorineural losses are caused by damage to the sensory hair cells of the inner ear or the nerves that supply it and usually do not improve with a hearing aid. Mixed hearing losses include those in which the problem occurs both in the outer or middle ear and in the inner ear. A central hearing loss results from damage to the nerves or brain.

Speech/Language disorders Speech and language disorders affect the way people talk and understand and may range from simple sound substitutions to the inability to use speech and language.

A child with a language problem may involve trouble expressing ideas coherently, learning new vocabulary, understanding questions and following directions, understanding or remembering information in a conversation, reading at a normal pace, comprehending, learning the alphabet, identifying sounds that correspond to letters, figuring out the correct order of letters in words, recalling information, or spelling.

Difficulties with speech may include being unable to be understood because of a motor problem or due to poor learning. A voice problem may cause hoarse, breathy, or harsh speech. Stuttering also affects speech intelligibility because the child's flow of speech is interrupted.

Evidence of a speech or language disorder may be seen when a person's speech or language significantly differs from that of others of the same age or background or when there is a marked problem in one's ability to express oneself.

Treatment Options and Outlook

Many communication problems can be improved by a variety of treatments. Because many speech problems are developmental and not caused by a physical problem, they can improve with remedial instruction. In the past, children with communication disorders were routinely removed from the regular class for individual intensive speech and language therapy, but today—unless the problem is quite severe—educators prefer to keep the child in the regular classroom as much as possible. In order to accomplish this goal, the teacher, speech and language therapist, audiologist, and parents all must work together to blend speech improvement and correction into the regular classroom curriculum and the child's home environment.

Although some problems may never be cured, students with problems such as stuttering or attention deficits can learn new ways to overcome their difficulties. Some children with mild problems, such as language delay, may be able to overcome their communication disorder as they grow older, while others may compensate by communicating via an augmentative communication device or hearing aid.

Children with hearing problems may be helped by hearing aids; those who still cannot hear well with these aids may require more intensive intervention. For deaf children, early, consistent, and conscious use of visible communication modes such as sign language, finger spelling, and cued speech and/or hearing aids and speech training can help reduce this language delay. However, the best way to educate a deaf child is extremely controversial. Some educators advocate a strict oral approach in which the child is required to use as much speech as possible, while others favor the use of sign language and finger spelling combined with speech (called *total communication*). Some advocates in the deaf community insist that sign language and finger spelling alone is quite sufficient. In any case, most experts now agree that whatever system works best for the child should be used.

Many children with hearing problems can attend a regular classroom with support services, hearing aids, captioned films, and high interest/low vocabulary reading materials. For most children with hearing problems, language acquisition and development are significantly delayed, sometimes leading to an incorrect estimate of low intelligence.

There is a strong relationship between good communication skills and academic success. The ability to use language and communicate effectively, and ultimate academic success, depend on whether students can match their communications to the learning-teaching style of the classroom.

comorbidity A medical term that refers to a relationship or association between one condition (such as ATTENTION DEFICIT HYPERACTIVITY DISORDER) and other psychological or LEARNING DISORDERS. For example, DYSLEXIA is comorbid with ADHD in as many as 40 percent of children with ADHD. ADHD may also be comorbid with substance abuse disorders, DEPRESSION, OBSESSIVE-COMPULSIVE DISORDER, and BORDERLINE PERSONALITY DISORDER.

The term suggests that one disorder may be linked with others in a relationship that is not fully understood. For effective treatment, a diagnosis must assess all possible learning and psychological problems. If more than one condition is present, treatment must take into account all of the existing conditions.

compensation A change in action, behavior, or attitude that is based on the influence of a disability or disorder. In learning, compensation is the development of skills or strategies to help strengthen a weak area or disability. Compensatory strategies can develop over time in order to learn successfully or more efficiently.

comprehension The ability to recognize and understand information. There are different types of comprehension (such as listening comprehension, reading comprehension, and picture compre-

hension), and an individual may perform differently in varying comprehension areas.

For example, an individual's listening comprehension may be stronger or weaker than his reading comprehension, and an individual with poor comprehension of verbal material may be much stronger in the area of social comprehension.

In academic settings, comprehension is often associated with intellectual potential and intelligence. However, comprehension involves a number of subcomponents, and it is important to be cautious in assessing the factors that may underlie comprehension problems. For example, listening comprehension difficulties may arise from problems in the area of auditory processing, rather than difficulties with reasoning. Likewise, problems with reading comprehension may be caused by underlying decoding problems and unfamiliarity with the material, or limited general knowledge.

Some learning disorders such as NONVERBAL LEARNING DISABILITIES may involve significant deficits in the area of social comprehension, resulting in large part from difficulties in processing visual-spatial information.

See also AUDITORY PROCESSING DISORDER.

comprehension monitoring A term that refers to how a student reads. The student writes down whether he or she is beginning to form a concept of the meaning of the passage, and adjusts the reading processes accordingly.

comprehension strategy In reading, a systematic sequence of steps for understanding text. However, there is little consensus in the research literature on what constitutes a comprehension strategy, which also may include teaching techniques such as MAPPING or diagramming, used to help students become strategic readers.

compulsion An irresistible urge to perform an action over and over.

computer assisted instruction (CAI) A form of individual learning that offers instruction, practice, and feedback delivered by software programs. CAI is a somewhat dated term that was used when computers were a relatively new phenomenon in classrooms. Now that most learning environments have integrated computer tools into instruction, the term is becoming obsolete.

CAI applies to any computer hardware or software that enhances learning, as opposed to ASSISTIVE TECHNOLOGY, which refers specifically to computer-based learning aids for people with various kinds of disabilities.

Computer assisted instruction can offer a useful means for practice of newly developed skills, and is most effective when facilitated by a skilled instructor. CAI can be a useful and motivating means of improving skills because of the graphic and interactive nature of most programs.

concentration   Focused attention. Someone who is concentrating on a task must both sustain ATTENTION over time and also hold information in active working MEMORY. Concentration requires a higher level of arousal than attention or vigilance, because of the requirement for processing in working memory on a continuing basis.

Although "concentration" is not a clinical term, it may be used in descriptions of task performance in order to describe the level of active processing of relevant information and a high level of filtering out distractions.

concept   A mental representation used to group things or ideas by their shared attributes. The term *concept* reflects a central element in COGNITION. Humans conceptualize information by first absorbing it and then organizing or classifying it.

A concept can be a concrete or abstract mental representation. The concept of "dog" is concrete—understanding that specific animals, although different in size, appearance, and behavior, can be grouped together as a "dog" category. Concepts are often understood to be abstract, as well, such as the concept of "justice." In understanding the term "justice," an individual must be able to apply a current use of the word to background knowledge and prior experience. While there may be no specific, agreed-upon mental representation or image for "justice," individuals store a range of information that allows them to retrieve an assortment of applications and meanings in order to help them understand.

Being able to form a concept is a cognitive process of abstraction. As individuals experience the world, they make inferences about the things in it. When a person perceives that qualities are similar and can be placed in the same class, concepts are formed. This process involves understanding a set of relevant features or qualifiers that can be used to represent a concept.

Concepts can be formed verbally or nonverbally—it may be easier to visualize a poodle than it is to describe a poodle. Verbal concepts are associated with ideas that are easier to describe with words than visually. Nonverbal concepts are easier to envision than to describe with words.

Individuals with LEARNING DISABILITIES can have difficulty with concept formation. They are likely to have difficulty if concepts are presented in a way not suited to their strongest learning style. If they are visual learners, they may have difficulty with concepts that are explained only verbally. Individuals with language-based learning difficulties may benefit from presentations that are more visual.

concept imagery   The ability to imagine the whole. Concept imagery is directly related to oral and written language comprehension and critical thinking.

See also CONCEPT IMAGERY DISORDER.

concept imagery disorder   A problem with visualizing related to language COMPREHENSION. The ability to imagine is directly related to oral and written language comprehension and critical thinking. Individuals with good comprehension report that they form mental images easily, but students with poor comprehension report that they see nothing when they read, or see only a few fleeting images. This means it is difficult to connect to the entire concept of what is read or heard.

Students with this problem grasp a few facts, but get lost after a few sentences when they read or listen. They can recall some specifics, but cannot generalize and create a "whole" from the information.

Symptoms of the disorder include

- poor reading comprehension
- poor oral language comprehension
- inability to follow oral directions
- weak expressive language

- weak higher order thinking skills
- poor problem solving

conceptual disorder Problems in thinking, memorizing, and organizing thoughts in relation to problem solving, following or producing logical sequences, or the ability to formulate and express concepts.

This problem may make it very hard for a student to understand written material or spoken information and seriously interfere with school performance. In general, conceptual disorders may be part of a specific learning disability, rather than an isolated learning problem.

Concerta See METHYLPHENIDATE.

concrete operational stage The third of the four stages in JEAN PIAGET's theory of cognitive development. This stage occurs from ages six or seven to about 11, during which the child learns to think logically about concrete events. During this period, the child will learn to consider several features of a task or situation rather than to focus on only the most obvious. At this stage children can mentally go through a series of steps to solve a problem and then reverse the series, returning to the beginning of the problem.

They are able to classify objects into subcategories and to place objects into a sequence based on a variety of qualities such as height, weight, or age. They also come to understand that objects remain the same in terms of mass and number when their shape or arrangement changes.

Research has confirmed that Piaget's sequence of the acquisition of various characteristics at this stage is generally accurate.

concrete thinking A type of thinking in which the individual is unable to understand the similarities between situations, seeing each situation as different.

conduct disorder Extremely severe, excessive, sustained aggressive behavior characterized by vandalism, theft, lying, property destruction, and drug use. Typically diagnosed in young boys, conduct disorders are characterized by antisocial behavior and patterns of "acting out" at home or at school. The child may have difficulty learning how to solve problems or to establish peer relationships.

Individuals with conduct disorder are more likely to attract attention from teachers and parents, to be referred for services, and to receive some treatment at an early age for their misbehavior.

There is a high correlation between conduct disorder and ATTENTION DEFICIT HYPERACTIVITY DISORDER (ADHD). Individuals with both disorders are particularly at risk for continuing social and emotional difficulties into adulthood. Other existing conditions include mood disorders anxiety, and substance abuse. Conduct disorder affects at least 6 percent of boys and 2 percent of girls under age 18.

Research suggests that the most severe cases of conduct disorder begin in early childhood, especially in the presence of inconsistent rules and harsh discipline, lack of enough supervision or guidance, frequent change in caregivers, poverty, brain damage, genetic vulnerability, school failure, trauma, neglect or abuse, or a delinquent peer group.

Symptoms and Diagnostic Path

Children with conduct disorder typically lack remorse for their actions or refuse to accept responsibility for them and engage in a repetitive and persistent pattern of behavior in which the basic rights of others or major age-appropriate societal norms or rules are violated. Typically, this includes at least three of the following symptoms over the course of one year, according to the *Diagnostic and Statistical Manual of Mental Disorders—Fourth Edition, Text Revision*:

- often bullies, threatens, or intimidates others
- starts physical fights
- has used a weapon, such as a knife or gun
- has been physically cruel to people
- has been physically cruel to animals
- has stolen something from a someone face-to-face
- has stolen items of value without confronting a victim (such as shoplifting)
- has broken into someone else's house, building, or car

- has forced someone into sexual activity
- has deliberately set a fire
- has deliberately destroyed someone else's property
- lies to obtain goods or favors or to avoid responsibilities
- often breaks rules to stay out at night, beginning before age 13 years
- has run away from home overnight at least twice while living at home (or once without returning for a long time)
- often skips class, beginning before age 13

Treatment Options and Outlook

Because antisocial behavior in children and adolescents is very hard to change after it has become ingrained, the earlier the problem is identified and treated, the better.

Treatment of children with conduct disorder can be difficult, especially because these children typically have an uncooperative attitude and distrust adults. Without treatment, many children with conduct disorder cannot adapt to the demands of adulthood and continue to have severe problems with relationships and responsibility. They often break laws or behave in an antisocial manner and frequently turn to criminal pursuits.

If begun early enough, intensive family therapy and behavior therapy may help the child learn how to express and manage anger. Some of the most effective programs deal with a variety of potential problems at home and at school, combining classroom social skills, a playground behavior program, parent training, and regular communication between parents and teachers. This has been shown to reduce short-term aggression and boost classroom skills.

In addition, the growing popularity of school programs that target bullying can be effective. These programs typically include coaching teachers to be more aware of the problem and how to handle it and intervene in specific problem cases.

Certain medications (including lithium, antipsychotic drugs, or stimulants) can be used to treat children with severe conduct disorder that has not responded to other treatments, although there has not been a great deal of research in this area. Studies have suggested that medications are only partly helpful in improving symptoms and must be combined with other types of treatment, such as psychotherapy, to be most effective.

confidential file In relation to SPECIAL EDUCATION, a confidential file is a limited-access file maintained by the school that contains evaluations and any other information related to special education placement. Parents have the right to know the information contained in a confidential file and to have copies of any materials.

configuration The visual shape of a word, including elements such as the height, depth, or width of various letters, and the overall length of the word. Word configuration may be used in sight-word reading as a cue in WORD-ATTACK SKILLS.

Connors Rating Scales—Revised (CRS-R) An instrument that uses observer ratings and self-report ratings to help assess ATTENTION DEFICIT HYPERACTIVITY DISORDER (ADHD) and evaluate problem behavior in children and adolescents. Various CRS-R versions offer different administration options while also providing the ability to collect varying perspectives on a child's behavior from parents, teachers, caregivers, and the child or adolescent. The three versions (parent, teacher, and adolescent self-report) all have a short and an alternative long form available. In addition, there are three screening tools that offer the option of administering a 12-item ADHD index or the 18-item *DSM-IV-TR* symptom checklist, or both.

The CRS-R tests are used for routine screenings in many different settings to help measure hyperactivity in children and adolescents and provide a perspective of the child's behavior from those who interact with the child on a daily basis. The test also can establish a base point before starting treatment and monitor how well treatment is working.

constructional apraxia The inability to assemble, build, draw, or copy accurately.

See also APRAXIA.

context clues Using information in a sentence or paragraph surrounding a new term to help the reader understand that term. There are several items to look for when searching for context clues, including

- a punctuation mark (such as a comma or dash) that may signal that information is being presented about the new term
- key words: words such as *or* and *that is* may signal that a definition is to follow
- definition: sometimes the meaning of a new term may be made clear by reading the entire paragraph in which it appears

Learning to use context clues to gain meaning is an important reading skill. A student who is able to use the context to identify an unknown word, grasp the meaning of a word, or comprehend a passage read, will become a good reader.

contextual reading   Reading that is performed using narrative text (paragraphs, stories, articles) rather than words in isolation. Assessing the way in which an individual reads contextually is essential to developing an accurate picture of the person's reading ability.

Determining a person's fluency is important in developing an overall reading program. Increasing the volume of reading (especially reading for pleasure) is considered essential to improving contextual reading abilities.

continuum of services   A range of services from least amount of change in a student's educational program to institutionalization. In the past, it was a common practice in many school districts either not to provide any SPECIAL EDUCATION at all or to provide only a very few placement options.

With the passage of the INDIVIDUALS WITH DISABILITIES ACT, schools were required to provide any necessary placement options such as resource classes, self-contained classes, or institutionalization.

contralateral   Relating to opposite sides. The human brain is contralateral in nature, since areas on one side of the brain are concerned with sensory and motor processes on the opposite side of the body. For example, left brain activity regulates physical movement on the right side of the body.

convergence   A way of thinking that combines existing information and knowledge to solve a problem in an analytical and rational manner. It is most useful for problems that can be solved algorithmically or that have a single correct answer.

convergent retrieval memory   The location of highly specific information in MEMORY on demand, such as in word-finding, spelling tests, or solving arithmetic equations. Trying to locate the precise word to describe a phenomenon, or attempting to recall the answer to a simple multiplication problem, are both examples of convergent retrieval memory at work. Individuals with LEARNING DISABILITIES often have trouble with these types of tasks.

Convergent retrieval memory is the opposite of divergent retrieval, in which there may be many possible appropriate responses.

coordination   The effective control of muscles in the body to perform smooth, voluntary, and complex movements. This is accomplished through regulating muscle groups by the motor control areas of the brain and the accompanying motor and sensory nerves.

Difficulties with the development of gross motor coordination in early childhood may be an early sign of a LEARNING DISABILITY; problems with fine-motor coordination may have a significant impact on some academic activities, such as the development of handwriting skills.

A coordination disability affects fingering, feeling, grasping, pinching, and handling. Tasks that may be impaired include typing, writing, eating, bathing, grooming, dressing oneself, telephoning, handling money—in general, any task that includes use of the hands for manipulation.

corporal punishment   Any intervention that is designed to, or likely to cause physical pain in order to stop or change behavior. In the United States, the most typical form of corporal punishment in schools is the striking of a student's buttocks with a wooden paddle by a school authority because the student disobeyed a rule.

More than half of all states ban the use of corporal punishment in schools because of its harmful physical, educational, psychological, and social effects on students. In states where it is allowed, many school boards voluntarily prohibit it. Yet, almost a half-million children are still being hit each year in public schools—a disproportionate number being minority children and children with disabilities.

Most experts agree that corporal punishment contributes to the cycle of child abuse and pro-violence attitudes of youth by teaching that it is an acceptable way of controlling the behavior of others. While discipline is important, effective alternatives are available to help students develop self-discipline.

The use of corporal punishment has been declining in U.S. schools because of waning public acceptance, increased litigation against school boards and educators, and legal bans.

Corporal punishment is a technique that can easily be abused and can lead to physical injuries. Evidence indicates that corporal punishment negatively affects the social, psychological, and educational development of students and contributes to the cycle of child abuse and pro-violence attitudes of youth.

Effective discipline includes programs and strategies for changing student behavior, for changing school or classroom environments, and for educating and supporting teachers and parents.

Alternatives for changing student behavior include

- helping students achieve academic success by identifying academic and behavioral problems and strengths
- behavioral contracting
- positive reinforcement of appropriate behavior
- individual and group counseling
- disciplinary consequences that are meaningful to students and have an instructional component
- social skills training

corpus callosum The broad, thick band of neural fibers that connect the left and right hemispheres of the brain, thus allowing both hemispheres to work together on complex functions. Because the callosum exchanges information between the two hemispheres, it allows the brain to be more effi-

cient. The two hemispheres can develop their own specialized functions, yet still take advantage of each other's benefits through the callosum.

The right side senses input, checks with the left side to see if there are rules to deal with this pattern of input, integrates the stored information, and reacts in a modified way.

Damage to any of these systems causes very poor, inappropriate responses. For example, if the corpus callosum cannot access the appropriate information quickly enough (or at all), then reaction to stimuli will be completely spontaneous, impulsive, and based solely on instinct.

Research suggests that the corpus callosum may be smaller in children with ATTENTION DEFICIT HYPERACTIVITY DISORDER (ADHD), and that both ADHD and DYSLEXIA may be linked to abnormalities in this part of the brain.

In the 18th century, the corpus callosum was considered the site of the soul, but by the early 20th century experts thought it existed merely to prevent the cerebral hemispheres from collapsing onto each other. It was not until the 1950s that scientists began to understand that the corpus callosum served to help transfer information between the two hemispheres. This was followed by the development in the early 1960s of a surgical intervention aimed at reducing the interhemispheric transmission of abnormal electrical discharges in epileptic patients.

corrective reading Supplemental, selective instruction for minor reading problems that is more specific than developmental reading but less intensive than remedial reading. Corrective reading instruction is often provided within a regular classroom by the regular teacher, aide, or a peer tutor.

criterion-referenced test A test that measures how thoroughly a student has mastered a specific skill or area of knowledge. It is based on the comparison of a student's specific knowledge to a predetermined level of mastery, rather than to another student's scores. The scores have meaning in terms of what the student knows or can do, rather than the relation to scores made by some external reference group. Such tests usually cover relatively small amounts of information and are closely related to instruction. Typically, a criterion-referenced test is subjective and relies on someone to observe and rate student work. Performance assessments are criterion-referenced tests.

Often, this type of ASSESSMENT is used to evaluate the acquisition of skills or knowledge based on a set of objectives or learning goals determined by a teacher or school system. It can also be used to evaluate a specific program of instruction or a system by examining the progress of individual students and then developing statistical profiles based on specified outcomes.

The opposite of a criterion-referenced test is a NORM-REFERENCED TEST, which is a type of assessment that compares scores of students in one school with a reference group. This reference group is usually other students in the same grade, called the "norm group."

cross-categorical   A system for grouping students with disabilities. Cross-categorical grouping places students with different kinds of disabilities into the same instructional setting at the same time.

cross dominance   Also known as mixed dominance or mixed laterality, this is a condition in which an individual prefers one side of the body for some activities and the other side for other activities. For example, a person who has cross dominance might be right-footed and right-eyed but left-handed.

cued speech   The use of hand gestures in conjunction with speech reading (lip reading) to distinguish between specific sounds. This method of communication was developed in 1966 as a speechreading support system that in English uses eight hand configurations and four hand positions near the mouth to supplement visible speech. The hand cue signals a visual difference between sounds that look alike on the lips, such as "p" and "b." These cues enable a deaf or hard-of-hearing person to see the phonetic equivalent of what others hear.

The hand configurations and locations are called "cues," not "cued speech" itself, which is the combination of the cues with speech. The cues are not readable alone.

It was developed primarily because some congenitally deaf people do not become good readers because they do not have an easy way to learn spoken language as young deaf children. Proponents of the system believe cued speech makes spoken language visually clear and solves the communication problem, and also helps youngsters learn a spoken language more easily. It is most successful when used consistently from childhood.

See also CUEING.

cueing   Providing additional verbal or nonverbal signals in order to help an individual retrieve, decode, or articulate words. It also may be used as a study strategy, through the development of MNEMONIC DEVICES or study cards, to help provide prompts or cues for remembering and retrieving information or specific language.

See also CUED SPEECH.

cultural determinant   A factor arising from racial, ethnic, or socioeconomic background that may systematically influence test performance on a specific ASSESSMENT instrument.

cumulative file   The general file containing all the educational records and information maintained for any child enrolled in a school. Parents have a legal right to inspect the file and have copies of any information contained in it.

cursive writing   A form of handwriting (sometimes called "script") in which letters are joined together in each word. Cursive writing may be useful for individuals with perceptual difficulties who frequently reverse letters. Cursive writing is typically introduced in third grade.

Cylert   See PEMOLINE.

D

decoding Understanding language through listening and reading. Decoding most often refers to the ability to recognize letter and word patterns and link them to the corresponding sounds. Decoding is different from COMPREHENSION, which implies an understanding of the material read.

Reading is a twofold process; decoding is the first step, but then students must be able to comprehend what the words mean once they have accurately decoded them from the text. Slow, single-word reading is the biggest predictor of poor reading comprehension skills.

Recent research on how children learn to read identifies decoding as a core problem for individuals with reading disorders. If a child has trouble learning sound-symbol relationships, there is a good chance that child will have a reading disability if not given early explicit PHONEMIC AWARENESS training.

Symptoms of poor decoding skills include slow, labored sounding out of words, frequent misidentification of familiar words (what/that or and/not), hesitant, stop-and-start reading, and frequent mispronunciations of words. An informal ASSESSMENT of decoding skills can be performed by having an individual read aloud. Decoding skills are also assessed by having students read nonsense words such as *dat, smop, thinkle.*

dementia The significant impairment of MEMORY, reasoning, personality, and intellect. Dementia is caused by brain injury or disease, including progressive forms of dementia such as Alzheimer's disease and some forms of Parkinson's disease. Generally, dementia involves some degree of language impairment, and in the case of progressive forms of dementia these impairments inevitably become more severe over time.

depression A mood disorder characterized by sadness, hopelessness, low self-esteem, fatigue, or agitation. Clinical depression is a serious disorder that responds well to medication and therapy. People with ATTENTION DEFICIT HYPERACTIVITY DISORDER (ADHD) and LEARNING DISABILITIES are at higher risk for developing depression because of the frustrations that go along with having ADHD.

Because it is not unusual for individuals with learning problems to feel despair and a loss of self-confidence, and because depression frequently co-exists with these disorders, it is essential that symptoms of depression be recognized and evaluated if they are persistent or severe.

Symptoms and Diagnostic Path

Major depression is almost always characterized by feelings of general sadness and total loss of pleasure for at least two weeks. There are a wide range of typical symptoms related to a clinical depression, including at least three of the following:

- deep sadness or crying jags
- gain or loss of weight
- chronic insomnia or excessive sleepiness
- outbursts of shouting and anger
- lost interest in hobbies and pleasure activities
- loss of interest in sex
- feelings of worthlessness, unattractiveness, guilt
- problems with concentration
- muddy, foggy thoughts
- anxiety, phobias, delusions, or fears
- restlessness
- slowed body movements
- suicidal thoughts

Treatment Options and Outlook

Depression can be successfully treated and responds best to a combination of therapy and medication with antidepressants. Today there are a wide range of antidepressants on the market, including the selective serotonin reuptake inhibitors (Prozac, Zoloft, and others), tricyclic antidepressants, MAO inhibitors, and structurally unrelated drugs. Doctors may need to try several antidepressants before finding one that is effective in alleviating depression.

developmental arithmetic disorder   See DYSCAL-CULIA.

developmental articulation disorder   A condition in which a child may mispronounce, have trouble controlling the rate of speech, or may be slower than classmates in learning to make speech sounds.

Developmental articulation disorders occur in at least 10 percent of children younger than age eight. Fortunately, articulation disorders are often outgrown or successfully treated with speech therapy.

In a typical substitution error, a child may say "y" for "L," as in "yamp" for "lamp," or "p" for "s," as in "pell" for "smell." The child may misarticulate only a couple of sounds but will mispronounce all words that contain that sound. This means that the child's speech could be virtually unintelligible depending on how often those error sounds appear when the child is talking.

In order to make speech sounds, a child must coordinate many muscles, including those of breathing, the vocal cords, the tongue, and the soft palate; the size and shape of teeth, the tongue, and the hard and soft palates also are important. If any one of these elements is abnormal, the child may develop an articulation disorder.

Children develop speech abilities at different ages and may be one or even two years behind another student. The vowels are the first group of sounds to develop, followed by the consonants, followed by the letters "r" and "s." Typically, 75 percent of all American children have developed all their sounds by the time they are four and a half years old.

The most common cause of articulation disorder is developmental delay, which can be caused by an ear infection or other hearing loss. Because the child cannot hear the slight differences between sounds, speech perception is inhibited. Articulation disorders also are associated with overall delayed language development.

APRAXIA of speech is generally associated with brain injury, leading to very slow, groping, or struggled speech. A developmental articulation disorder also may be caused by functional problems, such as having more than one language spoken in the home. Tongue thrust is a common organic and functional problem in which the child fails to develop a mature swallow, so that the pressure of the tongue against the front teeth pushes the teeth out of alignment and causes a lisp.

See also COMMUNICATION DISORDER; APHASIA; MIXED RECEPTIVE-EXPRESSIVE LANGUAGE DISORDER.

Developmental Disabilities Assistance Bill of Rights Act (PL 94-103)   A federal law enacted first in 1975 that created a "bill of rights" for people with developmental disabilities, funded services, added a new funding authority for university-affiliated facilities, and established a system of protection and advocacy organizations in each state. In 1987, amendments updated language, strengthened the independence of the state planning councils, strengthened authority of protection and advocacy systems to investigate allegations of abuse and neglect, and created separate line items for core funding and training for university-affiliated programs.

The act was totally rewritten in 1994, updating provisions pertaining to state planning councils and strengthening provisions pertaining to protection and advocacy systems, university-affiliated programs, and programs of national significance. Two years later, further amendments (PL 104-183) extended authority to fund developmental disabilities councils, protection and advocacy systems, university-affiliated programs, and projects of national significance.

Developmental Disabilities Council   A federally funded state organization, authorized in the DEVEL-OPMENTAL DISABILITIES ASSISTANCE AND BILL OF

RIGHTS ACT of 1990 to provide advocacy, policy analysis, and planning and to ensure comprehensive services for persons with DEVELOPMENTAL DISABILITIES. The council also has the responsibility of establishing a state plan, which must outline the major unmet needs of persons with developmental disabilities and identify services to be provided.

developmental disability   Any significant disability acquired before the age of 22. In actuality, however, "developmental disability" has also begun to replace the term MENTAL RETARDATION to describe the condition of individuals with severely impaired intellectual functioning from birth.

The term brings the description of mental retardation more in line with the general language used to define various types of difficulties; its focus on development rather than retardation provides a more accurate way of describing the actual nature of these difficulties.

However, the term also has a legal definition as it appears in the DEVELOPMENTAL DISABILITIES ASSISTANCE BILL OF RIGHTS ACT. In this law, the term *developmental disabilities* refers to severe, chronic disabilities of a person five years of age or older, which

- are caused by a mental or physical impairment
- occur before age 22
- are likely to continue indefinitely
- result in substantial functional limitations in at least three areas of self-care, language, learning, mobility, self-direction, ability to live independently, and economic self-sufficiency
- reflect the person's need for special long-term services

developmental expressive language disorder   A condition in which a child has problems using speech. This disorder can take many forms. For example, a four-year-old who speaks only in two-word phrases and a six-year-old who cannot answer simple questions both have an expressive language disorder.

Expressive language disorder affects between 3 and 10 percent of all school-age children. It is sometimes caused by brain damage or malnutrition, in combination with genetic factors. In fact, twin studies have established that genetic factors play a significant role in expressive language disorder without articulation difficulties (the most common expressive language disability) and expressive language disorder with articulation difficulties. In other cases, the cause is unknown.

Symptoms and Diagnostic Path
Symptoms of a developmental expressive language disorder include low-average vocabulary skills, improper use of verb tenses, difficulty in producing complex sentences, and trouble recalling words.

If this disorder is suspected, standardized expressive language and nonverbal IQ tests should be administered, along with testing for other LEARNING DISABILITIES.

Treatment Options and Outlook
Language and speech therapy aimed at increasing the quantity of phrases a child can use is the treatment of choice. How well a child recovers depends on the severity of the disorder.

developmental lag   A delay in some aspect of physical or mental development. For example, a student with a developmental lag in reading might be in the sixth grade but read like a third grader. If the student has the skills of a good third grade reader, the situation would be referred to as developmental lag, since there are no core issues like the ones a student with DYSLEXIA would have.

developmentally appropriate practice (DAP)   A set of guidelines ensuring that educational programs are appropriate for each child's age and developmental stage. The guidelines were recommended by the National Association for the Education of Young Children in 1990, requiring that early education programs be child centered and child directed with little effort to explicitly teach specific skills.

Developmentally appropriate practice has been debated by special educators who feel that early intervention and direct skill instruction are essential for children with LEARNING DISABILITIES to help them address their learning needs.

developmental reading disorder   Another term for DYSLEXIA.

developmental receptive language disorder A condition in which a child has trouble understanding certain aspects of speech. For example, a toddler who does not respond to his name or a first grader who consistently cannot follow simple directions most likely has a developmental receptive language disorder. Their hearing is fine, but they can not make sense of certain sounds, words, or sentences they hear. They may seem as if they are not paying attention, but in fact they simply can not understand certain types of speech. Because using and understanding speech are strongly related, many people with receptive language disorders also have EXPRESSIVE LANGUAGE DISORDERS.

developmental speech and language disorders People with developmental speech and language disorders have trouble producing speech sounds, using spoken language to communicate, or understanding what other people say. Speech and language problems are often the earliest indicators of a LEARNING DISABILITY. These speech and language disorders include DEVELOPMENTAL ARTICULATION DISORDER, DEVELOPMENTAL EXPRESSIVE LANGUAGE DISORDER, and DEVELOPMENTAL RECEPTIVE LANGUAGE DISORDER.

With a developmental articulation disorder, children may have trouble controlling their rate of speech, or they may lag behind their friends in learning to make speech sounds. These disorders are common, appearing in at least 10 percent of children younger than age eight. Fortunately, articulation disorders can often be outgrown or successfully treated with speech therapy.

Some children with developmental expressive language disorder have problems expressing themselves in speech—calling objects by the wrong names, speaking only in two-word phrases, or being unable to answer simple questions.

Some people have trouble understanding certain aspects of speech; this is developmental receptive language disorder. This explains the toddler who does not respond to his or her name or the worker who consistently cannot follow simple directions. While hearing is normal, these individuals cannot make sense of certain sounds, words, or sentences. Because using and understanding speech are strongly related, many people with receptive language disorders also have an expressive language disability.

Of course, some misuse of sounds, words, or grammar is a normal part of learning to speak. It is only when these problems persist that there is any cause for concern.

developmental spelling disorder A significant difficulty in learning to spell. This occurs in the absence of reading or other written language difficulties.

developmental writing disorder A condition in which a child with a writing disability, especially an EXPRESSIVE LANGUAGE DISORDER, may be unable to write complete, grammatical sentences. This problem involves several brain areas and functions that control vocabulary, grammar, hand movement, and MEMORY.

Dexedrine See DEXTROAMPHETAMINE.

dextroamphetamine/amphetamine (Adderall) A combination stimulant medication prescribed for ATTENTION DEFICIT HYPERACTIVITY DISORDER (ADHD) that can be used for children over age three to improve ATTENTION SPAN and decrease distractibility. Adderall also may decrease impulsivity, stubbornness, and aggression. The drug needs to be taken only once or twice a day, and although the effects may be noticed immediately, it may take up to six weeks to achieve its full benefit. This is why some parents stop giving this medication after only a few doses, thinking it is not working.

Adderall is usually prescribed as part of a treatment plan that includes educational and psychosocial treatment. It is sometimes prescribed in cases where Ritalin or other stimulant medications have not worked. Because it has a fairly slow onset of action, there may be less of a chance that it will cause or worsen tics.

Adderall had earlier been approved and marketed under a different name (Obetrol) as a weight control medication. When the manufacturer was taken over by another company, the product was renamed Adderall in 1994 and approved for treating ADHD in 1996.

Side Effects
Most common side effects include appetite and weight loss, insomnia, and headache. Less often, a

patient may experience dry mouth and nausea. Rare side effects include dizziness, irritability, stomach pain, increased heart rate, or hallucinations. As with most stimulants, there is the risk of growth suppression and the potential for triggering motor tics and TOURETTE'S SYNDROME. In rare cases, worsening of psychosis has been reported. College students have been known to grind the tablets and snort the powder to obtain a rush similar to Ecstasy.

As with all other stimulants in treating ADHD, one of the more troublesome side effects is a decrease in brain growth. Although there is a rebound effect once the child stops taking the drug, the rebound generally does not bring the child back to the same level on brain growth charts as prior to drug treatment.

Adderall should not be taken with antidepressant inhibitors monoamine oxidase (MAOI), because serious (even fatal) interactions can occur. At least 14 days must pass between stopping MAOIs and beginning Adderall. Acidifying agents such as guanethidine, reserpine, and fruit juices can interfere with the absorption of Adderall, whereas substance such as acetazolamide (Diamox) increase absorption. Tricyclic antidepressants such as Tofranil become more potent when taken with Adderall. Chlorpromazine (Thorazine), lithium, and haloperidoL (Haldol) can interfere with Adderall as well.

See also STIMULANT MEDICATIONS.

diagnosis The outcome of a clinical assessment. A diagnosis generally involves providing a specific label to a set of symptoms or phenomena exhibited by an individual, based on some standard diagnostic criteria, such as in the *DIAGNOSTIC AND STATISTICAL MANUAL OF MENTAL DISORDER—FOURTH EDITION, TEXT REVISION.*

Typically, a clinical diagnosis is reached after examining a range of factors, including performance on STANDARDIZED TESTS, reports of performance in classroom or home settings, and case history information derived from clinical interviews. Diagnostic criteria may vary and may change over time as new information develops through scientific research regarding specific disorders.

A diagnosis of LEARNING DISABILITIES can be reached in a variety of ways, due to the range of disabilities and deficits that can arise. Learning dis-

abilities can be suspected very early on in a child's development if there are significant deficits or a DEVELOPMENTAL LAG. In the primary years, a two-year delay in skills acquisition is considered significant. For some older children, learning disabilities may be suspected only after a considerable length of time in which the child has experienced progressive difficulty in school. In other words, the deficits may be subtle and not indicative of the gap between the child's performance and his or her potential for achievement.

Formal diagnosis of learning disabilities is made by a qualified expert using standardized tests that compare ability to what is considered normal for an individual of that age and intelligence.

Diagnostic and Statistical Manual of Mental Disorders—Fourth Edition, Text Revision **(DSM-IV-TR)** The primary manual of psychiatric classification, published by the American Psychiatric Association, which is used by a majority of practicing clinicians in the United States. Organized by categories of disorders (such as ANXIETY disorders or LEARNING DISORDERS), the text also provides diagnostic criteria and associated disorders for each listing.

The first edition was published in 1952; the revised fourth edition was published in 1994, significantly updating and adding listings from previous editions. It was followed in 2000 by the most recent revision known as *DSM-IV-TR.*

Because the interval between *DSM-IV* and *DSM-V* (12 years) is longer than the intervals between earlier editions (it was seven years between *DSM-III* and *DSM-III-R* and between *DSM-III-R* and *DSM-IV*), the information in the text was becoming more and more outdated. In order to bridge the span between *DSM-IV* and *DSM-V*, a revision of the *DSM-IV* text was designed to correct any factual errors that had been identified in the *DSM-IV* text, to review the *DSM-IV* text to ensure that all of the information is still current, and to change the *DSM-IV* text to reflect new information. The new version is *DSM-IV-TR* (text revision).

In order for a diagnosis to be made, the individual's behavior must match the criteria listed for a specific disorder in *DSM-IV-TR*. One criticism of the *DSM* is that there are no separate categories or criteria for the diagnosis of children. While the behavior may be slightly different, which is typically noted, children are essentially diagnosed using the same criteria as is used with adults. In addition, because a diagnosis from the *DSM* is typically required for health insurance coverage, some critics suggest that individuals, particularly children, may be prematurely diagnosed with serious disorders.

The *DSM-IV-TR* can be used for two purposes: as a source of diagnostic information to enhance clinical practice, research, and education; and to communicate diagnostic information to others.

Each revision of the *DSM* is the end result of a systematic, comprehensive review of the psychiatric literature, and contains the most up-to-date information available to assist the clinician in making a differential diagnosis.

The APA continues to update the *DSM* every 12 years. In the most recent update (*DSM-IV-TR*) the most important material remains exactly the same. The only things that have changed substantially are the text accompanying the diagnoses and some parts of the introduction and appendices.

diagnostic teaching   An instructional method of teaching that adapts lesson plans based on a student's specific needs and learning styles. While specific goals and objectives are first developed, diagnostic teaching focuses on determining the breakdown point of skills and providing appropriate instruction to individual students. In general the focus is on a teacher's own understanding of a student's strengths and difficulties within the classroom context.

A diagnostic approach to instruction is important for students with LEARNING DISABILITIES, who may acquire information and skills at a different rate from their peers, and who also may display unexpected patterns of strength and weakness that require careful adaptation of basic instructional plans. The errors displayed by individuals with learning disabilities on specific academic tasks may be caused by a wide range of underlying issues; for instruction to be effective, it must take into account the nature of these factors through a process of error analysis and comparison of performance on different types of academic tasks.

diagnostic test   Tests that provide information that will help reveal a student's particular learning style or disability. This type of evaluation is differ-

ent from other forms of ASSESSMENT because the goal is diagnosis, rather than solely the measurement of ability or of acquired knowledge.

See also DIAGNOSTIC TEACHING; EVALUATION.

diet and ADHD   One of the more controversial treatments for ATTENTION DEFICIT HYPERACTIVITY DISORDER is an additive-free diet (the most popular of which is the FEINGOLD DIET). Proponents of this diet, which promotes the elimination of most additives from food, assert that the plan will improve most (if not all) children's learning and attention problems.

However, many studies published in peer-reviewed journals have consistently failed to find support for these type of diets. While a few studies have reported some limited success with this approach, at best this suggests that there may be a very small group of children who are responsive to additive-free diets. On the other hand, these diets are not harmful, so there is nothing to be lost in trying to eliminate additives.

differential diagnosis   An ASSESSMENT that can differentiate between two different disorders or conditions. A differential diagnosis is required in any case where specific symptoms might be caused by more than one underlying condition, such as ATTENTION DEFICIT HYPERACTIVITY DISORDER (ADHD) or a LEARNING DISABILITY. A differential diagnosis is especially important in the case of symptoms that may be linked to ADHD because these symptoms may also be associated with other psychological problems.

dioxins   A group of some of the most toxic carcinogenic human-made chemicals in the world, which have been linked to developmental and learning disabilities. Exposure in childhood can cause lower IQ, result in withdrawn and depressed behavior, and increase hyperactivity and attention problems. Unborn children are even more acutely affected by exposure to dioxins because of the critical development that occurs during pregnancy, especially between the second and eighth week after conception.

Dioxin is the most harmful of all the chemicals in the dioxin group and is produced by burning plastics containing chlorine, incinerating household waste, and bleaching chlorine paper. It was first used as the toxic chemical in the weapon Agent Orange during the Vietnam War. Although some dioxins are produced naturally as a result of forest fires, most appear in the environment as an industrial by-product.

Dioxins are found everywhere in the environment, introduced into the air from incinerators and smokestacks, where they eventually settle on the ground, in the water, and on the food that livestock eat. Because dioxins do not decompose readily, they are stored in livestock fatty tissue. About 95 percent of human dioxin exposure occurs by eating traces in meat, dairy products, and fish.

Children are at a higher risk for both ingesting dioxins and being harmed because their diets usually have a higher concentration of animal fat in the form of dairy products.

direct instruction   The explicit teaching of specific tasks, including the teaching of rules and strategies, teacher modeling, and explicit practice of the steps involved in learning the skill. Clear and consistent feedback and error analysis is important.

Proponents of direct instruction believe that the approach requires teacher training, a highly structured learning environment, and explicit preparation for each lesson. Teachers must monitor student progress and plan lessons so that errors are corrected quickly.

For students with LEARNING DISABILITIES, direct instruction is one important approach that focuses on a drill and reward system that can help the student learn basic skills. Because children with learning disabilities can have a range of educational problems, no one approach is likely to meet the needs of all students, but strategies that emphasize planning, organizing, and reviewing work are helpful.

directionality   A person's sense of direction. The development of a sense of direction is an essential component of early childhood development. Directionality involves being able to distinguish left from right, as well as the ability to use visual cues to determine location and to find one's way to a familiar place. Difficulties in developing directionality are sometimes associated with learning disorders.

discrepancy   In the context of LEARNING DISABILITIES and SPECIAL EDUCATION, discrepancy refers to the traditional approach of identifying a specific learning disability by looking at a gap between performance on aptitude and achievement measures. In most states, a statistically significant discrepancy between ability and performance indicates a learning disability.

However, the discrepancy model has been questioned in recent years by research that focuses primarily on disability, such as phonological processing problems as the underlying factor in reading disabilities. Some experts argue that the discrepancy approach is not as effective a way of identifying learning disabilities as testing for underlying cognitive deficits. However, discrepancy formulas for determining learning disabilities are still deeply entrenched in law and in the procedures and regulations of state school systems, and are likely to continue to be a primary method for identifying schoolchildren who should receive SPECIAL EDUCATION services.

discrete trial training (DTT)   An intensive type of therapy that teaches a child how to learn through repetition of behavioral responses, developed by AUTISM expert Ivaar Lovaas at the University of California–Los Angeles. DTT requires one-on-one sessions with specially trained teachers for 40 hours a week over two to three years, which makes it a costly type of treatment—out of reach for many families. This therapy has been promoted as one of the most important treatments for autism, although critics point out that there is no comparative research to support the claim.

Modifications of Dr. Lovaas's theory have evolved into other forms of behavioral therapy, including applied behavior analysis. All of these therapies are begun in the preschool years in hopes of achieving kindergarten readiness with developmentally normal peers.

disinhibition   Lack of restraint in responding to a situation. A child exhibiting disinhibition reacts impulsively and often inappropriately. An individual who has problems with disinhibition may daydream during lectures, or respond impulsively rather than thoughtfully to a social cue. Problems with disinhibition may also have an affect on a person's ability to use effective strategies to perform a task. In general, behaviors and ideation related to disinhibition may be traceable to general difficulties in impulse control that are a large element in ATTENTION DEFICIT HYPERACTIVITY DISORDER (ADHD).

distractibility The shifting of ATTENTION from the task at hand to sounds or sights that normally occur in the environment. Distractibility is closely linked to DISINHIBITION because it relates to a person's difficulty in controlling impulses to unimportant distractions. A distractible person may not be able to filter out or ignore external distractions, such as random sounds. Distractibility primarily refers to a problem with controlling the focus of attention, which may shift to unimportant information such as a picture on a wall or a noise from outside a room.

Certain BEHAVIORAL RATING SCALES can measure distractibility, which can be an important way of determining whether an attention disorder is present.

dominant hemisphere Also known as cerebral dominance, this term refers to the side (or hemisphere) of the brain that usually controls a particular function.

Since language and logic are particularly important, the hemisphere that organizes and controls language is referred to as the dominant hemisphere. For most (99 percent) right-handed people, the left hemisphere is dominant. About 60 percent of left-handed people also process language and logic in the left hemisphere.

dopamine A chemical in the brain that has been linked to ATTENTION DEFICIT HYPERACTIVITY DISORDER (ADHD). It appears that certain receptors in the brain that normally respond to the neurotransmitter dopamine are not working properly. Most likely, dopamine is not being produced at normal levels in the brain.

Recent studies with adults who have ADHD point to a defect in an enzyme called dopa decarboxylase, which helps produce dopamine. This defect in dopamine production occurs in the ante-

rior frontal cortex, an area associated with cognitive processes such as focusing and ATTENTION.

Current treatments use medications to enhance dopamine production throughout the brain. However, these drugs also can cause adverse effects such as irritability, insomnia, and DEPRESSION.

Down syndrome A congenital form of MENTAL RETARDATION caused by an extra chromosome, characterized by distinct physical features as well as DEVELOPMENTAL DISABILITIES. Down syndrome affects people of all ages, races, and economic levels, occurring once in about every 800 to 1,000 live births. More than 350,000 people in the United States have Down syndrome.

The condition was first described in 1959 by French physician Jerome Lejeune, who discovered that instead of the usual 46 chromosomes present in each cell, there were 47 in the cells of individuals with Down syndrome. Because 95 percent of all cases of Down syndrome are caused by three copies of the 21st chromosome, it is also referred to as "trisomy 21."

While Down syndrome is usually caused by an error in cell division, two other types of chromosomal abnormalities (mosaicism and translocation) are also implicated in Down syndrome. Regardless of the type of Down syndrome which a person may have, all people with Down syndrome have an extra portion of the number 21 chromosome present in some of their cells. This additional genetic material alters the course of development and causes the characteristics associated with the syndrome.

Women age 35 and older have a significantly increased risk of having a child with Down syndrome: a 35-year-old woman has a one in 400 chance of conceiving a child with Down syndrome, which increases gradually to one in 105 by age 40. At age 46 the incidence is about one in 20.

Symptoms and Diagnostic Path
Most people with Down syndrome have some level of mental retardation ranging from mild to moderate, but most children with Down syndrome learn to sit, walk, talk, play, toilet train, and do most other activities. Because speech is often delayed, careful attention should be paid to the child's hear-

ing, as retention of fluid in the inner ear is a very common cause of hearing and speech difficulties.

Diagnosis during pregnancy   Pregnant women have access to both screening and diagnostic tests to find out if their unborn child has Down syndrome. Screening tests estimate the risk of the fetus having Down syndrome, whereas diagnostic tests tell whether or not the fetus actually has the condition.

Screening tests are typically offered between 15 and 20 weeks of gestation, and they can accurately detect only about 60 percent of cases. Many women who undergo these tests will be given false-positive readings, and some women will be given false-negative readings. Prenatal diagnosis of Down syndrome is by chorionic villus sampling (CVS), amniocentesis, and percutaneous umbilical blood sampling (PUBS).

Each of these procedures carries a small risk of miscarriage as tissue is extracted from the placenta or the umbilical cord to examine the fetus's chromosomes, but the procedures are about 98 to 99 percent accurate in the detection of Down syndrome. Amniocentesis is usually performed between 12 and 20 weeks of gestation, CVS between eight and 12 weeks, and PUBS after 20 weeks.

Diagnosis at birth   The diagnosis of Down syndrome is usually suspected after birth as a result of the baby's appearance. Among the most common traits are low muscle tone, a flat facial profile, an upward slant to the eyes, an abnormal ear shape, a single deep crease across the center of the palm, and an excessive ability to extend the joints. Other common symptoms include a fifth finger with one furrow instead of two, small skin folds on the inner corner of the eyes, too much space between large and second toe, and an enlarged tongue compared to the size of the mouth.

Treatment Options and Outlook

Early intervention services should begin shortly after birth to help children with Down syndrome develop to their full potential. These programs offer parents special instruction in teaching their child language, cognitive, self-help, and social skills, and specific exercises for gross and fine motor development (see GROSS and FINE MOTOR DEVELOPMENT). Research has shown that stimulation during early developmental stages improves the child's chances of developing to his or her fullest potential. Continuing education, positive public attitudes, and a stimulating home environment also have been found to promote the child's overall development. Quality educational programs and good medical care enable people with Down syndrome to become contributing members of their families and communities.

Because people with Down syndrome respond well to their environment, those who receive good medical care and are included in community activities can attend school, make friends, find work, participate in decisions that affect them, and make a positive contribution to society.

Over the past few decades, beginning with Section 504 of the REHABILITATION ACT OF 1973, continuing with the EDUCATION FOR ALL HANDICAPPED CHILDREN ACT OF 1975, and culminating with the passage of the AMERICANS WITH DISABILITIES ACT in 1991, people with Down syndrome have been granted equal protections under federal law.

Because of these individual differences among these children, it is impossible to predict their future achievements. However, it is important for families and the school not to place limitations on potential capabilities. It may be effective to emphasize concrete concepts rather than abstract ideas. Teaching tasks in a step-by-step manner with frequent reinforcement and consistent feedback has been proven successful. Improved public acceptance of persons with disabilities, along with increased opportunities for adults with disabilities to live and work independently in the community, have expanded goals for individuals with Down syndrome. Independent Living Centers, group shared and supervised apartments, and support services in the community are important resources for those with Down syndrome.

due process hearing   A remedy provided in the INDIVIDUALS WITH DISABILITIES ACT in which parents can protest decisions that have been made about SPECIAL EDUCATION services for their child.

The first type of due process hearing occurs at the local level, where all parties present their arguments and a specially trained hearing officer makes a decision about the disagreement. For example, if parents believe their child needs an interpreter who will sign instruction, but the school district representatives do not agree to provide one, the hearing officer could rule in two ways. He or she could agree with the school district and rule that the student is not entitled to an interpreter, or side with the parents and require the school district to provide one.

After the local hearing officer has rendered a decision, the losing party may appeal the decision in a state-level due process hearing. At this hearing, a state hearing officer follows the same procedures as in the local hearing and renders a decision regarding the dispute. After the state-level hearing officer has rendered a decision, the losing party has the option to seek a legal remedy through the courts.

Dursban   An extremely toxic organophosphate pesticide used widely in homes, schools, hospitals, and agriculture. One of 37 similar chemicals, it is produced as granules and designed to kill insects by damaging the nervous system. Dursban has been produced and used for more than 20 years but is currently being phased out of production because of its toxicity. Dursban exposure early in life can lead to harmful changes in the nervous system and in normal learning behavior. Exposure during pregnancy may lead to MENTAL RETARDATION and brain defects.

Dursban has been found in very high concentration in the breast milk of animals in studies. It can be found almost everywhere outside—on the ground, on plants, in dirt, in water, in parks and lawns, and in the fat of animals. It is also an indoor air pollutant and is found in dust, on floors, on vegetables, in dog and cat flea collars, and in the air near the floor.

Humans eat, drink, and breathe Dursban; the danger of exposure depends on how recently Dursban has been used and in what concentration. In addition to the learning problems in children, acute exposure to Dursban and other organophosphates can cause nausea, headaches, twitching, dizziness, teeth grinding, increased sweating, and salivation. It is a severe skin irritant and has the ability to cause intestinal cramps, diarrhea, sleeplessness, and nightmares. Dursban and organophosphates depress an enzyme in the bodies after long-term exposure, which can cause neurobehavioral effects.

dysarthria   A speech problem caused by damage to or disease of the muscles controlling the voice appa-

ratus. Unlike APHASIA, patients with this condition have no problems with the speech center of the brain. They can select and write out words and sentences; they simply cannot form vocal expressions.

The condition may be caused by a stroke, brain tumor, or damage to a particular nerve controlling the structures of speech.

There is no specific treatment, although medication or surgery may restore the ability to speak by treating the underlying problem. Speech therapy also may help.

dyscalculia   A significant LEARNING DISABILITY involving mathematics that affects between 2 percent and 6 percent of school-age children in the United States. Dyscalculia is a medical term associated with brain dysfunction that is presumably present at birth. Many students identified as having a specific learning disability or attention disorder may have associated problems with learning or applying mathematical concepts, functions, and procedures.

It may relate to a variety of more basic disorders such as confusion or deficits in perception, spatial skills, sequencing, and so on. It is sometimes referred to as ACALCULIA, which is technically a total inability to do arithmetic.

Because problems with arithmetic and mathematics may arise from widely varying causes, it is important to understand the underlying sources of the learning difficulty in this area before deciding what educational remedies to choose.

Symptoms and Diagnostic Path

There are a variety of symptoms with this condition, including normal or advanced language and other skills and often good visual memory for the printed word. This is accompanied by poor mental math ability, often with problems in using money (such as balancing a checkbook, making change, and tipping). This may develop into an actual fear of money and its transactions.

In addition, a person with dyscalculia has problems with math processes such as addition, subtraction, or multiplication, as well as with math concepts (such as sequencing numbers). The student may have trouble retaining and retrieving concepts, or have problems grasping math rules.

This is combined with a poor sense of direction, as well as trouble reading maps, telling time, and grappling with mechanical processes. There is difficulty with abstract concepts of time and direction, schedules, keeping track of time, and the sequence of past and future events.

Common mistakes in working with numbers include number substitutions, reversals, and omissions. Students also may have trouble learning musical concepts, following directions in sports that demand sequencing or rules, and keeping track of scores and players during games such as cards and board games.

Treatment Options and Outlook

Individuals with dyscalculia need help in organizing and processing information related to numbers and mathematical concepts. Since math is essentially a form of language using numbers instead of words as symbols, it is important to communicate frequently and clearly with a child as to what is needed to do a mathematical problem. While the condition is lifelong, performance can be improved with intensive intervention. The child should have real-life exposure to how to use math as a part of everyday life: counting ingredients in a cake, how to make change, and so on.

Parents and teachers should work together to determine helpful strategies, such as using graph paper to help with alignment on a page or a calculator to check work. Textbooks, workbooks, or computer programs may give students more opportunities to practice skills. A tutor or a learning center may provide additional enrichment opportunities.

dysfluency Difficulties in processing oral or written language fluently, in a continuous and consistent sequence. Dysfluency may occur in reading, speaking, or writing. It may arise from a range of potential sources, and is primarily a descriptive term for specific behaviors that arise from other learning problems, rather than a specific category of learning difficulty in itself.

dysgraphia See WRITTEN EXPRESSION, DISORDERS OF.

dyslexia A specific learning difficulty, usually with spelling and writing, and sometimes with reading and numbers. It is characterized by problems in coping with written symbols, despite normal intelligence. Dyslexic children and adults may have problems putting things in order, following instructions, and may confuse left and right. The word *dyslexia* comes from the Greek meaning "difficulty with words."

Experts estimate that dyslexia is estimated to occur in about 8 percent of the population. It is a permanent disability that is often accompanied by strengths in areas such as creativity or physical coordination. Each dyslexic person's difficulties are different and vary from slight to very severe disruption of the learning process.

Its cause has not been fully established, but the effect creates neurological anomalies in the brain. These anomalies trigger varying degrees of difficulty in learning when using words and sometimes symbols. Children or students who are dyslexic have trouble sorting out the sounds within words, which is why they have problems with reading, writing, and spelling. Most children with dyslexia have difficulty with text, memory, and basic mathematics.

Children are either born with dyslexia or acquire the difficulty during early childhood, but it is when they begin to learn using words and sometimes other symbols that it becomes a noticeable problem.

Modern experts believe dyslexia may be caused by differences in brain structure and function present since birth, with a strong genetic component. A number of studies have indicated a strong heritability for dyslexia, predominantly among boys within a family. In general, the ratio of males to females identified with dyslexia is about four to one. Because of this, the role of the hormone testosterone before birth is being investigated as a possible cause of inherited dyslexia.

The reading difficulties associated with dyslexia are not related to intelligence or motivation; students often possess unusual talents, especially in areas that require visual, spatial, and motor skills. This disorder is not due to a physical disability, such as a visual problem. Instead, it is a problem in how the brain processes the information as the individual is reading.

Traditional definitions of dyslexia have relied on an unexpected gap between learning aptitude and achievement in school, particularly in the area of reading. However, contemporary research has indicated that difficulties or delays in developing awareness of sounds and processing abilities play a primary factor in the development of the reading problems associated with dyslexia. Word-finding difficulties are a second factor in the case of some individuals with severe reading difficulties.

Some research links it to low levels of the brain chemical DOPAMINE.

Symptoms and Diagnostic Path

Dyslexia may include a variety of reading problems, such as

- lack of understanding what is read
- lack of awareness of sounds that make up words, often including a difficulty with blending sounds to make words
- problems with spelling
- problems with the order of letters in words
- trouble rhyming words
- difficulty with pronouncing words
- delay in speaking
- delay in learning the alphabet, numbers, days of the week, months, colors, shapes, and other basic information
- difficulty understanding subtleties of language such as jokes or slang

Dyslexia is diagnosed with a formal evaluation of intellectual ability, information processing, language processing, and academic skills. The results of these tests will determine a child's eligibility for SPECIAL EDUCATION services as described in federal law and will be used to make educational recommendations.

A child may be tested for dyslexia at any age; even very young children may be tested for phonological processing, receptive and expressive language abilities, and the ability to make associate sounds and symbols.

Instead of one specific dyslexia test, a child is given a series of tests to measure word recognition in isolation or lists, word attack skills, reading speed, and spelling. Extra tests also may be given to assess reading COMPREHENSION, written expression, and math reasoning and calculation.

Trained school experts or outside specialists can conduct the testing, but the expert or team should have experience in psychology, reading, language, and education. The tester also must understand how children learn to read and be able to recommend appropriate reading interventions.

After the test, a written report with test scores as well as an explanation of the results, including the child's strengths and weaknesses, should be prepared. Specific recommendations would be made at that time.

Treatment Options and Outlook

Although dyslexia is a lifelong condition, with appropriate instruction individuals with dyslexia may largely overcome their reading difficulties. Individuals with a reading disability most often benefit from a language program that provides direct instruction in understanding the letter-sound system. A child with dyslexia should be taught the basic sounds and the letters that represent them slowly and carefully and also how to put these together and take them apart. The earlier this instruction is given, the greater the chance the person will become a fluent reader.

Typically, the more senses that can be used when learning something, the better the person will learn. For individuals with reading disabilities, it is important to learn as much as possible by seeing, hearing, writing, and speaking. For example, a teacher of students with this disability can provide a written outline of the day's lecture in addition to giving the lecture itself.

The school will probably suggest academic modifications to help a child succeed, such as being given extra time to complete in-class writing assignments, modifying homework requirements, giving alternative assignments, allowing children with dyslexia to record notes instead of writing them down, and giving taped tests. Students also may be given audio books-on-tape and be allowed to compose most assignments and tests on a computer.

Parents of children with reading disabilities can encourage their children to read by providing reading materials on subjects in which they have an interest.

Several decades of teacher-based and clinical research support the need for a multisensory, sequential, phonetic-based approach to reading instruction as the essential foundation for the development of reading skills. For example, a student learning the consonant blend "bl" might listen to the sound while looking at the letters, then say it aloud while tracing the two letters on a roughboard. This method of instruction increases the chance that the information will be stored and retained in long-term MEMORY.

There is no total cure, but the effects can be eased by skilled, specialist teaching of phonics, sequencing, and techniques to raise the person's self-esteem. Given proper support, dyslexic students are able to go on to college and pursue successful careers.

See also LEARNING DISABILITY.

dysnomia A specific form of APHASIA that involves problems in finding words as a result of the inability to recall and express the names of objects or concepts. Individuals with this condition may substitute a general term like *thing* for a word that they cannot recall, substitute another word in place of the target word, or use circumlocution— talking around the word that they are trying to remember and express. The condition is not as severe as ANOMIA (the complete loss of the ability to recall words, as the names of objects, persons, activities). This problem may be particularly noticeable if a person with dysnomia is asked to answer a question and is expected to give an immediate answer. However, when the person speaks spontaneously, without prompting, the speech appears perfectly normal.

Dysnomia rarely occurs by itself, but is associated with other difficulties, including EXPRESSIVE-LANGUAGE DISORDERS and, in some cases, attention disorders. It often occurs with a language or learning disability.

dysphasia The partial or total loss of the ability to speak, read, and write. It is a term for a disorder of communication that may be caused by damage to the brain due to stroke, head injury, or disease. Dysphasia may potentially affect understanding, speaking, reading, or writing. The type and severity of the language problems depends on the part of the brain that has been affected.

Symptoms and Diagnostic Path

A person with dysphasia may have trouble understanding word meaning, telling the difference between sounds, comprehending reading material, or remembering or grasping long, complex sentences. They may have trouble recognizing or understanding individual letters or words or recalling details from long stories. People with dysphasia may have trouble speaking, so that they struggle to think of the right word, or have trouble forming grammatically correct sentences, explaining things clearly, saying the word in the right form, and using language correctly in a variety of situations. There also may be writing problems, so that the person has trouble forming letters, spelling, knowing the right word to write, or sequencing ideas.

Treatment Options and Outlook

Speech therapists can develop individualized treatment programs and recommend aids such as communication boards or electronic devices. They also can provide support for individuals with communication disorders and their families.

There are ways to help a person with dysphasia who is struggling to communicate. First, it is important to communicate in a quiet, relaxed environment that does not have many distractions. All forms of communication should be encouraged and accepted, including gestures, pointing, and writing. The person should be encouraged to communicate, even if it takes a long time.

To make sure the affected person understands, other speakers should attract the person's attention before speaking, talk slowly using short sentences, and accompany instructions with actions. Sentences should be clear and simple, with familiar words. The speakers should avoid discussing complex matters and check that the person has understood, repeating or rephrasing if necessary. The person with dysphasia may not be able to easily understand sarcasm, jokes, or other abstract language.

dysphonia A subtype of DYSLEXIA characterized by specific reading-spelling error patterns. Dysphonetic readers typically have a functional albeit limited sight word vocabulary, but they lack phonic word analysis skills. Their most striking error is the substitution of a word similar in meaning to the original word but unlike it phonetically (such as "sheet" for "quilt").

Their misspellings are phonetically inaccurate and include such errors as extra letters, omitted syllables, reversed syllables, letter-order errors, and other sequencing mistakes.

dyspraxia A general term used to describe a range of different conditions involving difficulty with learned patterns of movement without any muscle or nerve damage. In some cases, dyspraxia is used to describe coordination problems and gross-motor and fine-motor body movements. It is related to an underdevelopment of the brain in which messages are not properly transmitted to the body, producing a number of problems in physical and thinking areas. It affects at least 2 percent of the population in varying degrees; 70 percent of those affected are male. Dyspraxia can be subtle or more pronounced, and often a person's disability is not readily apparent.

The term is also commonly used in the field of speech-language therapy to describe the condition of developmental verbal dyspraxia, in which a child has significant problems in producing speech sounds and sequencing sounds into words. This condition may also be accompanied by a difficulty in making and coordinating the physical movements required to produce speech (oral dyspraxia). There are many other types of dyspraxia, including

- ideomotor: inability to perform single motor tasks, such as combing hair or waving goodbye
- ideational: difficulty with multilevel tasks, such as taking the proper sequence of steps for brushing teeth
- dressing: problems with dressing and putting clothes on in order
- constructional: difficulty with spatial relations
- verbal: problems and delay with expressive language

Symptoms and Diagnostic Path

Dyspraxia causes a range of symptoms such as coordination problems (awkwardness, clumsiness,

trouble with hopping, skipping, throwing and catching a ball, or riding a bike). There may be confusion about which hand to use for tasks, problems with holding a pen or pencil properly, and sensitivity to touch (the child may find some clothes uncomfortable; there may be an intolerance to having hair or teeth brushed, or nails and hair cut). In addition, there may be problems with short-term MEMORY, trouble with reading and writing, poor sense of direction, speech problems, phobias, or obsessive behavior.

While older children may be verbally adept, they may not develop the social skills to get along with their peers. While children with dyspraxia can be of average or above average intelligence, they often have immature behavior. Logic and reasoning may be challenging.

Treatment Options and Outlook

There is no cure for dyspraxia, but the earlier a child is treated, the greater the chance of improvement. Occupational therapists, physiotherapists, and ACCOMMODATIONS at school can all help a child to cope with the condition. A child with dyspraxia wants to communicate, but often cannot, so pressuring such a child will lead only to further inhibition. Repetitive verbal activities can help develop language skills, including songs, poems, nursery rhymes, and so on. A child who has trouble communicating can use sign language or a communication board to supplement speech temporarily. To improve motor function, the child should practice tasks to learn the correct sequence of movements that must be followed. Physical activities should be encouraged to strengthen a child's overall performance and coordination, beginning with simple physical tasks and leading up to more complicated tasks involving multiple steps.

dyssemia Difficulty in using and understanding nonverbal signs and signals; a nonverbal communication deficit.

dystaxia Difficulty controlling voluntary movements.

See also ATAXIA.

early childhood assessment   Testing that identifies early developmental and learning problems in preschool and primary grade children. Early childhood assessment practices allow for accurate and fair identification of the developmental needs of infants, preschoolers, and young children.

Sound early childhood assessment should involve a multidisciplinary team including school psychologists with specialized training in the assessment of the young child who work together with parents and caregivers.

Early assessment of potential problems is essential because of a child's broad and rapid development. An early childhood assessment should examine all aspects of the child's development, including how the child plays, moves, eats, talks, and listens. This development can be affected by a variety of things, such as the child's health and temperament, the daily family routines, and the family's values, beliefs, and traditions.

The assessment will also note how well the child listens to the parents or other people and how much attention is paid to an interesting toy. How the child gets what he or she wants, or how the child gets the parents to help him or her, also will be assessed.

The assessment should give a clear picture of the baby or child in different situations. This information can be provided by interviews with family and friends; by looking at baby books, health records, baby calendars, and so on; or by viewing photographs and home videos.

Typically, an early childhood assessment begins when the professional interviews the parents about the child's strengths and weaknesses. Parents describe their child in their own words as professionals listen carefully. Next, the child is observed at home or in a familiar setting, as he or she plays with parents or caregivers. This is one of the most important parts of the developmental assessment, as the expert observes the young child interacting with someone the child trusts.

After the assessment, the professional should provide a report to discuss with the parents, which should identify the child's strengths and abilities, plus any areas that will help the child develop further.

Standardized assessment procedures should be used with great caution in educational decision making because such tools are inherently less accurate when used with young children. Multidisciplinary team assessments must include multiple sources of information, multiple approaches to assessment, and multiple settings in order to yield a comprehensive understanding of children's skills and needs. Therefore, assessments should center on the child in the family system and home environment, both substantial influences on the development of young children.

early intervention program   A program designed to identify and provide intervention for infants and young children who are developmentally delayed and at high risk for school failure. The purpose of this type of program is to help prevent problems as the child matures.

These programs address the needs of young children from birth to the beginning of school with a collaborative effort from parents and medical, social services, and educational professionals. The pre-academic skills that may need help include self-concept, fine and gross motor skills, awareness of sounds, visual discrimination, communication and language development, thinking skills, and social skills. Nationally recognized early intervention programs include Project Head Start and Reading Recovery.

See also INDIVIDUALIZED FAMILY SERVICE PLAN; EARLY CHILDHOOD ASSESSMENT.

educable mentally handicapped (EMH)   See MILD MENTAL RETARDATION.

educational consultant   A term used to describe an individual with a variety of backgrounds and areas of expertise. For example, some educational consultants may specialize in college placement, while others may provide testing and specialize in primary or secondary school placement or consultation. An educational consultant may or may not have a background in LEARNING DISABILITY. Consultants who specialize in SPECIAL EDUCATION should have a background in assessment.

An educational consultant may provide counseling to help student and family choose a school, college, or other program that will foster academic and social growth. Educational consultants can provide a student and family with individual attention, firsthand knowledge of hundreds of educational opportunities, and the time to explore all of the options. Consultants may specialize in college admission, boarding school, summer programs, troubled teens, international students, or learning disabilities.

educational evaluation   An educational evaluation is typically part of the process of defining an INDIVIDUALIZED EDUCATION PROGRAM. Educational evaluation may involve administration of standardized academic tests, ASSESSMENT of performance in different academic classes, and observation of classroom performance. To be effective, evaluation should encompass a number of different types of measures, and involve the entire range of academic skill areas.

See also INDEPENDENT EDUCATION EVALUATION.

educational therapist   A professional who evaluates and treats learning problems in young children, adolescents, and adults. These problems may include DYSLEXIA; ATTENTION DEFICIT DISORDER; reading, writing, LANGUAGE, or math problems; academic SELF-ESTEEM and motivation; social skills; and organizational and study skills.

An educational therapist is skilled in

- formal and informal education assessment
- synthesis of information from other specialists and parents
- development and implementation of appropriate remedial programs for school-related learning and behavioral problems
- strategies for addressing social and emotional aspects of learning problems
- forming supportive relationships with the client and those involved in the client's educational development
- improving communication among the client, family, school, and other professionals

In a remediation session, the educational therapist works with a client on activities chosen especially for that person based on results from formal and informal testing. The educational therapist, who keeps extensive notes on each session, provides activities with an appropriate level of challenge and watches the client's response to those activities to assess their approach to the task and how they process information. This is a key element of progress during treatment.

Educational therapists plan and carry out treatment using educational situations, equipment, and methods to rehabilitate patients. Some educational therapists participate in the rehabilitation of blind patients. Educational therapists try to diminish emotional stress of clients, provide a sense of achievement, and channel energies into acceptable forms of behavior.

Education Department General Administrative Regulations (EDGAR)   Regulations for managing projects funded by grants awarded by the Department of Education. As is generally the case with the Code of Federal Regulations, specific regulations falling within EDGAR define, specify, and provide the framework for implementing laws about education.

Education for All Handicapped Children Act of 1975 (PL 94-142)   This significant legislation was renamed the INDIVIDUALS WITH DISABILITIES

EDUCATION IMPROVEMENT ACT in 1990 and requires the provision of a free and appropriate public education to children with disabilities.

elaboration The process of discussing or going over new information in order to form connections with familiar information, a process that helps MEMORY and affects depth of processing. There is a great deal of evidence in support of the idea that the more details are processed and repeated, the more likely they are to be retrieved from long-term memory.

electroencephalogram (EEG) A graphic record of the electrical activity at the surface of the brain obtained by attaching small electrodes to the scalp. This allows the regular electrical potential of the brain to be amplified and recorded on an oscillograph in wave patterns. It can be recorded in graphic form by an electroencephalograph.

Characteristic changes in type and frequency of the waves can provide different information about the brain and how it is functioning. These wave patterns can be used to diagnose specific disorders, diseases, and injuries. For example, EEG studies have shown that children with ATTENTION DEFICIT HYPERACTIVITY DISORDER (ADHD) have more theta (slow wave) activity and less beta (fast wave) activity compared with normal controls. (Theta activity is associated with daydreaming and other distractions.)

Some experts have used this information in an attempt to treat ADHD by training patients in biofeedback using EEGs (called neurofeedback). This training allows children to decrease theta activity. Proponents of neurofeedback believe that the child's ability to change brain activity is the direct result of EEG neurofeedback training. However, other experts point out that it is unclear how much of the improvement is due to EEG neurofeedback and how much is due to other factors.

Most experts believe that neurofeedback research results in patients with ADHD are inconclusive. Well-controlled scientific studies have not been published either to support or refute the effectiveness of EEG neurofeedback for children with ADHD.

eligibility The criteria for whether or not a student is eligible for SPECIAL EDUCATION services is determined by the INDIVIDUALIZED EDUCATION PROGRAM team. The team should consider qualitative and quantitative information from the assessment process.

Many states continue to determine eligibility by a DISCREPANCY formula, which is a mathematical equation that shows a significant discrepancy between a student's achievement (ACHIEVEMENT TEST scores) and potential (IQ score).

However, recent studies discourage the practice of determining eligibility solely on discrepancy of test scores, and encourage the consideration of other significant factors such as the observations and experiences of teachers and parents.

See also INTELLIGENCE QUOTIENT.

eligibility committee See MULTIDISCIPLINARY TEAM.

emotional and behavioral disorder A condition in which behavioral or emotional responses of a student interfere with performance in self-care, social relationships, personal adjustment, academic progress, classroom behavior, or work adjustment. Therefore, early identification and intervention for students with emotional and/or behavioral problems is essential.

EBD is more than a transient, expected response to stress in the child's environment; the problem persists even with individualized interventions, such as feedback, consultation with parents, and modification of the educational environment.

Assessment EBD must be exhibited in at least two different settings, at least one of which is school related. It can coexist with other handicapping conditions, such as schizophrenia, affective disorders, ANXIETY disorders, or other disturbances.

It is important that the ASSESSMENT identify both the strengths and needs of the individual and those with whom the student interacts. The assessment should ensure that the child's difficulties are not primarily due to transient developmental or environmental variables, cultural or linguistic differences, or influences of other handicapping conditions. Referral for special services should not be used as a disciplinary action or an effort to resolve conflicts.

The results of the assessment should provide information about

- environmental factors: the relationship between the instructional, social, and community environment and the student's specific problems
- strengths: identify the resources of the student, family, teacher(s), and school setting
- history: duration of the difficulties, their relationship to specific developmental or situational stressors and previous attempts to resolve the difficulties
- intensity: how severe the problems are in affecting school achievement, social skills, or interpersonal relationships within the school setting
- pervasiveness: the number of settings in which difficulties occur in the school, family, or community
- persistence: the extent to which difficulties have continued despite the use of well-planned, empirically based and individualized intervention strategies provided within lesser restrictive environments
- developmental/cultural data: the extent to which the student's behavior is different from the behavior expected for children of the same age, culture, and ethnic background. Information should be obtained from a variety of sources that can provide data about the child's difficulties across various settings.

The assessment should gather information about a child's behavioral and emotional functioning, developmental history, areas of significant impairment in school adaptive behavior and achievement, impairment outside the school setting in areas such as vocational skills, and social skills or interpersonal relationships. Because biological and neurological factors may contribute to, cause, or trigger problem behaviors, consultation with medical care providers and consideration of relevant student and family medical history is important.

Formal methods for gathering information may include behavior checklists, standardized self-reports, structured interviews, rating scales, and other appropriate assessment techniques. Informal methods, such as behavior observation and analysis of work samples, can also be useful.

Treatment Options and Outlook

Eligibility for services under the category of emotional/behavioral disorders should not automati-cally imply placement in a categorical special education program. Since emotional and behavioral disorders have many influences, interventions for children with these disorders must be comprehensive. Interventions should be planned by a team that includes the parent, the child, the school psychologist and other teachers, administrators, and community service providers. Intervention plans should take into account the strengths of the child, the family, the child's teachers, and the school.

Most schools exist primarily as an educational setting rather than a treatment setting, so children with significant emotional or behavioral disorders may need treatment outside school.

Individualized academic and curricular interventions   Children with emotional or behavioral problems frequently achieve below-grade expectations in academic areas. Academic problems often seem less important than a student's behavioral difficulties. Students may benefit from adaptations to the curriculum, alteration of the pace of delivery, improvements to the instructional and organizational ecology, and instruction in learning and study skills.

Consultation with teachers   Teachers may benefit from a discussion of the needs to the student and the most effective strategies to help the child improve behavior. Teachers will also benefit from the psychosocial support component of consultation in dealing with the frustration and isolation that often are present when working with children with significant problems.

Consultation and partnership with parents   Parents will benefit from consultation directed at understanding their child's difficulties, developing and implementing effective behavior management strategies, and working collaboratively with other caregivers. The parent may also need assistance with negotiating the array of services available in the community.

Individual and group counseling   Counseling may help the student more readily improve social skills and school adjustment. Students often need help in dealing with the stress in their environment, and understanding responsibility and self-directedness.

Social skills training   Students with emotional and behavioral disorders often have problems with social skills, so social skills training in the child's multiple environments is often helpful.

Crisis planning and management Crises should be anticipated and plans for dealing with crises should be a part of the student's intervention plan.

Specialized educational settings By law, children must be provided services in the least restrictive environment that meets the student's academic, psychological, and social needs. Many students' needs can be effectively addressed through consultation with teachers and parents, short-term counseling, and interventions in the regular classroom setting.

Job and transitional planning Career exploration, pre-vocational and vocational skills development, and transition to the after-high school world should be included for all adolescents with emotional and behavioral disorders.

emotional-behavioral tests A psychological test that measures how parents, teachers, and the child rate the child's behavior, attitude, and feelings at home and at school. They include

- Behavior Assessment System for Children
- CONNORS PARENT-TEACHER RATING SCALES—REVISED
- Achenbach
- Reynolds Child Depression Scale
- Piers Harris Self-Concept Scales
- Differential Test of Conduct and Emotional Problems
- Assessment of Interpersonal Relationships
- Depression and Anxiety in Youth Scale
- Multidimension Depression Inventory

emotional disturbance Emotional disorders that can interfere with a child's ability to learn. "Emotional disturbance" is defined under the INDIVIDUALS WITH DISABILITIES EDUCATION IMPROVEMENT ACT.

Experts are not sure what causes emotional disturbance, but various factors such as heredity, brain disorder, diet, stress, and family functioning have been suggested as possible causes.

Symptoms and Diagnostic Path

Many children who do not have emotional disturbances may act out occasionally, but when children have serious emotional disturbances these behaviors continue over long periods of time. Some of the characteristics and behaviors seen in children who have emotional disturbances include

- short attention span, impulsiveness
- acting out, fighting
- withdrawal, excessive fear or anxiety
- immaturity (inappropriate crying, temper tantrums, poor coping skills)
- learning difficulties (academically performing below grade level)

Children with the most serious emotional disturbances may experience distorted thinking, excessive anxiety, bizarre behavior, or abnormal mood swings.

Emotional disturbance is a condition exhibiting one or more of the following characteristics over a long period of time and to a severe degree

- an inability to learn that cannot be explained by intellectual, sensory, or health factors
- an inability to build or maintain satisfactory relationships with other children and teachers
- inappropriate types of behavior or feelings under normal circumstances
- a general unhappiness or DEPRESSION
- a tendency to develop physical symptoms or fears associated with personal or school problems

Treatment Options and Outlook

Educational programs for students with a serious emotional disturbance must include attention to mastering academics, developing social skills, and increasing self-awareness, SELF-ESTEEM, and self-control. Academic and vocational education) is also an important part of secondary education and should be a part of every teenager's transition plan in the INDIVIDUALIZED EDUCATION PROGRAM (IEP).

Students eligible for SPECIAL EDUCATION services under the category of "serious emotional disturbance" may have IEPs that include psychological or counseling services as a related service. These must be provided by a qualified social worker, psychologist, or guidance counselor.

Behavior modification is one of the most common treatment methods for children with emotional disturbances.

encoding   The process of expressing messages through speaking or writing.

English as a Second Language (ESL)   Instruction in which individuals are taught English with minimal emphasis on their native language. (Adult English for Speakers of Other Languages, or adult ESOL, is alternately used in various parts of the United States.) As the number of ESL students in regular classrooms increases, instruction of these students has become more controversial. While some promote a bilingual approach to instruction for individuals for whom English is a second language, others suggest an immersion approach is more efficient.

Adult ESL programs vary in scope and content. Some programs, especially those for recent arrivals, including refugees, emphasize survival or life skills in the curriculum and focus on improving listening and speaking abilities. Others stress work-related topics, citizenship and civics education, family literacy, or academic or GED preparation. Learners who lack literacy skills in their native language and those who are new to the Roman alphabet may be placed in classes that focus on developing basic literacy skills. Classes are provided by local educational agencies, community colleges, local businesses and unions, community-based organizations, volunteer groups, churches, and for-profit language schools.

ESL teachers use a variety of approaches to teach adult learners to speak, read, and write English. Some approaches focus on language functions such as asking for assistance and expressing likes and dislikes, still others focus on the knowledge and skills needed to function in the United States, such as giving and following directions on the job. Some approaches focus on discussing and writing about issues in the learners' lives. Finally, some emphasize teaching the grammar rules of the language. However, a mix of approaches is usually necessary to effectively teach English as a second language.

Some techniques developed for use with second language learners have been useful for teaching individuals with LEARNING DISABILITIES, such as the use of manipulatives.

See also BILINGUAL APPROACH.

Enright Diagnostic Inventory of Basic Arithmetic Skills   This test, designed for elementary and middle school grades, provides a task analysis of the student's computation errors using whole numbers, fractions, and decimals. It also identifies areas in which the student demonstrates mastery.

environmental factors   Factors that affect normal development of children, such as parental substance abuse, extreme poverty, disturbed parent-child interaction, and neglect. For a student to be identified with a LEARNING DISABILITY, it must be first determined that environmental factors are not the primary cause of the learning problems.

environmental toxins   Harmful substances that may lead to LEARNING DISABILITIES by disrupting childhood brain development or the central nervous system, both of which are highly vulnerable during gestation through the first years of life. While learning disabilities are clearly caused by complex interactions among genetic, environmental, and social factors, there is sound scientific evidence indicating a much stronger link between toxic exposures in the environment and learning and other developmental disabilities than experts had realized in the past. In fact, a recent report from the National Research Council concluded that 3 percent of developmental disabilities are the direct consequence of neurotoxic environmental exposures and that another 25 percent are caused by the interaction between environment and individual genetic susceptibility.

Children are much more susceptible to the risks of exposure to dangerous environmental toxins than adults because of their smaller size and closeness to the floor, their faster metabolic rate, and their tendency to put their hands into their mouths.

Some of the most common toxic substances that may be linked to learning disabilities in children include heavy metals such as LEAD or MERCURY; chemicals such as DIOXINS, FLAME RETARDANTS, or PCBs; solvents such as ALCOHOL; pesticides such as DURSBAN or LINDANE; and toxic black MOLD.

Lead   Lead is the most well-studied environmental toxin known to interfere with learning—decreasing IQ, interfering with the ability to pay attention, and influencing disruptive classroom behavior. Exposure to lead in the early years has been linked to failure to graduate from high school, violent tendencies, addictive behaviors, and other behavioral and emotional problems. Because of this wide range of effects in children, researchers are also studying whether lead exposure may be involved in a diagnosis of ATTENTION DEFICIT HYPERACTIVITY DISORDER (ADHD). However, while some studies have shown significant relationships between lead levels and attention-deficit behaviors, the extent to which lead contributes to a diagnosis of ADHD or may interfere with genetic, social, familial and cultural factors is still unclear.

Mercury   Mercury is a naturally occurring metal that, once ingested or inhaled, can cause mental retardation, developmental disabilities, and brain damage. It is found in the ground and in oceans, lakes, rivers, and streams—and thereby also in tuna, shellfish, shark, tilefish, and king mackerel. Mercury also is used in dental fillings, fluorescent lights, batteries, and thermometers, and in other forms in some cosmetic creams. Humans most typically ingest mercury when eating fish, although it is also possible to be exposed through dental and medical procedures, some vaccines (thimerosal), or broken thermometers. In addition, mercury passes from mother to child through the placenta and breast milk. In newborns, exposure can cause mental retardation, brain damage, lack of coordination, blindness, seizures, and the inability to speak. For this reason, the government recommends that pregnant women eat no more than two cans of tuna per week and limit their intake of other possibly contaminated fish.

Dioxins   DIOXINS are a group of some of the most toxic human-made chemicals in the world. In addition to being known carcinogens, dioxins have been linked to developmental and learning disabilities.

Dioxin itself is the most harmful of all of the toxins in the dioxin group and is produced by burning chlorine-containing plastics, incinerating household waste, and bleaching chlorine paper. Dioxins are found just about everywhere in the environment, but humans most often are exposed by eating them in the fat of meats, dairy products, and fish. Some dioxins also can be inhaled.

Flame retardants (PBDE)   PBDE stands for a group of chemicals called polybrominated diphenyl ether that are chemically similar to PCBs (polychlorinated biphenyls), which were banned decades ago because of human toxicity.

The main differences between the two chemical groups are that PBDEs contain bromine instead of chlorine, and unlike PCBs, PBDEs are not chemically bound to plastic. What this means is that it is not necessary to burn or chemically change a product containing PBDE for it to get into the environment. Most humans are exposed by eating contaminated fish or by breathing vapors indoors around electronic equipment. Babies are exposed through breast milk, since PBDEs accumulate in fat and mother's milk. There have been drastic increases of PBDEs in human breast milk in the past 30 years. The effects on a child's developing system are much more drastic than in an adult's and include potential harm to the developing brain as well as possible hormone disruption that could lead to unknown results.

Polychlorinated biphenyls (PCBs)   These toxic chemicals also interfere with learning and attention and were used as electrical insulators until their U.S. ban in 1976. PCBs are a particular concern because they persist for such a long time in the environment and in human tissue. Children may be exposed to PCBs before birth, via breast milk, or by eating fish, shellfish and other fatty foods that contain high concentrations. In the United States, eating fish has been the most common route of exposure and has been associated with poor brain developmental function in infants. Studies have found that exposure to PCBs can result in decreased intellectual function and lower IQ scores. Although no human studies have examined whether prenatal exposure to PCBs is a risk factor for clinically diagnosed ADHD, a rat study found a link between PCB exposure through a mother's milk and hyperactive behavior.

Alcohol   Alcohol exposure to the fetus can cause devastating, lifelong damage and is the leading cause of preventable mental retardation. Drinking during pregnancy can cause FETAL ALCOHOL

SYNDROME (FAS), a pattern of facial abnormalities, growth retardation, and brain damage that occurs only in babies whose mothers drank during pregnancy. Even when fetal alcohol exposure does not result in full-blown FAS, it can cause FETAL ALCOHOL EFFECT, a less serious but still debilitating, lifelong condition of lowered intelligence, hyperactivity, and behavioral disorders.

Alcohol appears in breast milk shortly after the mother takes a drink. There is no known safe level of alcohol consumption during pregnancy. For this reason, most experts advise pregnant women and women likely to become pregnant to abstain from alcohol altogether.

Dursban This extremely toxic organophosphate pesticide is used widely in homes, schools, hospitals, and agriculture. One of 37 similar chemicals, it is produced as granules and its primary function is to kill bugs by damaging their nervous systems. Dursban has been produced for more than 20 years but is currently being phased out of production because of its toxicity.

Some studies show that Dursban exposure early in life results in adverse changes in the nervous system and in normal learning behavior. Exposure during pregnancy may lead to mental retardation and brain defects.

Humans eat, drink, and breathe Dursban, which also has been found in very high concentration in the breast milk of animals. The danger depends on how recently Dursban has been used and in what concentration. Children are affected much more severely by pesticides than adults because they play in the grass, in the garden, and close to the floor, and they also place their hands and toys in their mouths regularly.

Lindane This solid organochloride pesticide evaporates quickly in the air and does not occur naturally in the environment. It is primarily use to kill head lice, body lice, and scabies and was used for 50 years in agriculture to kill insects on fruits and vegetables. Although there has been little study on human exposure to lindane during pregnancy, animal studies suggest that lindane can damage the central nervous system of the unborn child, leading to developmental, behavioral, and learning disabilities.

Lindane is being phased out of production and use in the United States but is still widely used in imported products from countries without such bans. It accumulates in the fat of fish and has been found in human breast milk. Although it is a common ingredient in head lice treatments, lindane products are no longer recommended for children.

Toxic black mold Molds are fungi that grow in damp, dark places; although many are harmless, toxic black mold can be harmful to health. Children who are exposed to molds may exhibit symptoms and behaviors similar to learning disabilities, having trouble focusing or remembering. They may be tired or complain of headaches or stomachaches.

Mold's toxic effects come from its spores, which grow on the surface of a mold and can be blown into the air or carried home on clothes and shoes. They grow quickly in moist places—especially in damp or porous things like wood, paper, cardboard, and ceiling tiles. They also grow well in drywall, upholstery, carpets, and wallpaper. Humans breathe air and dust that contain mold spores, and poor ventilation in buildings increases the likelihood of growth and therefore exposure.

epilepsy A chronic brain disorder marked by recurrent seizures. Epilepsy may express itself in major (grand mal) seizures causing unconsciousness, or in minor (petit mal) seizures. It is sometimes associated with other conditions, including specific LEARNING DISABILITIES, AUTISM, or attention disorders. In epilepsy, the normal pattern of brain cell activity is disturbed, causing strange sensations, emotions, and behavior or sometimes convulsions, muscle spasms, and loss of consciousness.

Symptoms and Diagnostic Path

It is not unusual for children with epilepsy to develop behavioral and emotional problems, sometimes the consequence of embarrassment and frustration or bullying, teasing, or avoidance in school. Seizures may include convulsions, brief stares, muscle spasms, odd sensations, or episodes of automatic behavior and altered consciousness.

Epilepsy is a disorder with many possible causes. Anything that disturbs the normal pattern of neuron activity—from illness to brain damage to abnormal brain development—can lead to seizures. Epilepsy may develop because of an abnormality in brain wiring, an imbalance of nerve signaling chemicals called neurotransmitters, or some combination of these factors. Having a seizure does not necessarily mean that a person has epilepsy. Only when a person has had two or more seizures is epilepsy diagnosed.

A doctor can diagnose epilepsy from a number of different tests. Which tests are ordered may vary, depending on how much each test reveals, but they may include

- a detailed medical history
- a thorough physical examination, especially of the nervous system
- blood tests
- electroencephalogram (EEG)
- brain scans (magnetic resonance imaging [MRI]) and/or computed tomography (CT) scans

Treatment Options and Outlook

Once epilepsy is diagnosed, it is important to begin treatment as soon as possible. Seizures can be controlled with modern medicines and surgical techniques in about 80 percent of patients. In 1997, the FDA approved the vagus nerve stimulator for use in people with seizures that are not well controlled by medication.

The goal of all epilepsy treatment is to prevent further seizures, avoid side effects, and make it possible for the patient to lead a normal, active life.

Most epilepsy medicines are taken by mouth in the form of tablets, capsules, sprinkles, or syrup. The drugs act on the brain to prevent the seizures from getting started, by reducing the tendency of the brain cells to send excessive and confused electrical signals. They may include

- carbamazepine (brand names: Tegretol, Tegretol-XR, Carbatrol)
- clonazepam (Klonopin)
- ethosuximide (Zarontin)
- phenobarbital
- phenytoin (Dilantin)
- primidone (Mysoline)
- valproic acid (Depakene)
- divalproex sodium (Depakote)

- felbamate (Felbatol)
- gabapentin (Neurontin)
- lamotrigine (Lamictal)
- levetiracetam (Keppra)
- oxcarbazepine (Trileptal)
- tiagabine (Gabitril)
- topiramate (Topamax)
- zonisamide (Zonegran)

Other new drugs are in development. A rectal gel form of diazepam (Diastat) may be prescribed to stop cluster seizures or prolonged seizures. Some doctors may prescribe diazepam (Valium), lorazepam (Ativan), or clonazepam (Klonopin) for the same purpose. A steroid drug (ACTH) may be injected to treat children with a type of epilepsy called infantile spasms, or for severe seizures that cannot be controlled with other drugs.

The particular drug that is prescribed depends on what kind of seizure a person is having, since different drugs control different types of seizures. People also react to these medicines in different ways. Some experience side effects, others may not. Some people's bodies break down medicines at a faster or slower rate than the average person. Some people's seizures will respond well to a particular drug while someone else will have seizures that continue. This is why it may take some time to find exactly the right dose of the right drug for each person who has a seizure disorder.

In addition to medications, brain surgery can be a successful way of treating epilepsy. Surgery is most likely to be considered when someone with epilepsy has already tried the standard medicines without success (or has bad reactions to them), has seizures that always start in just one part of the brain, and has seizures in a part of the brain that can be removed without damaging important things like speech, memory, or eyesight.

Surgery for epilepsy is a delicate, complicated operation that must be performed by an experienced surgical team. In addition to operations that remove a small part of the brain where seizures begin, other procedures may be done to interrupt the spread of electrical energy in the brain.

Most people with epilepsy lead normal lives, although many people with epilepsy believe that the risk of seizures restricts their independence (some states refuse a driver's license to people with epilepsy). People with epilepsy are at special risk for two life-threatening conditions: status epilepticus and sudden unexplained death.

episodic memory That part of MEMORY that stores the events an individual experiences in life. Episodic memory enables a person to remember personal experiences, to be consciously aware of an earlier experience in a certain situation at a certain time. According to some psychologists, there are at least five major human memory systems for which evidence is now available. They include episodic, semantic, procedural, perceptual representation, and short-term memory.

Episodic memory operates together with SEMANTIC MEMORY, which stores concepts about the world in the broadest sense, and makes it available for retrieval. Remembering the contents of a dinner consumed last evening would require episodic memory. Remembering that a foot has 12 inches or that the Sun is at the center of the solar system involves semantic memory.

Episodic memory is more easily impaired than semantic memory, perhaps because rehearsal or repetition tends to be minimal.

error analysis An approach to ASSESSMENT that goes beyond test performance to examine the nature of the errors and to discern patterns in types of errors. Error analysis may be used either with formal tests or in informal academic settings, for example, as when a teacher examines a written composition to identify specific patterns of mechanical or grammatical errors.

Analyzing errors of decoding performance is an important first step to defining appropriate educational interventions. Determining which sound-symbol patterns are involved in specific patterns of reading mistakes provides a starting point for reading instruction.

evaluation Testing of an individual for the purpose of diagnosis or treatment. In educational settings, an evaluation is a required part of a plan for SPECIAL EDUCATION services, usually called an INDIVIDUALIZED EDUCATION PROGRAM (IEP). For the eval-

uation of a DEVELOPMENTAL DISABILITY or LEARNING DISABILITY, multiple assessments are required, including intelligence and achievement tests.

A parent can ask the school to test a child, or the school may ask parents for permission to do an evaluation. If the school thinks a child may have a disability and may need special education and related services, it must evaluate the child before providing these services. This evaluation is free to the family.

Step 1: Checking What's Already Known
An evaluation will tell the parents and the school if a child has a disability—and what kind of special help the child needs in school. The evaluation will be done by a group of people, including parents, who will begin by checking the child's school file and recent test scores and interviews with parents and teachers. This initial survey will provide information to decide if a child has a disability and what kind of special help may be needed. However, if a child is being evaluated for the first time, the initial review may not provide enough information.

Step 2. Collecting More Information
Before the school can conduct additional testing, staffers must ask the parents for permission, and describe what tests will be used and any other ways in which the school will collect information about the child.

The group involved in a child's evaluation will include

- at least one of the child's regular education teachers

- at least one of the child's special education teachers or service providers

- parents

- a school administrator expert in special education policies, children with disabilities, the general curriculum, and available resources

- an expert who can interpret the evaluation results and talk about what instruction may be necessary

- individuals (invited by parents or the school) with knowledge or special expertise about the child

- the child, if appropriate

- representatives from other agencies responsible for paying for or providing transition services
- other qualified professionals such as a school psychologist, occupational therapist, speech therapist, physical therapist, medical specialists

Although tests are an important part of an evaluation, they are only part of the process. The evaluation should also include the observations of professionals who have worked with the child, the child's relevant medical history, and the parents' ideas about the child's experiences, abilities, needs, and behavior.

It is important that the school evaluate a child in all areas of possible disability. For example, the tests should evaluate

- language skills (speaking and understanding)
- thoughts and behavior
- adaptability to change
- school achievement
- intelligence
- movement, thinking, learning, seeing, and hearing function
- job-related and other post-school interests and abilities

Tests must be given in the child's native language or by other means of communication (for example, sign language, if the child is deaf). Tests must not be biased, and the tests must be given correctly. Evaluation results will be used to decide if a child is a "child with a disability" and to determine what kind of educational program is needed. These decisions cannot be made based on only one procedure, such as a single test.

Step 3. Assessing Eligibility
The next step in the evaluation process is to decide if the child is eligible for special education. This decision will be based on the results of the child's evaluation and local policies about eligibility for these special services. Based on the evaluation results, the committee will decide if the child is eligible for special education and related services. Under the IDEIA, parents have the right to be part of any group that decides a child's eligibility for special education and related services.

The IDEIA lists 13 different disability categories under which a child may be eligible for services:

- AUTISM
- deaf-blindness
- deafness
- hearing impairment
- MENTAL RETARDATION
- multiple disabilities
- orthopedic impairment
- other health impairment (such as having limited strength, vitality, or alertness that affects a child's educational performance)
- serious emotional disturbance
- specific learning disability
- speech or language impairment
- TRAUMATIC BRAIN INJURY
- visual impairment, including blindness

Parents have the right to receive a copy of the evaluation report and to receive a copy of the paperwork about the child's eligibility for special education.

Step 4. Developing an IEP
If the child is eligible for special education and related services (such as speech therapy), parents then meet with the school to discuss special educational needs and to create an individualized education program for the child. The IEP is a written document that parents and school personnel develop together to describe a child's educational program, including special services.

If a child is not eligible for special education and related services, the school must inform parents in writing and must provide information about an appeal if the parents disagree with this decision. Parents have the right to disagree with the eligibility decision.

executive functions Mental activities associated with self-control, attention, focus, or concentration that allow an individual to achieve specific goals. Problems in executive function are associated with dysfunction of the frontal part of the brain. Mild or nonspecific deficits of executive functions are common in the general population. Executive functions also may be impaired by injury to the brain, fatigue, DEPRESSION, schizophrenia, ANXIETY, and various psychological disorders, including LEARNING DISABILITY and ATTENTION DEFICIT HYPER-ACTIVITY DISORDER (ADHD).

Problems with attention, self-regulation, planning, and impulse control may be connected to differences in the processing of neurotransmitters, particularly dopamine, in the brain.

Executive functions control four kinds of mental activities. *Working memory* is essential to the problem-solving process. Information must be held in mind and internalized while a task is being completed. *Internalized* or *private speech* allows people to use complex sets of rules in problem solving. These include rules for using sets of rules. Third is the *control of emotions and impulses,* which allows an individual to remain focused and to continually return to a path of progress toward a desired goal. This allows an individual to set aside the attraction of immediate gratification. The achievement of deferred greater gratification is the product of this kind of self-regulation. Fourth is *reconstitution,* a process of observing behaviors and then synthesizing components of what has been observed into new combinations. This function is essential to problem solving and survival in a complicated world.

Individuals with ADHD and learning disabilities may have problems in reading long assignments or completing writing projects, since these tasks require executive functions. These difficulties may be connected to differences in the way certain brain chemicals are processed in the prefrontal lobes.

Some individuals with executive function difficulties are also very impulsive, having a hard time considering alternatives and consequences before they act. In solving problems, they are likely to select the first alternative without weighing other possibilities. They often speak out without thinking of the consequences of their statements. Some students with these problems get so fidgety that it is hard for them to sit through a 50- or 90-minute class session.

Many individuals with executive function difficulties experience problems with time. Understanding the passage of time and planning for the future or the completion of a task by a particular point in time, can be a challenge. These individuals may frequently arrive late to appointments or classes. Long-term academic projects are among the greatest challenges for students who have executive function difficulties.

experiential learning   Learning based on experiences rather than lectures or reading. Experiential learning, also referred to as hands-on learning, can be especially helpful to students with a LEARNING DISABILITY since it allows them to learn without being hindered by difficulties in reading or writing. An experiential approach to education and learning is based on the belief that students are more motivated and will remember concepts better when they have a direct physical experience.

Experiential learning also may have a strong basis in the nature of memory, especially for individuals with learning disabilities or ATTENTION DEFICIT DISORDERS. For many students, learning techniques that incorporate sight and touch are much easier for them to remember and retrieve. Evidence suggests that many individuals with learning disabilities or attention deficit hyperactivity disorder have a hard time remembering concepts, rules, and verbal information (semantic memory), while finding it much easier to remember events, people, places, and experiences (episodic memory).

To some degree, experiential learning activities may provide a means for bridging these two basic forms of memory, and for enabling individuals to use strengths in one area to compensate for weaknesses in the other.

explicit direct instruction   Structured, sequential, and cumulative instruction that is presented in a way that follows a logical sequence, without assuming any prior skills or language knowledge.

explicit memory   Type of memory used to reorganize or recall presented materials.

expository writing   A term that refers to informational writing typically given during the first year of college to prepare first-year students for academic writing. Generally, entering first-year students will take at least one semester of expository writing. Some colleges require a two-semester sequence of expository writing courses.

In some cases, students with writing problems may be required to complete developmental or basic writing courses before they can enter the expository writing course.

Expository writing includes description, comparison/contrast, definition, classification, argument, process analysis, and cause-and-effect. These types of writing or rhetorical strategies may be taught using models and examples, and as ends in themselves, or as strategies to use within informational essays that include a number of different patterns.

In general, the goal of teaching these types of writing patterns is to provide a foundation for the kinds of text-based writing required in specific academic disciplines.

Expository writing may be contrasted with expressive writing or the personal essay, in which students are allowed to focus on their own experience, perceptions, and memories. Much more than expressive writing, expository writing may pose problems for individuals with LEARNING DISABILITY who may find it difficult to organize ideas, support main ideas with details, or apply paragraph and essay structures.

See also RHETORICAL PATTERNS.

expressive language A type of communication involving speaking and writing. The process of producing spoken language is called *oral expressive language*. Listening and reading are considered to be RECEPTIVE LANGUAGE.

expressive language disorders An impairment in the ability to express ideas through language, characterized by problems with vocabulary, grammatical structures, word order, and overall language development. Expressive language disorders may have a severe impact on an individual's ability to generate spoken language and may be associated with other language-based LEARNING DISORDERS, such as reading disability or WRITTEN EXPRESSION DISORDER. Three to five percent of all school-age children have expressive language disorder.

There are a number of disorders relating to expressive language. DYSNOMIA refers to the inability to remember and express specific words. Individuals with dysnomia may "talk around" a word in order to express an idea without finding the appropriate words. For example, someone with dysnomia might say "that thing you eat that is yellow and long" when attempting to say "banana."

Because of a general cultural bias toward associating intelligence with communication, individuals with an expressive-language disorder may often be seen by others as less capable and intelligent than they actually are, even when nonverbal measures indicate extremely high intellectual potential.

Although the cause of this disorder is unknown, brain damage and malnutrition have been associated as underlying factors. The condition can be present at birth or acquired before age four.

Symptoms and Diagnostic Path

Expressive language disorders also include those patients who can remember the word they want to say, but cannot physically manipulate their speech muscles to produce the word. This disorder is called APRAXIA. Disorders in oral expressive language are called expressive APHASIA. Students would be considered aphasic if they have problems expressing themselves orally but have no difficulty understanding language spoken to them and are successful with nonverbal tasks.

Expressive language disorders are diagnosed by tests of discrepancy between verbal performance and nonverbal and receptive measures of potential performance.

Treatment Options and Outlook

Expressive language disorders are treated by speech-language pathologists. The best treatment approach combines direct speech-language therapy with psychotherapy. In addition to special classroom instruction at school, students with expressive language disorders benefit from individualized tutoring. Psychotherapy is recommended for children because of the possibility of an emotional or behavioral problem associated with expressive language disorder.

externalization The attribution of specific behaviors or feelings to causes outside the self. Externalization is common in school settings when students experience repeated failure and have poor SELF-ESTEEM. In these cases, many will blame these problems on teachers or institutions, rather than on their own actions or lack of ability.

extrinsic phonics PHONICS taught as a supplemental learning aid rather than as an integral part of the program of reading instruction, often in separate workbooks during special time periods.

eye-foot coordination The ability to control and direct movements of hands (and arms) and feet (and legs) in accordance with visual stimuli. Examples of eye-foot coordinated activities are operating a foot-drive potter's wheel, or driving a car.

eye-hand coordination A combination of fine motor skills of the hand and visual skills. Eye-hand coordination is required for many daily activities such as handwriting, drawing, typing, and many sports such as basketball, baseball, and javelin. Individuals with dysgraphia often have poor eye-hand coordination, resulting in poor control of handwriting.

See also VISUAL MOTOR SKILLS; FINE MOTOR SKILLS.

Family Educational Rights and Privacy Act (FERPA) This act, also known as the Buckley Amendment, outlines procedures and guidelines for maintaining and disclosing student records.

Under this law, parents and students over 18 years of age have the right to review education records within 45 days of their application, and to request a change of records that the parent or student believe to be inaccurate or misleading.

Individuals also have the right to request disclosure of records that contain personally identifiable information.

Under the act, such information also may be disclosed without consent to school officials with a legitimate educational interest. (The definition of "school official" includes individuals employed by a school district as an administrator, supervisor, teacher, or support staff member, and may also include other individuals performing official functions, such as school board members.)

FERPA is important legislation for parents of children with learning disabilities who seek services under INDIVIDUALS WITH DISABILITIES EDUCATION ACT because it governs the circumstances under which information related to a child's academic performance and learning needs may be made available to others.

family history An important component of a thorough ASSESSMENT that identifies development factors that may have had an impact on the individual, together with family events, trends, and other conditions. A family history may point toward potential genetic links between an individual's condition and that of parents or other family members, and it may also discern factors in the family dynamic that have an impact on an individual's case.

family therapy A type of behavioral therapy that involves the entire family in treatment. In many cases, behavioral problems affect the entire family as well as the person with a LEARNING DISABILITY. In family therapy, the child with a learning disability, together with parents and siblings, is supported emotionally and guided to find better ways to handle disruptive behaviors and to promote change.

far point copying The ability to see and copy from a distance, typically used in the context of being able to read from a chalk or whiteboard and to copy the written or diagrammed information.

Federal Register A daily publication of the U.S. government that contains amendments to federal regulations and other legal and legislative information.

Feingold diet A special diet that eliminates synthetic colorings and flavorings, certain preservatives, and salicylates (chemicals similar to aspirin), advocated by pediatrician and allergist Benjamin Feingold. Dr. Feingold believed that these substances are linked to HYPERACTIVITY, LEARNING DISABILITIES, and ATTENTION DEFICIT HYPERACTIVITY DISORDER in some children.

In studies where different levels of salicylates were investigated, some researchers found a link between salicylates and additives in some hyperactive children. Some proponents believe that as many as 10 percent to 25 percent of all children may be sensitive to salicylates. The success of the Feingold diet, they say, may depend on the degree of a person's sensitivity to salicylates and food additives and the amount of additives present in foods.

According to the Feingold Association, children under six years of age respond within one week of following the diet, whereas children over six may need to follow the diet for two to six weeks to achieve positive results.

However, the diet is not universally accepted. Critics argue that other studies show that salicylates are not an underlying cause of hyperactivity. However, since this diet is not generally seen as harmful, many pediatricians do not object to families trying the diet to see if it improves the child's condition.

The basis of the diet is to limit salicylates by avoiding foods and substances containing them, including almonds, apples, apricots, aspirin, berries, cherries, cider vinegars, cloves, coffee, cucumbers, oil of wintergreen, oranges, peaches, bell or chili peppers, pickles, plums, prunes, raisins, tangerines, tea, tomatoes, or wine. In addition to salicylates, a number of ingredients and additives should be avoided as well. These may be found not only in foods but also in cleaning supplies, art supplies, and toiletries.

They include BHA (butylated hydroxyanisole), BHT (butylated hydroxytoluene), benzoates (including sodium benzoate and benzoic acid), carminic acid, cochineal, and a number of artificial colorings, including tartrazine (Yellow No. 5), quinoline yellow, yellow 2G, sunset yellow FCF, carmoisine (red), amaranth (Red No. 2), ponceau (Red No. 4), erythrocine (Red No. 3), red 2G, allura red 2C, patent blue, indigo carmine (Blue), brilliant blue FCF, black, vegetable carbon (banned in the United States), brown FK, and chocolate brown HT. The diet also recommends avoiding concentrates, corn syrup, flavoring, hydrolyzed vegetable protein (HVP, may contain MSG), monosodium glutamate (MSG), natural coloring (may contain salicylates), natural flavoring (may contain salicylates or MSG), nitrites oil (may contain the preservatives BHA, BHT, or TBHQ), and sulfur. Also prohibited are sulphites, including sodium sulfite (sulphate), sodium bisulfite (bisulphate), sodium metabisulfite (metabisulphite), potassium bisulfite (bisulphate), and potassium metabisulfite (metabisulphite). Finally, the diet also forbids TBHQ (tertiary butyl hydroquinone) and vitamin A palmitate (can contain the preservatives BHA, BHT, or TBHQ).

fetal alcohol effect (FAE) A combination of mild defects in an infant caused by excessive alcohol intake by a pregnant woman; it is less severe than FETAL ALCOHOL SYNDROME (FAS). Symptoms include LEARNING DISABILITIES and other brain difference that do not become evident until well after birth.

While individuals with this condition may lack the outward physical appearance of people with fetal alcohol syndrome and generally have higher IQs, the internal damage to the brain and other organs can be just as serious as in FAS. Because FAE individuals "look normal," they are expected to perform normally. These issues lead to secondary disabilities—those that develop as a result of failure to properly deal with the primary disabilities.

fetal alcohol syndrome (FAS) A condition that describes the physical and mental birth defects in a child caused by the mother's consumption of ALCOHOL during pregnancy. Maternal use of alcohol during pregnancy may have been a factor for a substantial number of children receiving SPECIAL EDUCATION services.

More than 10 percent of children have been exposed to high levels of alcohol before birth, which may cause effects ranging from mild LEARNING DISABILITIES to major physical, mental, and intellectual impairment. It takes very little alcohol to cause serious damage; research has shown that even a single exposure to high levels of alcohol can cause significant brain damage in an unborn child.

Approximately 10 percent of pregnant women used alcohol, and approximately 2 percent engaged in binge drinking or frequent use of alcohol, according to a 2002 survey by the Centers for Disease Control and Prevention (CDC). The CDC results further indicated that more than half of women who did not use birth control (and therefore might become pregnant) reported alcohol use, and 12.4 percent reported binge drinking. As a result, the CDC recommends that women who are pregnant or who might become pregnant should abstain from alcohol use.

Alcohol in a pregnant woman's bloodstream circulates to the fetus by crossing the placenta, where it interferes with the baby's oxygen and nourishment needed for normal cell development in the brain.

Symptoms and Diagnostic Path

A variety of problems are typically associated with FAS, including

- central nervous system problems: small brain; faulty arrangement of brain cells and connective tissue; MENTAL RETARDATION, usually mild to moderate but occasionally severe; learning disability; short ATTENTION span; irritability in infancy; HYPERACTIVITY in childhood; poor body, hand, and finger coordination

- small body size and weight

- slower than normal development

- deformed ribs and sternum; curved spine; hip dislocations; bent, fused, webbed, or missing fingers or toes; limited movement of joints; small head

- facial abnormalities: small eye openings; skin webbing between eyes and base of nose; drooping eyelids; nearsightedness; failure of eyes to move in same direction; short upturned nose; sunken nasal bridge; flat or absent groove between nose and upper lip; thin upper lip; opening in roof of mouth; small jaw; low-set or poorly formed ears

- organ deformities: heart defects; heart murmurs; genital malformations; kidney and urinary defects

Early diagnosis can help prevent secondary disabilities such as mental health problems, dropping out of school, trouble with the law, and substance abuse. After diagnosis, parents often find that their ability to cope with the child's behavior changes dramatically when they understand that the problems are most likely based on organic brain damage, rather than the child's choice to be inattentive or uncooperative.

Treatment Options and Outlook

FAS is a lifetime disability with no cure; a child will not outgrow the problem. However, early and intensive intervention can make an enormous difference in the prognosis for a child. Interventions should begin before age 10 or 12, since this is the period of greatest development of neural pathways.

Risk Factors and Preventive Measures

FAS is preventable if a woman refrains from alcohol use during pregnancy. Studies suggest that drinking a large amount of alcohol at any one time may be more dangerous to the fetus than drinking small amounts more often. The fetus is most vulnerable to various types of injuries, depending on the stage of development in which alcohol is encountered.

Because a safe amount of drinking during pregnancy has not been determined, health experts agree that women should not drink at all during pregnancy. Unfortunately, women sometimes wait until a pregnancy is confirmed before they stop drinking. By then, the embryo has gone through several weeks of critical development, a period during which exposure to alcohol can be very damaging. Therefore, experts urge women who are pregnant or anticipating a pregnancy to abstain from drinking alcoholic beverages.

figurative language Forms of communication that use nonliteral ways of conveying meaning, such as comparisons, analogies, and exaggeration. Common forms of figurative language include metaphors (such as "the moon was a ghostly galleon") or similes ("my love is like a red, red rose"). Figurative language is common in literature, but it is also used in everyday speech: "I could eat a horse." Difficulty with understanding or using figurative language may cause significant problems for an individual.

figure-ground deficits Difficulty telling the difference between foreground and background images or sounds. Individuals with this deficit may have trouble with printed words on a page; identifying important visual information in pictures, photographs, graphs, or charts; or following conversation in a crowded room.

It is important to eliminate competing visual distractions and noise for a child with figure-ground deficits. Using the mute button or turning off noisy appliances can be very helpful. The child should have a study area free from auditory and visual distractions.

Children who have figure-ground deficits may benefit from sitting near the front and center of the classroom to keep distractions to a minimum but allow the child to remain part of the regular seating. The child should be kept away from auditory and visual distractions such as open windows, pencil sharpeners, doorways, air conditioners, computers, and learning centers. The best seating is in the quietest place in the room that still allows the child to be close to classroom instruction. The classroom may be sound-treated to reduce background noise by adding drapes, carpets, and sound-absorbing materials.

See also FIGURE-GROUND DISCRIMINATION.

figure-ground discrimination The ability to visually distinguish between foreground and background. Individuals with deficits in this area cannot easily identify the predominant image or design in a picture from other objects and background. Figure-ground discrimination can also refer to the auditory discrimination involved in understanding what a person is saying when there are other sounds, including other people speaking in the same room.

See also FIGURE-GROUND DEFICITS.

fine motor skills The use of small muscle groups for specific tasks such as handwriting. Fine motor abilities are developmental, with children generally improving in their ability to use writing or drawing implements as they enter elementary school and are introduced to the concept of writing and copying. Deficits in fine motor function can have a detrimental effect on the development of writing skills.

finger agnosia The inability to recognize and interpret sensory impressions with fingers (usually the finger tips); caused by an impairment in the brain.

fluency Fluid or unrestricted movements or abilities. Often, fluency refers to learned or practiced ability in oral language. Individuals are said to be fluent in a language when they can speak in an uninterrupted fashion and convey meaning easily.

Individuals with speech difficulties such as STUTTERING are said to have *dysfluent* language abilities.

In reading development, fluency refers to the development of an automatic reading process in which words are effortlessly decoded and understood.

fluent aphasia A language disorder characterized by clear articulation, normal rhythm, long phrases having nonsensical content, and incorrect words or sounds. This type of APHASIA includes Wernicke's aphasia and anomic aphasias.

fluoxetine (Prozac) An antidepressant medication that is sometimes used to treat ATTENTION DEFICIT HYPERACTIVITY DISORDER in patients who are (ADHD) also depressed, both alone and in conjunction with METHYLPHENIDATE (Ritalin). Results of trials with this medication suggest that Prozac may be helpful in the treatment of ADHD, although the first-line therapy for ADHD is still Ritalin, Strattera (atomoxetine), or DEXTROAMPHETAMINE (Dexedrine).

Introduced in 1988, Prozac was the first of a new class of antidepressants known as selective serotonin reuptake inhibitors (SSRIs), which increases the levels of a neurotransmitter called serotonin. Many people who are depressed have low levels of this chemical, and therefore their depression lifts when serotonin levels rise.

As with other pharmaceutical interventions for ADHD, Prozac is usually prescribed as part of a treatment plan that includes educational and psychosocial interventions. Prozac and other antidepressant medications in the SSRI class (such as Zoloft) are sometimes prescribed when individuals with ADHD do not respond to stimulant medication, or when they have other coexisting conditions such as DEPRESSION or OBSESSIVE-COMPULSIVE DISORDER.

As all antidepressants, Prozac takes one to three weeks to achieve its full effect.

Studies suggest that younger people respond to Prozac with very small doses, and that a sizable portion of young people who do not respond to other antidepressants do respond to Prozac.

Side Effects

All antidepressants carry side effects, but Prozac and the other SSRIs cause fewer, less uncomfortable problems than older antidepressants. Most common side effects include sexual problems, nausea, headache, insomnia, diarrhea, nervousness, and ANXIETY. Less common side effects include dry mouth, appetite loss, tremor, upper respiratory infection, and dizziness.

Studies suggest that younger people experience slightly different side effects, including restlessness and sweating as the most common complaints, followed by drowsiness, dry mouth, and tremors.

In 2004, evidence appeared that suggested a possible connection between starting antidepressant treatment and an increase in suicide risk. An analysis of records of 3 million British patients of all ages, published in July 2004 in the *Journal of the American Medical Association*, showed that there was four times the risk of suicidal behavior and 38 times the risk of actual suicide patients in their first nine days on an antidepressant compared with patients who had been taking antidepressants for three months or longer. Although there were no suicides among patients ages 10 to 19, their increased risk of suicidal behavior was similar to that of the group as a whole.

Researchers are not sure why antidepressants have this effect, but some believe that these antidepressants quickly reverse the lethargy associated with depression but take several weeks to ease the depression itself. This gives patients the energy to contemplate or carry through suicide attempts.

In March 2004, the FDA asked the makers of 10 major antidepressants to warn doctors and patients to watch for increased suicidal tendencies in children and adults in their first weeks on the medicines, or when the dose changes. The agency is now gathering more evidence on the issue, as other studies, although inconclusive, suggest younger people are not more likely to commit suicide while taking SSRIs.

formal operational stage   The fourth and final stage in psychologist Jean Piaget's stage theory of cognitive development that occurs some time after the age of 11. Preadolescents gradually become capable of abstract logic and hypothetical reasoning, and become able to generate many possible solutions to problems. They can use deduction to draw conclusions based on observations, and can debate moral dilemmas and detect inconsistencies in the behavior of others. All these cognitive abilities have important social consequences as children become adolescents.

See also PIAGET, JEAN.

fragile X syndrome   The most common inherited form of MENTAL RETARDATION, caused by a mutation in a single gene that can be passed from one generation to the next. Fragile X appears in families of every ethnic group and income level.

Fragile X syndrome occurs when the mutated gene cannot produce enough of a protein that is needed by the body's cells, especially cells in the brain, to develop and function normally. The amount and usability of this protein, in part, determine how severe the effects of fragile X are.

The gene for fragile X (called the *FMR1* gene) is carried on the X chromosome. Because both boys (XY) and girls (XX) have at least one X chromosome, both can pass on the mutated gene to their children. A father with the altered gene for fragile X on his X chromosome will pass that gene only to his daughters. He passes a Y chromosome to his sons, which does not transmit the condition. Therefore, if the father has the altered gene on his X chromosome, but the mother's X chromosomes are normal, all of the couple's daughters would have the altered gene for fragile X, while none of their sons would have the mutated gene.

Research indicates that a father can pass on the premutation form of the *FMR1* gene only to his daughters. In other words, if a daughter inherits the mutated *FMR1* gene from her father, she will get only the premutation from him, not the full mutation. Even if the father himself has a full mutation, it appears that sperm can carry only the premutation. A summary of research conducted by the Centers for Disease Control and Prevention in 2001 estimated that approximately one in 3,500 to 8,900 boys is affected by the full mutation of the *FMR1* gene and that one in 1,000 boys has the premutation form of the *FMR1* gene. This study also estimated that one in 250 to 500 girls has the premutation and that one in 4,000 girls is affected by the full mutation.

Symptoms and Diagnostic Path

More than 80 percent of boys with fragile X have an IQ of 75 or less; the effect of fragile X on INTELLIGENCE is not as devastating in girls. Some girls are mentally retarded, some have LEARNING DISABILITIES, and some have a normal IQ.

People with fragile X syndrome also share medical problems and common physical characteristics, such as large ears, a prominent jaw, and a long face. In addition, having fragile X is often associated with problems with sensation, emotion, and behavior.

Treatment Options and Outlook

As a developmental disorder, fragile X syndrome cannot be cured. Standard treatment includes SPECIAL EDUCATION; speech, occupational, and sensory integration training; and BEHAVIOR MODIFICATION programs.

Other treatment is symptomatic and supportive. Folic acid has been found to improve hyperactivity and attention deficits in some preadolescent males with fragile X syndrome. Surgical correction of heart defects may be needed.

Preventive Measures

Genetic counseling may be helpful for families of affected persons.

free appropriate public education   SPECIAL EDUCATION and related services—provided at public expense, under public supervision and direction, and without charge—that meet the standards of the state's department of education and are based on an INDIVIDUALIZED EDUCATION PROGRAM.

Under Public Law 94-142 and IDEIA (the INDIVIDUALS WITH DISABILITIES EDUCATION IMPROVEMENT ACT), children with disabilities who fall under the act must be provided with "a free appropriate public education which emphasizes special education and related services. . . ."

Under the act, states are required to provide the minimum services that assure equal access to educational services, but are not expected to provide all of the services that may be required for students to reach their full potential.

See also EDUCATION FOR ALL HANDICAPPED CHILDREN ACT OF 1975.

frontal lobe   One of four major areas of the cerebral cortex in the brain that lie just behind the forehead and extend back to the central fissure. This area includes the prefrontal lobes and the motor cortex. It is involved in producing speech, voluntary movement, making plans and judgments, and MEMORY. The prefrontal area involves the ability to concentrate and pay attention and provide elaboration of thought. It is considered to be the seat of judgment, inhibition, personality, and emotional traits.

Damage to the frontal lobes can impair a person's ability to plan and organize, and can cause problems with impulsivity and motor control. Damage also can impair recent memory, and lead to inattentiveness, an inability to concentrate, behavior disorders, difficulty in learning new information, inappropriate social or sexual behavior, a lack of emotion, and expressive APHASIA.

Problems in the frontal lobes, which are responsible for integrating information in the brain, may be linked to certain types of LEARNING DISABILITIES, including ATTENTION DEFICIT HYPERACTIVITY DISORDER (ADHD).

Experts believe that physiological differences in this area of the brain also account for much of the normal individual variation in FINE MOTOR SKILLS.

full inclusion   A placement in which a SPECIAL EDUCATION student receives instruction within the regular classroom setting for the entire school day.

Gall, Franz Joseph (1758–1828) One of the founders of phrenology, the belief that IQ is related to bumps on the skull. Gall was born in Baden, now a part of Germany, on March 9, 1758. He is best known for identifying a set of organs in the brain that he associated with 35 affective and intellectual faculties, believing that the size of these organs in the brain could be detected by cranial bumps. This idea was widely popular at the turn of the 19th century and had many advocates.

Gall studied medicine in Vienna, Austria, where he became a renowned neuroanatomist, physiologist, and pioneer in the study of the localization of mental functions in the brain.

At the turn of the 19th century, he developed "cranioscopy," which was a method to divine the personality and development of mental and moral faculties on the basis of the external shape of the skull. Cranioscopy was later renamed "phrenology" (*phrenos,* "mind," and *logos,* "study") by his followers.

His revolutionary concepts on brain localization offended religious leaders and scientists alike. The church considered his theory blasphemous (they did not approve of the idea that the mind, which was created by God, should have a physical seat in the brain). Established science also condemned him for a variety of reasons, including the fact that Gall could not provide scientific proof of his theory.

Because of this disapproval, Gall was forced to leave Austria in 1805 and go to France, where his theories were likewise pronounced invalid by politicians and scientists alike. Despite all this, Gall was able to live comfortably from his phrenological theories and practices. They were best accepted in England, where the ruling class used his beliefs to justify the so-called inferiority of colonial subjects, including the Irish. Phrenology also became very popular in the United States from 1820 to 1850.

Despite his misguided theories, he also made many true scientific contributions, such as his discovery that the gray matter of the brain contained cell bodies (neurons) and the white matter contained fibers (axons). Gall's most important contribution involved his discovery of the localization of specific behaviors to areas in the brain. His ideas led to further study in attempts to correlate specific intellectual or psychological deficits to areas in the brain through the examination of diseased brains.

Gall died in Paris, on August 22, 1828.

Gallistel-Ellis Test of Coding Skills (G-E Test) This ASSESSMENT for grades two through six is designed to test a child's ability to decode and spell the basic phonetic patterns in the English language. Reading and spelling of irregular patterns are also tested. G-E Test results can be helpful in planning reading remediation.

gender differences Statistics from schools and research show that boys are diagnosed with LEARNING DISABILITY up to four times more often than are girls, although recent research suggests that there may be as many girls with learning disabilities as boys. Many factors, such as biological and cultural reasons, may explain the prevalence of identifying boys with learning disabilities. Biological research indicates boys may be more vulnerable to learning disabilities. Other studies show that boys are referred for SPECIAL EDUCATION more frequently because they exhibit more disruptive behaviors. Yet some other studies attribute the disproportionate number of identified boys to increased academic pressure, making boys more likely to buckle under stress.

general education Regular instruction provided to most students. Placing SPECIAL EDUCATION students in general education classes is considered the LEAST RESTRICTIVE ENVIRONMENT, but special considerations must be made to ensure students are able to achieve academically and socially in this environment.

genetic factors In both DYSLEXIA and ATTENTION DEFICIT HYPERACTIVITY DISORDER (ADHD), research has identified genetic factors that appear to make an individual more predisposed to having the condition.

Genetic factors have mainly been identified through family studies that highlight groups of family members who have experienced similar conditions. In addition, some genetic research has begun to identify specific genes and chromosomes that may be involved in the genetic transmission of dyslexia or ADHD. Research that indicates a genetic component or genetic factors underlying these two disorders also supports a neurological basis for understanding their nature and underlying factors.

Gerstmann's syndrome A neurologic condition characterized by four groups of symptoms: a writing disability (AGRAPHIA or dysgraphia), a lack of understanding of the rules for calculation or arithmetic (ACALCULIA or DYSCALCULIA), an inability to distinguish right from left, and an inability to identify fingers (FINGER AGNOSIA). The disorder should not be confused with Gerstmann-Sträussler-Scheinker disease, a type of transmissible spongiform encephalopathy.

This is a fairly rare syndrome (sometimes called developmental Gerstmann's syndrome), and the cause is not known. Most cases are identified when children reach school age and begin to be challenged with writing and math exercises.

Symptoms and Diagnostic Path
Children with the disorder typically have poor handwriting and spelling skills and trouble with adding, subtracting, multiplying, and dividing. They also may be unable to differentiate right from left and to discriminate among individual fingers.

In addition to the four primary symptoms, many children also suffer from an inability to copy simple drawings, known as constructional APRAXIA. Often there is also an impairment in reading. The condition affects children of all ranges of INTELLI-GENCE, from those who are very bright to those with brain damage.

Treatment Options and Outlook
There is no cure for Gerstmann's syndrome. Occupational and speech therapies may help diminish the dysgraphia and APRAXIA, and calculators and word processors may help school children cope with the symptoms of the disorder. As children reach adulthood, many of the symptoms diminish.

gifted and talented The definition and ASSESSMENT of giftedness varies from state to state and even from school district to school district. Most definitions of giftedness include characteristics such as extraordinary inquisitiveness, creativity, spontaneity, and emotionality. Many of these characteristics can be found in students with a LEARNING DISABILITY; therefore, students with learning disabilities may also be gifted in certain areas.

Both types of learners require stimulation. When a gifted student's learning needs are not met, the student may display disruptive behaviors or signs of depression.

Academic accommodations for the gifted may range from supplementing regular education programs with acceleration and enrichment activities, to self-contained programs. Suggested features of such programs would include teaching thinking skills and independent projects. The identification of gifted students and implementation of special services largely depend on how the school defines giftedness.

Gillingham, Anna (1878–1963) A gifted psychologist and educator with a superb mastery or language; well known in the field of LANGUAGE DISABILITIES. Together with neuropsychiatrist Samuel Orton, she helped develop techniques for remediating reading and language processing problems in children with DYSLEXIA, helped train teachers in the method, and compiled and published instructional materials.

Over the past 50 years, the ORTON-GILLINGHAM APPROACH has been the most influential, widely used, and respected program for teaching reading, and is still in use today.

See also ORTON, SAMUEL TORREY.

global aphasia   Loss of all language function.

grade equivalent   A score that expresses a student's performance as the average performance for a particular grade. These scores are expressed in grades and tenths of grades (for example, 6.4 is grade six and four months).

Grade-level equivalent scores are determined by giving a test that is developed for a particular grade to students in other grades. For instance, test designers establish grade-equivalents for a fourth grade test by giving that same test to students who are in the sixth and the second grades.

Grade-level equivalent scores are often misunderstood. If a fourth grader received a seventh grade equivalent score on a fourth grade reading achievement test, the child is not ready for seventh grade material. Actually, the score means that the child reads fourth grade material as well as the average seventh grader.

Grandin, Temple (1947–)   An associate professor of animal science at Colorado State University and a well-known person with AUTISM who has written books about her experiences with the condition. Grandin is the author of *Emergence: Labeled Autistic and Thinking in Pictures* and a designer of livestock handling facilities. (Half of the cattle in North America are handled in facilities she has designed.)

A popular speaker at colleges and autism conferences, she obtained her B.A. at Franklin Pierce College, her M.S. in animal science at Arizona State University, and her Ph.D. in animal science from the University of Illinois in 1989. Today she teaches courses on livestock behavior and facility design at Colorado State University and consults with the livestock industry on facility design, livestock handling, and animal welfare.

She has appeared on television shows such as *20/20, 48 Hours,* and CNN's *Larry King Live,* and has been featured in *People* magazine, the *New York Times, Forbes, U.S. News and World Report,* and *Time.* She has written more than 300 articles in both scientific journals and livestock periodicals on animal handling, welfare, and facility design.

grapheme   The written letter symbol that represents a sound (phoneme). For example, the grapheme "c" represents the sounds "k" and "s."

graphic organizer   A device that helps an individual understand and recall concepts by visually displaying how ideas are connected. Venn diagrams, flow charts, and mind maps are all examples of visual organizers. Using graphic organizers is a useful strategy with learning disabled students because it makes related ideas more meaningful by utilizing vision, which can aid in recall.

Research has shown that using visual organizers has increased reading comprehension by mapping out main ideas and details. In the context of writing, visual organizers can be useful in generating and organizing ideas.

graphomotor ability   Handwriting skills or drawing figures in replication of models or in response to specific prompts. Graphomotor ability is linked to FINE MOTOR SKILLS but can be distinguished from them because of the role that MEMORY plays—for example, memory for the forms of letters, which must be called into play in various ways in copying tasks, writing from dictation, and in independent writing.

Problems with graphomotor skills may exist by themselves, but they are also frequently linked to ATTENTION DISORDERS or LEARNING DISABILITIES.

graphophonemic knowledge   The understanding that words are made of sounds and sounds are written with letters in the right order. Students who understand this can blend sounds associated with letters into words and can separate words into component sounds for spelling and writing.

Students should be assessed to determine if they can hear sounds in spoken language prior to letter-sound instruction.

Gray Oral Reading Test-Diagnostic (GORT-D)   The GORT-D measures a child's speed and accuracy when reading out loud, COMPREHENSION, ability to sound out and blend nonsense words that follow English structural patterns, ability to find smaller words within larger words, word identification and comprehension skill, and the ability to deal with compound words, contractions, and inflectional endings. Because many of the subtests do not use traditional formats, the score may not reflect a student's classroom performance.

gross motor skills   Skills in which the large muscles are used in the neck, torso, and arms and legs. The development of gross motor skills involves activities such as rolling over, crawling, sitting, walking, running, catching, and jumping.

Early development of gross motor skills appears to be largely inbred, while later gross motor abilities (used for such skills as swimming, bicycling, skiing, and so on) are largely learned.

There is little relationship between gross motor abilities and INTELLIGENCE.

guided reading   Reading instruction in which the teacher provides the structure and purpose for reading and for responding to the materials read. Most basic reading programs have guided reading lessons.

hand-eye coordination   Ability of the hand and eye to perform together.

handicap   A term that refers to a disadvantage or impairment based on a disabling condition. Federal legislation, such as Public Law 94-142: the EDUCATION FOR ALL HANDICAPPED CHILDREN ACT OF 1975, uses *handicap* to identify the disadvantageous status of an individual with specific impairments as compared to others without such impairments.

However, the term *handicapped* is no longer used to mean disability of disorder, as it places an emphasis on social status or on defining an individual, rather than suggesting a particular difference. In the same manner that many individuals challenge the use of the word *disability* because it by definition focuses on a negative condition, *handicap* is best used in a legal context rather than in a social one.

haptic sense   A person's sense of touch. Haptic recognition tests involve blindfolded subjects feeling geometric shapes, then choosing the picture corresponding to the shape from a limited set. Many people with language-based disabilities have a difficult time with these tasks.

hard neurological signs   Physical signs of brain injury that can be identified medically, such as muscle wasting or reflex changes.

See also SOFT NEUROLOGICAL SIGNS.

Head Start   An EARLY INTERVENTION PROGRAM established under the Economic Opportunity Act of 1964 in order to provide preschool educational opportunities to disadvantaged children. In 1972, Project Head Start was amended to include chil-

dren with disabilities. This program has proven to be the most influential national early childhood program; it allowed comprehensive studies to be done on the effect of early intervention and school success.

Since the inception of the program in 1965, Head Start has benefited more than 20 million at-risk children and their families. In 2002, Head Start and Early Head Start programs worked with more than 900,000 children through 2,590 local programs that serve families in communities across America. Today, Head Start serves only three out of five eligible three- and four-year-old children.

Project Head Start was established by Congress in 1965, part of President Lyndon B. Johnson's War on Poverty and the 1964 Economic Opportunity Act. Head Start is the only national program of its kind to use a comprehensive service approach to early childhood education. First established as a summer program for low-income preschool children and their families, Head Start has grown to include full-day, full-year programming and services for children from birth to three years of age, their families, and pregnant women. By 2003 there were 1,900 Head Start programs affecting a million children.

Head Start has received strong bipartisan support through many presidential administrations and has been consistently acknowledged for its effectiveness in helping children become successful in school and later life. The program's hallmark has been its strong emphasis on families, recognizing that parents are the first and primary educators, nurturers, and advocates of their children. The program survived a 2004 attempt by the Bush administration to dismantle it turning over Head Start funds to individual states as part of a block grant. However, deeper funding cuts, according to the Head Start Association, are making it increasingly hard to extend services to the children who need them.

Ever since its inception, Head Start has taken a strong community advocacy approach, recognizing that communities must be supportive for healthy families and children.

It provides comprehensive prekindergarten experiences (education, health care, nutrition, and social services) to almost 18 million of the nation's poorest children. Research demonstrates that Head Start can help children build the confidence and skills they need to succeed in school and to become the leaders, taxpayers, and productive citizens of the future.

A national review of 36 studies on the long-term impact of early childhood education programs found that low-income children who participated in such programs were less likely to be held back in school or to be placed in SPECIAL EDUCATION classes, more likely to succeed in school and to graduate, and more likely to be rated as behaving well in class and being better adjusted in school.

The typical child completing Head Start has the knowledge and skills in early literacy and numbers and the skills that signify a readiness to learn more in kindergarten, such as listening and comprehension skills. Children also acquire a variety of social skills important for kindergarten, such as following the teacher's directions, using free time in acceptable ways, and helping put work materials away.

Head Start children perform higher on cognitive tests than children from other low-income families who have not attended center-based preschool programs, according to a comparison between the results of the Head Start study and earlier studies.

hearing problems "Hearing impairment" and "deafness" are two of the categories under which children with disabilities may be eligible for SPECIAL EDUCATION and related services under the INDIVIDUALS WITH DISABILITIES EDUCATION IMPROVEMENT ACT (IDEIA).

While the term *hearing impairment* is often used to describe a wide range of hearing loss, including deafness, the regulations for IDEIA define hearing loss and deafness separately.

Hearing impairment is defined by IDEIA as "an impairment in hearing, whether permanent or fluctuating, that adversely affects a child's educational performance." *Deafness* is defined as "a hearing impairment that is so severe that the child is impaired in processing linguistic information through hearing, with or without amplification." Thus, deafness may be viewed as a condition that prevents an individual from receiving sound in all or most of its forms. In contrast, a child with a hearing loss can generally respond to auditory stimuli, including speech.

Hearing loss and deafness affect individuals of all ages and may occur at any time from infancy through old age. More than 70,000 students aged six to 21 (or 1.3 percent of all students with disabilities) received special education services under the category of "hearing impairment" during 1998. However, the number of children with hearing loss and deafness is undoubtedly higher, since many of these students may have other disabilities as well.

Hearing problems can exist in only one ear or in both ears, and may be described as slight, mild, moderate, severe, or profound, depending upon how well a person can hear the intensities or frequencies associated with speech. Generally, only children whose hearing loss is greater than 90 decibels (dB) are considered deaf for the purposes of educational placement.

There are four types of hearing loss: *conductive* hearing loss is caused by diseases or obstructions in the outer or middle ear. A person with a conductive hearing loss usually is able to use a hearing aid well or can be helped medically or surgically. *Sensorineural* hearing loss is caused by damage to the delicate sensory hair cells of the inner ear or the nerves that supply it. These hearing losses can range from mild to profound, so that a hearing aid may not help. A *mixed* hearing loss refers to a combination of conductive and sensorineural loss and means that a problem occurs in both the outer or middle and the inner ear. A *central* hearing loss is caused by damage to the nerves of the central nervous system, either in the pathways to the brain or in the brain itself.

Education

Hearing loss or deafness does not affect a person's intellect or ability to learn, but children who are either hard of hearing or deaf generally require some form of special education services, including

- regular speech, language, and auditory training from a specialist
- amplification systems
- services of an interpreter for those students who use manual communication
- favorable seating in the class to facilitate speechreading
- captioned films/videos
- assistance of a notetaker, who takes notes
- instruction for the teacher and other students in alternate communication methods such as sign language
- counseling

Children who are hard of hearing may find it harder to learn vocabulary, grammar, word order, idiomatic expressions of verbal communication. For children who are deaf or have severe hearing losses, early, consistent, and conscious use of visible communication modes such as sign language or fingerspelling—or oral training—can help reduce this language delay.

By age four or five, most children who are deaf are enrolled in school on a full-day basis and do special work on communication and language development.

higher cognitive functions A term that usually refers to complex thinking skills such as judgment, abstraction, problem-solving, and planning.

See also HIGHER ORDER THINKING.

higher order thinking Advanced intellectual abilities that go beyond basic information processing. Higher order thinking involves such abilities as concept formation, understanding rules, problem-solving skills, and the ability to look at information from multiple perspectives.

Students exercise their higher order thinking abilities when they analyze, synthesize, and evaluate materials to which they have been exposed. The construction or creation of new material also requires higher order thinking.

In general, abilities in the area of higher order thinking are closely linked to intellectual capacity. However, individuals with LEARNING DISABILITIES who have underlying information-processing deficits may appear to have difficulties with higher order activities. This may be especially true with higher order tasks involving a verbal component for students with language-based learning problems.

holistic assessment An approach to ASSESSMENT of academic skills and performance using a variety of methods, with an emphasis on the quality of the information rather than the quantity.

Methods of holistic assessment include

- observing the student in various settings
- interviewing parents, teachers, and the student
- academic, developmental, and medical history of the student
- educational testing and writing samples

hyperactivity Constant and excessive movement and activity. A child with hyperactivity may not be able to stop an action when directed to, or to sit still for any period of time. Hyperactivity often occurs with inattentiveness and impulsivity. An affected child might have trouble sitting still, fidgets excessively, and moves about excessively even during sleep. Onset occurs before the age of seven years. Behaviors are chronic (present throughout the child's life), present throughout the child's day, and are not due to other factors such as anxiety or depression.

In older children, symptoms of hyperactivity may be more subtle, displaying themselves in restlessness, fidgeting, a tendency to interrupt in class, or in conflict-seeking behaviors with peers and family members.

See also ATTENTION DEFICIT HYPERACTIVITY DISORDER; HYPERKINESIS.

hyperkinesis A condition of abnormally increased muscle movement; often associated with ATTENTION DEFICIT HYPERACTIVITY DISORDER in children. It is often used interchangeably with HYPERACTIVITY.

hyperlexia A complex condition that includes an ability to read words at a far earlier developmental stage than is typical and often an intense fascination with symbols such as letters and numbers. These world-calling skills are high in the presence of poor reading COMPREHENSION. It also involves a significant difficulty in understanding verbal language and problems with social skills, including difficulty interacting appropriately with peers and family members.

The term *hyperlexia* was first used in 1967, although the condition was described in the 1940s. There is no consensus concerning either the cause or significance of the condition. Hyperlexia has been reported in populations of children with varying cognitive abilities, including some with severe mental retardation. Intellectual level by itself does not therefore seem to be a definitive factor in the condition. Hyperlexia is considered by some researchers to be a unique type of language disorder and a condition occurring with another reading disability. Others report that children with hyperlexia demonstrate a profile opposite from that shown by children with classic dyslexia on certain tests.

Hyperlexia shares similar characteristics with AUTISM, behavior disorders, LANGUAGE DISORDERS, emotional disorders, attention deficit disorder, hearing impairment, giftedness, and paradoxically, METAL RETARDATION.

Symptoms and Diagnostic Path

Some children with hyperlexia may also develop expressive language skills in unusual ways, echoing what they hear without understanding the meaning, and failing to develop the ability to initiate conversations. They often exhibit a powerful need to maintain routines and ritualistic patterns of behavior, and have trouble with transitions and handling external sensory stimuli.

Children with hyperlexia often display very strong auditory and VISUAL MEMORY, but may have trouble understanding and reasoning in abstract rather than concrete and literal terms. Often, their approach to listening to others may be highly selective, and they can appear to be deaf.

To develop effective teaching strategies and more typical childhood development, it is important to differentiate hyperlexia from other disorders. A thorough ASSESSMENT by a speech and language pathologist who is familiar with hyperlexia is the first step. Psychological tests that emphasize visual processes rather than verbal skills can also help identify hyperlexia. Hearing, neurological, psychiatric, blood chemistry, and genetic evaluations can be performed to rule out other disorders, but are not needed to identify hyperlexia.

Treatment Options and Outlook

The future of a hyperlexic child depends on developing language expression and comprehension skills. Intensive speech and language therapy and early intervention programs can help. The child's reading skills should be used as a primary means of developing language.

It is also important to teach the child appropriate social skills by providing opportunities for the child to interact with others whose behavior is more socially appropriate. Parent, teachers, and other professionals should work together to develop programs for each child.

hypoactivity A medical term for lethargy. Some individuals with a LEARNING DISABILITY, ATTENTION disorders, or other conditions affecting learning may suffer from hypoactivity, making it more difficult to complete school work.

ideation A mental representation of thoughts or visual images, or a combination of linguistic and visual representations.

illiteracy The inability to read or write a language.

illiterate Unable to read or write.
See also ILLITERACY.

implicit memory MEMORY without awareness, which occurs when information that was encoded is subsequently expressed without conscious recollection.

impulse control Current research suggests that lack of impulse control is a major underlying factor in attention disorders. The onset of the ability to control impulses is a significant element of child development. Individuals with impulse control problems also may have trouble sustaining a train of thought.

Individuals with impulse control disorders suffer from recurrent failure to resist impulsive behaviors that may be harmful to themselves or others. The disorders include intermittent explosive disorder, explosive disorder, kleptomania, pathological gambling, pyromania (setting fires), and trichotillomania (pulling out one's hair).

impulsivity Difficulty in controlling or monitoring speech or actions, often a primary element in ATTENTION DEFICIT HYPERACTIVITY DISORDER (ADHD). An individual who has problems with impulsivity may blurt out responses without thinking, make take excessive risks, or may act in socially inappropriate ways.

Impulsivity also may affect school performance in more subtle ways. For example, a student may respond impulsively to questions on a multiple-choice test, choosing answers before considering all alternatives. Likewise, an impulsive individual might answer an essay question before having thought through a response.

Impulsivity is often poorly understood in school, and may be judged harshly in social or interpersonal contexts, rather than seen as arising from underlying difficulties in IMPULSE CONTROL.

inattention Difficulty in focusing on important information in the immediate environment. It is a major constituent in ATTENTION disorders, and may have a pervasive negative effect on academic or social functioning.

independent education evaluation (IEE) An evaluation of a student conducted by a qualified examiner who does not work for the school district. According to Public Law 94-142 (amended to the INDIVIDUALS WITH DISABILITIES EDUCATION IMPROVEMENT ACT), parents have the right to have their child independently tested either to seek a more comprehensive assessment than is sometimes provided in a school setting, or because they fear a school-based evaluation is biased or inaccurate.

An IEE would include the same elements as a school-mandated evaluation, focusing on measures of aptitude and achievement. Parents may obtain an evaluation at school district expense if they disagree with the evaluation arranged for by the school district.

If the parent wants the school district to pay for the tests, the district may ask (but not require) the parents to explain the reason why they object to the district's evaluation. The school district also may ask for an impartial hearing to show that its evaluation is appropriate. If the impartial hearing officer finds that the district evaluation is appropriate, parents still have the right to obtain an IEE—but the district does not have to pay for it. The school district may not unreasonably delay either providing the test or calling an impartial hearing to defend the district's own evaluation.

Individualized Education Program (IEP)   A written educational prescription developed for each child with a LEARNING DISABILITY, describing what SPECIAL EDUCATION the child needs and what will be done to address those needs. School districts are required by law to develop these programs, sometimes called an Individualized Education Plan, in cooperation with parents. An IEP must be created for each exceptional child, according to the INDIVIDUALS WITH DISABILITIES EDUCATION IMPROVEMENT ACT (IDEIA, formerly PL 94-142).

An IEP is prepared by a team including parents, the child, the child's teacher, educational specialists, and a representative of the public agency that oversees special education.

An IEP includes information about the child's current level of academic performance; annual goals and short-term educational objectives; specific educational services to be provided; a definition of the extent to which the student will take part in regular educational programs; and a timetable for providing services. The IEP also defines procedures for measuring how well the educational objectives are being met.

An IEP must contain

- the child's present levels of educational performance
- annual and short-term educational goals
- the specific special education program and related services that will be provided
- the extent to which the child will participate in regular education programs with non-handicapped children
- a statement of when services will begin and how long they will last
- provisions for evaluating the effectiveness of the program and the student's performance at least once a year

- statement of transition services for students 14 years of age or older

Individualized Education Program Committee   A group of people who meet to create an INDIVIDUAL EDUCATION PROGRAM for a child who has been identified as learning disabled by a multidisciplinary team.

The committee should include a representative of the public school, the student's teacher, one or both parents, the student (when appropriate), and any other individuals deemed relevant by the school or parents such as an educational psychologist, speech teacher, legal expert, or adviser.

Individualized Family Service Plan   A written plan developed with teachers and parents to outline special services to be provided to children of preschool age.

As stated in Public Law 99-457, Part H, families play a crucial part in a child's development from birth to age two; therefore, the individualized family services plan is written to address the special needs of the child and the family.

According to the INDIVIDUALS WITH DISABILITIES EDUCATION IMPROVEMENT ACT (IDEIA), the plan must include

- present levels of the child's development (cognitive, physical, language/speech, psychosocial, and self-help)
- family resources and concerns regarding the child's development
- expected outcomes for the family and child, including criteria, timelines, and assessment procedures
- specific intervention services necessary to meet the needs of the family and child
- projected start and end dates of services
- name of case manager
- steps needed for smooth transition from early intervention program to preschool program

See also EARLY INTERVENTION PROGRAM.

individualized reading   An approach to reading instruction developed in the 1950s as an alternative to basic reading programs; emphasizes student selection of reading materials and self-pacing in reading. With this method, the teacher adjusts instruction to student needs during small-group work and in individual conferences.

Individuals with Disabilities Education Improvement Act (IDEIA) A revised law that provides children with disabilities access to a free, appropriate public education, and to improve the educational experience of such children. IDEIA was first enacted as the EDUCATION FOR ALL HANDICAPPED CHILDREN ACT OF 1975 (Public Law 94-142), renamed the Individuals with Disabilities Education Improvement Act (IDEIA) in 1990 (Public Law 101-476) and amended (Public Law 102-119) in 1991, and again in 2004. On December 3, 2004, President George W. Bush signed the revised IDEIA legislation. The revision is an attempt to update and improve the criteria for identifying a specific LEARNING DISABILITY by easing the requirement that students must exhibit a severe discrepancy between ability and achievement in order to be found eligible for services under IDEIA (regardless of age). This requirement had been part of the IDEIA federal regulations since 1977 and, according to a 2000 survey conducted by the National Association of State Directors of Special Education, all 50 states have *required* a severe discrepancy between ability and achievement for purposes of learning disability SPECIAL EDUCATION eligibility. There is widespread agreement that such policies require students to experience failure for several years in order to show the requisite degree of discrepancy. Despite the fact that clinical judgment, curriculum-based ASSESSMENTS, discrepant results on achievement assessments, parental information, and other factors might all point to the presence of a learning disability, before the IDEIA revision, a student could not have been found eligible under the specific learning disability category if this severe discrepancy did not exist. Under the IDEIA, money is given to local school systems to educate children up to age 22; local schools are required to comply with the act as a condition of receiving funds.

Before IDEIA's implementation in 1975, about 1 million children with disabilities were shut out of schools and hundreds of thousands more were denied appropriate services. Since then, IDEIA has changed the lives of these children. Many are learning and achieving at levels previously thought impossible, graduating from high school, going to college, and entering the workforce as productive citizens in unprecedented numbers.

Previously, 90 percent of children with developmental disabilities were housed in state institutions; today they are no longer institutionalized. Today three times as many young people with disabilities are enrolled in colleges or universities, and twice as many of today's 20-year-olds with disabilities are working.

IDEIA covers students with a specific learning disability as defined within the act. Both DYSLEXIA and ATTENTION DEFICIT HYPERACTIVITY DISORDER are covered by IDEIA. IDEIA also includes students who have MENTAL RETARDATION; hearing, vision, orthopedic, speech, or language impairments; serious emotional disturbance, AUTISM, TRAUMATIC BRAIN INJURY, or other health impairments.

The 2004 revisions to IDEIA maintain the definition of specific learning disabilities that is contained in the original IDEIA, including the disorders that are not included under this definition, such as a learning problem that is primarily the result of visual, hearing, or motor disabilities; of mental retardation; of emotional disturbance; or of environmental, cultural, or economic disadvantage.

The IDEIA provides that children covered by the act have access to a FREE APPROPRIATE PUBLIC EDUCATION. In general, students receiving services under IDEIA will take part in regular educational programs to some degree, and also receive special education services as described in their INDIVIDUALIZED EDUCATION PROGRAM.

Most students who fall under the IDEIA are served within their own public school system, although in some cases students may attend a private educational institution, with the school district assuming the cost.

inferential thinking A primary element in high order thinking and an essential factor in academic success, involving the ability to examine factual information and make predictions. These predictions might involve estimating likely behavior based on the characteristics of a figure in a story or film, deducing expected outcomes, or determining the nature or meaning of an event from an analysis of surface elements.

Some individuals with a LEARNING DISABILITY may struggle with inferential thinking, especially if such reasoning processes require the ability to reason verbally or understand texts. At the same time, with appropriate support, individuals with learning disabilities may demonstrate strength in this area of cognitive performance.

information processing disorders   A problem in any of the ways in which an individual processes information: VISUAL DISCRIMINATION, visual FIGURE-GROUND DISCRIMINATION, VISUAL MEMORY, VISUAL MOTOR COORDINATION, visual closure, understanding spatial relationships, AUDITORY DISCRIMINATION, AUDITORY FIGURE-GROUND DISCRIMINATION, and AUDITORY MEMORY.

A person's senses of sight, smell, hearing, taste, and touch are constantly providing information, which is stored in short- and long-term MEMORY. For each of the hundreds of things people do each day, they need to quickly decide what information to use to complete the task. Managing all of the stored information and using it effectively is called "information processing."

Symptoms and diagnostic path   A child with an information processing disorder may have trouble with one or more of the information processing skills, which interferes with using information efficiently, solving problems, or completing tasks. The inability to process information efficiently often causes frustration and learning failure.

Visual discrimination   The ability to visually compare the features of different items to distinguish one from another. Children with this condition may find it hard to notice the small differences between some letters and numbers, certain colors, or between similar shapes and patterns.

Visual figure-ground discrimination   The ability to separate a shape or printed character from its background. Children with problems in this area may find it hard to find the specific bit of information they need from a printed page or computer screen filled with words and numbers.

Visual memory   Long-term visual memory is the ability to recall something seen a long time ago, while short-term visual memory is the ability to remember something seen very recently. Visual memory often depends upon the nature of the information being processed. For example, most people find it easier to remember what an object looked like four weeks ago if the object is associated with a special event. Children with problems in this area may find it hard to describe a place they have visited, remember the spelling of a familiar but irregularly spelled word, dial a telephone number without looking carefully at each of the numbers and letters on the telephone, or use a calculator, typewriter, or computer keyboard with speed and accuracy.

Visual motor processing   The kind of thinking needed to use feedback from the eyes to coordinate the movement of other parts of the body. For example, eyes and hands need to work together to write with a pen or pencil. Children with problems in this area may find it difficult to write neatly or stay within the margins or on the lines of a page, use scissors, sew, move around without bumping into things, place objects on surfaces so they will not fall off, participate in sports that require well-timed and precise movements in space.

Visual closure   The ability to know what an object is when only parts of it are visible. Children with problems in this area may find it difficult to recognize a picture of a familiar object missing some parts, or to identify a word when a letter is missing.

Spatial relationships   How objects are positioned in the space. People use their ability to recognize and understand spatial relationships as they interact with their surroundings and also when they look at objects on paper. The ability to recognize and understand spatial relationships helps people understand whether objects are near or far, on our left or right, or over or under other objects. This skill is needed to learn to read, write, count, and think about numbers. Children with problems in this area may find it hard to find their way from one place to another, or write intelligibly.

Auditory discrimination   The ability to notice, compare, and distinguish the distinct and separate sounds in words. In order to read efficiently, students must be able to isolate sounds, especially those that match letters in the alphabet. Children with problems in this area may find it difficult to learn to read or understand spoken language, follow directions, and remember details.

Auditory figure-ground discrimination   The ability to pick out important sounds from a noisy background. Children with problems in this area may find it hard to separate meaningful sounds from background noise.

Auditory memory   Like visual memory, there are two kinds of auditory memory. Long-term auditory memory is the ability to recall something heard long ago, whereas short-term auditory memory is the ability to remember something heard very recently. Children with problems in this area may find it difficult to remember people's names, memorize and recall telephone numbers, follow multistep spoken directions, recall stories they have been told, or remember lines from songs.

Treatment Options and Outlook

There are things that can be done to help someone make it easier to process information. These include

- simplify directions
- maintain eye contact while speaking
- speak slowly, especially when providing new information
- ask for repetitions

People with LEARNING DISABILITIES often have strong preferences for one type of information processing over another. These preferences are sometimes referred to as learning or working styles. Something as simple as giving instructions both orally and in writing can be of enormous help to some individuals with learning disabilities.

information-processing model   A theory of learning and MEMORY that examines the way people take in, store, and retrieve information based on a computer model. This theory can be reduced to a three-step process:

1. input or encoding (taking in information)
2. storage (transferring information into long-term memory)
3. retrieval (taking information out of long-term memory and expressing it)

A person's senses of sight, smell, hearing, taste, and touch are constantly providing information, which is stored in short- and long-term memory. For each of the hundreds of things people do each day, they need to quickly decide what information to use to complete the task. Managing all of the stored information and using it effectively is called "information processing."

See also INFORMATION PROCESSING DISORDERS.

inhibition   The ability to defer responses to unimportant distractions. The ability to control inappropriate responses or strategies while developing more effective or appropriate ones is essential to success in both academic and social settings.

Individuals with ATTENTION DEFICIT HYPERACTIVITY DISORDER (ADHD) often have difficulty with inhibition, and because of this may express themselves in ways that are impulsive or inappropriate, or may experience difficulty with internal distractibility.

See also DISINHIBITION.

initial blend   The joining of two or more consonant sounds, represented by letters, without losing the identity of the sounds, as in the "bl" sound in *black*. An initial blend also involves the joining of the first consonant and vowel sounds in a word, as "b" and "a" in *baby*. Many experts believe this process is a crucial step in learning phonics.

insertions   Words or letters that an individual incorrectly includes in a sentence when reading orally. An example might be reading "blank" for "bank" or, instead of reading "It was night," reading "It was a dark night."

instructional reading level   The reading ability or grade level of material that is challenging, but not frustrating, for the student to read successfully with normal classroom instruction and support. Although this may vary, a student should score better than 95 percent word-identification accuracy and better than 75 percent COMPREHENSION in order to be considered as reading at this level.

intelligence   As commonly used, intelligence refers to the level of intellectual functioning and capacity of an individual—the ability to learn or understand.

Recently some experts have suggested that intelligence is not a single phenomenon, but that there exist "multiple intelligences"—a number of discrete "intelligences"—and that an individual will possess a unique pattern of strengths and abilities across this range of intellectual functions.

In the context of a LEARNING DISABILITY, the concept of intelligence is important for two reasons. First, there can often be significant discrepancies between intellectual ability and academic performance. Second, learning disabilities have often been misunderstood as a sign of lower intelligence despite extensive research and the achievement of many notable individuals with learning disabilities.

Intelligence is measured by intelligence tests, which provide an INTELLIGENCE QUOTIENT, a measure of intellectual development that is the ratio of a child's mental age to his chronological age, multiplied by 100.

intelligence quotient (IQ)   A measurement of INTELLIGENCE based on performance on INTELLIGENCE TESTS. Use of intelligence testing remains controversial because of the limitations of testing for specific abilities and knowledge, and because of possible cultural bias in the design of tests.

Nonetheless, IQ is used in educational and psychological settings in combination with other types of tests in order to evaluate an individual's mental capacity and to recommend appropriate remediation or treatment.

For individuals with a LEARNING DISABILITY, IQ scores can demonstrate superior intelligence despite weak language skills or poor academic performance. Conversely, poor performance on intelligence tests can inaccurately reflect true ability and potential, with many capable individuals outperforming the level of achievement their IQ scores might have predicted.

IQ is generally based on a mean of 100, with scores ranging in classification from mentally retarded at the low end to very superior at the high end.

The concept of intelligence has existed for centuries, but it was not until this century that scientists began testing it—and debating whether or not they should. Intelligence testing was developed in the late 19th century as France's Alfred Binet began work on tests of individual differences, which led him to study "subnormal" children in Paris schools. Several years later, Binet and Paris physician Theodore Simon recommended that an accurate diagnosis of intelligence be established for schoolchildren. The result was the Simon-Binet test of intelligence, which first appeared in 1905 and was revised in 1908.

Binet thought of the test as a tool for selecting students who needed special remedial teaching, not as a measure of absolute and innate ability. The test was translated into English for the American audience in 1908 by Henry H. Goddard and revised several times, but it was not until 1916 that the test was standardized with the revision by Lewis M. Terman in the form known as the Stanford-Binet test.

In 1911, William Stern developed the idea of relating mental age to chronological age with his formulation of the Intelligence Quotient. This simple formulation of $IQ = MA/CA \times 100$ gave a number to stand for the performance of the child. This allowed the IQ to be manipulated within statistical tests and to be used for prediction of later performance.

During World War I, the first massive use of psychological tests of intelligence was begun with the testing of military recruits. Hundreds of psychologists and graduate students in psychology were recruited to administer the tests to recruits. After the war, critics were outraged to find that the army test suggested that southern and eastern Europeans were inferior to northern Europeans, and that blacks were inferior to whites. Some believe it was these test results that prompted restrictive immigration policies in America in 1924 and fanned the flames of racial prejudice against blacks and other minorities.

David Wechsler developed his tests in response to many of the criticisms of the Binet tests. In 1939, he introduced his WECHSLER ADULT INTELLIGENCE SCALE (WAIS), the first of a stable of tests still much in use.

Since that time there have been many intelligence tests produced, some specifically aimed at reducing cultural and background effects on pencil-and-paper tests. In 1969, the debate about the inherent versus the environmental bases of intelligence exploded with an article by psychologist Arthur Jensen in which he argued for the inheritance of racial differences in intelligence. The debate continued into the last decade of the 20th century in response to further controversial work on intelligence and class structure in American life. In recent years, influential books by psychologist Howard Gardner and others have supported multiple intelligences over a single global factor in intelligence.

intelligence test   A test used to determine a person's INTELLIGENCE QUOTIENT (IQ) in relation to others the same age. There are many IQ tests used today, but critics still argue about whether these tests measure a person's true intelligence or whether they simply assess only certain abilities in a culturally biased way.

The most popular intelligence tests for children is the WECHSLER INTELLIGENCE SCALE FOR CHILDREN—IV (WISC-IV), the third revision of psychologist David Wechsler's classic 1949 test for children modeled after army IQ tests developed during World War I. Average test results range from 90 to 110; a score below 70 indicates MENTAL RETARDATION. A score above 130 is usually considered gifted, although different programs set different levels for this classification. A score of 165 or higher is usually considered genius.

The first IQ tests were developed by psychologist Alfred Binet, who used a standardized test to identify learning-impaired Parisian children in the early 1900s. Since that time, IQ tests have become one of the most important ways of identifying children with mental retardation and LEARNING DISABILITIES. Since the administration of the original SCHOLASTIC APTITUDE TEST (SAT) in 1926, it has led to the development of a variety of aptitude and achievement tests that directly affect the college careers of millions of high school students.

Unfortunately, education experts point out that there is still a serious gap between the theories and tests that have been developed in the past 20 years and the way intelligence tests are actually used. Testing experts have argued that IQ tests unfairly divide students by race, gender, class, and culture and minimize the importance of creativity, character, and practical know-how. Many educators also disagree with the idea that a person is born with a static number that illustrates an unchanging intellectual potential that can be used to determine a person's success in life.

Since the 1970s, researchers have been trying to address those concerns by tinkering with the makeup of the IQ tests. They have updated the WISC and the STANFORD-BINET INTELLIGENCE SCALE (now in its fifth edition) to take into consideration test takers' cultural and linguistic backgrounds. They also have developed new and better ways of creating and interpreting those tests. As a result, many of the previous biases have been lessened, and new tests are available that, unlike traditional intelligence tests, are based on modern theories of brain function.

interim alternative educational setting (IAES) Because students with disabilities must not be suspended for longer than 10 days, when such a student needs to be disciplined, an IAES is an alternative to suspension.

Most students with disabilities are disciplined as are any other students, but in certain extraordinary circumstances, a suspension longer than 10 days would require education in an IAES. School officials may place students with disabilities in an alternative educational setting with or without parental consent. The interim alternative educational setting is determined by the INDIVIDUALIZED EDUCATION PROGRAM COMMITTEE and allows the student to continue to participate in general educational programs and receive special services as outlined on the INDIVIDUALIZED EDUCATION PROGRAM. If suspension is necessary for a longer period, an IAES must be put into place for up to 45 days.

internalization The incorporation of external information within an individual's thought processes, emotions, and behavior. Internalization may be positive, such as when an individual internalizes positive feedback and forms a more positive self-image. Internalization may also be used to denote the process of acquiring specific skills or strategies, such as keeping a daily schedule or automatically proofreading written work.

Often, however, internalization refers to taking in negative feedback and self-images, as when a student who struggles to succeed in school internalizes the notion that academic failure is inevitable and lies beyond his or her control.

intervention   See EARLY INTERVENTION PROGRAM.

invented spelling   An attempt to spell an unknown word based on a child's knowledge of the spelling system and how it works. Invented spellings are often used as an instructional strategy in beginning writing, as the child moves toward controlled use of conventional spelling of words. For example, invented spelling for the word "because" may look like: bekuz, bcus, or beekuz.

The concept of invented spelling is controversial, however. Proponents believe invented spelling is a natural development of writing, and that by encouraging students to use invented spelling, they are freed from the burden of perfection so they can express their thoughts more easily. Critics believe invented spelling should not be encouraged because it may interfere with learning proper spelling from reading, or with learning specific spelling rules.

inversion   A confusion in the directionality of letters or numbers. For example: "m" for "w" or "6" for "9," in reading, spelling, or mathematics.

IQ   See INTELLIGENCE QUOTIENT.

itinerant teacher   A SPECIAL EDUCATION teacher who works in several schools within an area or district. It is not an uncommon practice for special services to be spread across a district, especially when part-time personnel are employed. For small schools, itinerant teachers may include district music, art, and physical education teachers, who may visit each school once a week.

For students with special learning needs, special educators are an important part of the child's INDIVIDUAL EDUCATION PROGRAM. Special services are mandated by the local and federal agencies, and must be reevaluated periodically. This creates fluctuations in staffing and the services provided in each school on an annual basis.

While itinerant teachers can provide the necessary special instruction for each student, it is more difficult for children to develop ongoing relationships with such teachers, depending on the contact hours, if the teachers are not available more informally. This type of service provision can also make children more self-conscious about their learning differences, as it calls attention to their need for special instruction by teachers who visit the school for the sole purpose of providing direct services and participating in IEP conferences.

Kaufman Test of Educational Achievement   This test for children in grades one through 12 measures decoding of letters and individual words, spelling, reading COMPREHENSION, math computation, and the ability to answer math reasoning questions. The test is most useful in students beyond first grade, since there are too few lower level questions to adequately assess a first grader with poor skills.

Key Math Diagnostic Arithmetic Test-Revised This test is designed for students from age five through 15 years, 11 months, to assess their knowledge of basic mathematical concepts such as numbers, fractions, decimals, percentages, geometric shapes, principles, addition, subtraction, multiplication, division, mental computation, measurement, time and money estimation, interpretation, and problem solving.

kinesthetic   One of the body's senses that refers to the acquisition of information from body movements. Like other forms of learning, kinesthetic learning involves the input of stimuli to specific channels in the brain, in this case through the motion of joints and muscles. Kinesthetic learning is best understood through movements that have been made automatic through practice and repetition, or made unconscious and automatic, such as throwing a baseball or driving a car.

For individuals who are good kinesthetic learners, reinforcement of learning in basic skill areas can be supplemented with a kinesthetic approach, such as walking or dancing movements used to represent concepts or steps in a sequence, to aid recall.

Kurzweil reading machine (KRM)   A device that provides both sound and visual presentation of scanned text and images on a computer screen; considered to be the world's first consumer product to successfully incorporate artificial intelligence technology. Text can be imported into the program by scanning or typing directly into the machine. Once text is in the program, users can adjust features such as reading speed, reading units, highlighting, and voices to preferred settings.

Additional study features such as highlighters, note creation, and built-in dictionary make the device a powerful active reading tool.

The first Kurzweil reading machine, which was introduced in 1976, was basically a scanner that contained a camera that could move in both vertical and horizontal directions. As the camera automatically moved back and forth scanning each line of print, it transmitted the image electronically to a minicomputer in a separate cabinet. The minicomputer recognized the characters, grouped them into words and computed the pronunciation of each word. To accomplish this last task, several hundred pronunciation rules were programmed in, along with several thousand exceptions. The resulting string of sounds (phonemes) was sent to a speech synthesizer, which articulated each word.

Subsequent models of the KRM were substantially improved, but they are organized in a similar way.

Today, the user simply places a document facedown on the machine, presses start, and listens. The KRM can control the movement of the scanner, back it up, make it reread sections or spell out words, and provide a variety of other functions.

Within 10 years, the technology is expected to improve so that a full print-to-speech reading machine will be produced that can fit in a pocket. The device will simply be held over the page to be scanned, and snap a picture of the page. All of the electronics and computation will be inside this small camera-sized device. The student can then listen to the text being read from a small speaker or earphone.

It also should be possible to snap a picture and read a poster on a wall, street sign, soup can, an ID badge, or an appliance LCD display—and many other examples of real-world text. This reading machine should cost less than a thousand dollars and will ultimately come down to a few hundred dollars.

Landau-Kleffner syndrome (LKS) A childhood disorder that leads to the gradual or sudden loss of the ability to understand and use spoken language. All children with this condition have abnormal electrical brain waves that can be documented by an electroencephalogram (EEG), a recording of the electric activity of the brain. LKS is sometimes called infantile acquired APHASIA, acquired epileptic aphasia, or aphasia with convulsive disorder. This syndrome was first described in 1957 by doctors William M. Landau and Frank R. Kleffner, who identified six children with the disorder. More than 160 cases have been reported from 1957 through 1990.

No one knows what causes LKS, and some experts think there is more than one cause. All of the children with LKS appear to be perfectly normal until their first seizure or the start of language problems. Because there have been no reports of children with a family history of LKS, the condition does not appear to be an inherited disorder.

Symptoms and Diagnostic Path

The condition often begins in normally developing children between ages three and seven, often preceded by an epileptic seizure that usually occurs at night. They begin to have trouble understanding what people are saying to them—a symptom known as word deafness. The auditory AGNOSIA may occur either slowly or very quickly, and parents often think their child is developing a hearing problem or has become suddenly deaf. However, hearing tests reveal normal hearing.

Eventually, the inability to understand language begins to affect the child's spoken language, which may progress to a complete loss of the ability to speak. Children who have learned to read and write before the beginning of the auditory agnosia

can often continue communicating through written language. Some children develop a type of gestural communication or sign language. The communication problems may lead to behavioral or psychological problems, but INTELLIGENCE usually appears to be unaffected.

About 80 percent of children with LKS have one or more epileptic seizures that usually occur at night, but these seizures usually stop by the time the child enters adolescence. Behavioral disorders such as HYPERACTIVITY, aggressiveness, and DEPRESSION can also accompany this disorder, and children may appear to be autistic or developmentally delayed. All LKS children have abnormal electrical brain activity on both the right and left sides of their brains.

Treatment Options and Outlook

Medication is available to control the seizures and abnormal brain wave activity, but the drugs do not usually have any effect on language ability. Corticosteroid therapy has improved the language ability of some children, and sign language instruction has benefited others.

There have not been many long-term follow-up studies of children with LKS. This lack of evidence, along with the wide range of differences among affected children, makes it impossible to predict the outcome of this disorder. Although complete language recovery has been reported, language problems usually persist into adulthood. The continued language problems can range from difficulty following simple commands to no verbal communication. If recovery takes place, it may occur at any time from within days to years. Most children outgrow the seizures, and electrical brain activity on the EEG usually returns to normal by age 15.

No relationship has been found between the extent of the language impairment, the presence or absence of seizures, and the amount of language recovery. Typically, however, the earlier the disorder begins, the poorer the language recovery.

language An organized system of symbols that represents objects, actions, feelings, processes, and relationships. Every language has rules that govern how that language is used.

language delay A lag in the development of communication skills, progressing more slowly than would be expected based on age, environment, or specific deprivation or disease. Children with a LEARNING DISABILITY are likely to have LANGUAGE delays. Language delay includes the diagnostic subgroups of language disorder, language and learning disability, MENTAL RETARDATION, and AUTISM.

language development Changes in the features of a LANGUAGE over time because of contact with other languages or technological advancements, as the growth of technical terms in English after the Industrial Revolution.

language disabilities A range of deficits in linguistics, whether related to expressive LANGUAGE, written or oral, receptive language, or auditory processing, the processing of sounds and meaning.

language disorder A developmental disorder involving disabilities of reception, integration, recall, and/or production of LANGUAGE. Language disorders may be spoken, written, or both.

See also LEARNING DISABILITY; COMMUNICATION DISORDER.

language processing disabilities The most common type of LEARNING DISABILITY; children with this problem have trouble with the spoken word, which usually interferes with reading and writing when these children first start school. They may have trouble with any aspect of language, such as

- hearing words correctly
- remembering verbal material
- understanding the meaning of words
- communicating clearly

This learning problem may range from mild to extremely severe—so difficult that these children may find that coping with reading and writing is like learning a foreign language. They may be slow in learning to speak, and speak in brief sentences, and their memory for verbal directions may be poor.

Many children with this problem may speak in a garbled fashion because their brains may have trouble sorting out the right sounds; these children may pronounce "elephant" as "efelunt." They may have a poor grasp of grammar and trouble with word sequencing in a sentence, and may confuse words that sound alike. These types of errors usually get worse if they must speak in public or before an authority figure.

laterality The awareness of both sides of one's body.

See also LATERAL PREFERENCE.

lateral preference The development of a preference for one side of the body, also sometimes called "lateral dominance" or "lateralization." This preference develops very early in life, and is expressed most prominently in "handedness" (the dominant hand that a child uses for activities such as writing or throwing a ball).

In some cases, lateralization is not clear, and an individual will express a mixed lateral preference—writing with one hand, for example, and throwing a ball with the other.

lead poisoning One of the most common preventable accidents in the United States. More than 434,000 children between ages one and five had harmful lead levels in their blood in 2004. Repeated exposure to low levels of lead can lead to a LEARNING DISABILITY.

The brain is most sensitive to lead during the first six years of life, when the brain cells are rapidly developing. Nearly 1 million U.S. children have lead levels in their blood that are high enough to cause irreversible damage to their health.

Lead can be ingested from dust, soil, and lead-based paint flecks in old homes. In fact, more than 80 percent of homes built before 1978 have lead paint, and the older the house, the more likely it is to contain lead-based paint. In public playgrounds and in yards, the dirt where children play may contain high lead levels. For decades, peeling exterior building paint, air emissions from leaded car exhaust, and pollution from smelters and other industries have been significant sources. The highest levels of lead in soil usually are found close to foundations of homes painted with exterior leaded paint.

In addition, lead is still found in low levels in some drinking water as a result of a lead-based solder on old water pipes. The Environmental Protection Agency estimates that drinking water is the source of about 20 percent of Americans' lead exposure. Even after lead pipes were banned, leaded solder was legal for use on drinking water lines until the 1980s and is still for sale in hardware stores. Faucets and plumbing fittings may legally contain up to 8 percent lead. The greatest risk is to infants using formula mixed with contaminated water.

Lead-glazed pottery that has not been properly fired also can allow lead to leach into whatever comes into contact with it, and lead can be found in some folk remedies, "health foods," and cosmetics.

Because young children are often crawling and mouthing objects, they are more likely to ingest lead; moreover, a child's smaller body size means a higher dose of lead per exposure. At the same time, a child is not as capable of clearing lead from the body, so the body's concentration builds up.

Symptoms and Diagnostic Path

The symptoms of low levels of lead poisoning are low IQ scores, decreased attention span, poor hearing, speech delays, and other developmental problems.

While the symptoms of severe lead poisoning are obvious, repeated exposures to small amounts can also cause poisoning but may not be as easily detectable. There may be no visible symptoms of lead poisoning in this instance that would alert parents to seek medical care.

There is evidence that lead poisoning is harmful at blood levels once thought safe. Lower IQ scores, slower development, and more attention problems have been observed in children with lead levels as low as 10 micrograms per deciliter. (Micrograms per deciliter, written µg/dL, indicate the amount of lead in a deciliter of blood.)

If a thumb-prick blood test reveals a high lead level, a blood sample taken from a vein must be tested before chelation therapy begins.

Screening The Centers for Disease Control and Prevention (CDC) recommends testing every child at 12 months of age and, if resources allow, at 24 months. Screening should start at six months if the child is at risk of lead exposure (for example, if the child lives in an older home built before 1960, which has peeling or chipping paint). Decisions about further testing should be based on previous blood-lead test results, and the child's risk of lead exposure. In some states, more frequent lead screening is required by law. The Centers for Disease Control and Prevention in 1991 identified a number of reasons for testing a child for lead poisoning, including

- child lives or regularly visits a house built before 1960 and being renovated, or that has peeling, chipped paint
- sibling or classmate is being treated for lead poisoning
- child lives with someone whose hobby or work includes exposure to lead, such as making pottery or stained glass and working in auto repair or bridge or highway construction
- child lives near industry likely to release lead
- child received treatment for foreign object in ear, nose, or stomach
- child often swallows nonfood items
- any child under six with unexplained developmental delays, hearing problem, irritability, severe ATTENTION deficit, violent tantrums, or unexplained anemia

The test identifies how many micrograms of lead are found in one deciliter of the child's blood. Based on what is known today, children should have less than 10 micrograms per deciliter (10 µg/dL) of blood lead concentration. If higher levels are found, there are certain steps that can be taken.

At 10–19 µg/dL, a child has mild lead poisoning and should be retested in a few months. The home and all the places the child spends time should be checked for lead sources, and identified lead hazards should be controlled. Frequent wet cleaning and handwashing will help reduce lead dust. Good nutrition can help the child fight lead.

A blood lead level between 20 and 44 means the child has moderate lead poisoning. Sources of lead in the child's environment must be removed, and the child may need chelation therapy to remove lead from the body. Chelation therapy means the child is given a drug capable of binding lead and reducing its acute toxicity. All drugs have potential side effects and must be used with caution.

A blood lead concentration of 45 to 69 is severe lead poisoning. A child with this concentration needs both medical treatment and lead removed from the environment.

A blood lead level over 70 is an acute medical emergency. The child may stay in the hospital for treatment and not be released until he or she can return to a lead-free, safe home.

Risk Factors and Preventive Measures

To prevent further lead poisoning, parents should keep children away from peeling or chipping paint and chewable surfaces painted with lead-based paint, especially windows, windowsills, and window wells. Parents should wet mop and wet wipe hard surfaces, using trisodium phosphate detergent (found at hardware stores) or automatic dishwasher soap and water. Hard surfaces should not be vacuumed because this is believed to scatter dust. If inspection shows a house has lead-based paint, the family should not renovate or attempt to remove the paint themselves. Work should be done by someone who knows how to protect workers, the family, and the environment. The family should not be in the home during renovations or paint removal.

Parents should wash children's hands and faces before meals and wash toys and pacifiers frequently. Children should eat regular nutritious meals, since more lead is absorbed on an empty stomach. Children's diets should contain plenty of iron, such as liver, fortified cereal, cooked beans, spinach, and raisins. Calcium is also important (including foods like milk, yogurt, cheese, and cooked greens).

If soil around the home is likely to be contaminated (if a home was built before 1960 or near a major highway), parents should plant grass or other ground cover. If lead-based paint is the source of soil contamination, most lead will be near painted surfaces such as exterior walls. In such cases, par-

ents should plant bushes next to the house to keep children away. If the soil is contaminated with lead, parents should provide a sandbox with a solid bottom and top cover, and clean sand for children to play and dig in.

If the lead content of tap water in the home is higher than the drinking water standard, parents should let the water run for several minutes (until the temperature changes) before using. Only fully flushed water from the cold-water tap should be used for drinking and cooking. To conserve water, parents should collect drinking water in bottles at night after water has been fully flushed from the tap. This procedure will help if the source of lead is from the home's plumbing, but it will not help if the city water supply is contaminated.

Parents should not store food in open cans (especially imported cans), nor in pottery that is meant for decorative use, or in lead crystal or china.

If members of the family work with lead, they should make sure children are not exposed to any lead-contaminated clothing or scrap material brought home.

learned helplessness   A conditioned response that creates problems in thinking, motivation, and emotions in children with LEARNING DISABILITIES. The theory of learned helplessness was developed in the 1960s after researchers observed the phenomenon in dogs. During their research, scientists used electric shocks when the dogs tried to leave their cage. Later, when the dogs were provided a way out, they made no effort to escape. This "giving up" after a period of negative consequences was termed *learned helplessness.*

Symptoms and Diagnostic Path

Many studies have suggested that children with a learning disability develop learned helplessness in academic settings as a result of continual failure in school. This failure also leads to withdrawal, unwillingness to approach new tasks, DEPRESSION, and a lack of persistence. Like the dogs in the study, students who have developed learned helplessness may apply this maladaptive behavior to new situations where they should be capable of academic success, but instead believe their efforts are useless. Learned-helpless children see failure as permanent—it is caused by lack of ability, about which they can do nothing. They also believe failure is present in everything they do.

Other factors have been shown to contribute to this learned academic helplessness, including

- grouping students with a variety of disabilities under one teacher
- too much external reinforcement
- lack of early identification of learning disabilities
- belief that intelligence cannot be changed
- lack of reward for individual effort

The concept of learned helplessness is tied to the idea of control. Individuals who may be defined as having learned helplessness essentially believe that their performance is outside their control—that no matter what they do, they will fail. As a result of continual academic failure, some students with learning disabilities come to expect failure regardless of their effort. This expectation can erode motivation. Often, students who exhibit learned helplessness also tend to believe that the responsibility for learning rests entirely with the teacher.

The cure for learned helplessness is not the rediscovery of the power of positive thinking; positive statements alone, without first dealing with underlying negative beliefs, will have little effect. If a student is to conquer learned helplessness, the individual must change the destructive things said to oneself when failing.

Treatment Options and Outlook

It is what the child thinks about failure and its cause that leads to learned helplessness. In other words, it is not just the failure, but the way the child sees the failure, that is important. This is one of the reasons why it is possible to treat learned helplessness.

Cognitive behavioral training teaches a child to recognize his automatic negative thoughts and then to change these thoughts by gathering evidence to the contrary. The child should be taught to

- make different explanations (reattributions) and use them to dispute automatic thoughts
- distract himself or herself from the thoughts that depress one

- change unrealistic, demanding assumptions to realistic, flexible ones

Research has shown that the most productive learners are those who believe INTELLIGENCE can be changed and that effort is just as powerful as ability in achieving success.

learning centers An instructional part of a classroom organized by tables, in which a teacher arranges learning materials such as worksheets or games. Learning centers are also known as "teaching stations" or "instructional stations." Children can complete these activities on their own to supplement their other classroom learning experiences.

learning disability (LD) A neurobiological disorder in which a person's brain works or is structured differently, affecting one or more of the basic processes involved in understanding or using spoken or written LANGUAGE. Such a disability may result in a problem with listening, thinking, speaking, reading, writing, spelling, or doing mathematical calculations. Experts believe that children with learning disabilities have a problem with the way the brain handles information, which in turn hinders the normal learning process.

Learning disabilities affect one in seven people, and represent a national problem of enormous proportions. Every year, more students are diagnosed with learning disabilities, a diagnosis now shared by 2.9 million schoolchildren in the United States. Many thousands more are never properly diagnosed or treated, or do not get treatment because they are not considered eligible for services. Half of all students receiving SPECIAL EDUCATION services in public schools have learning disabilities. However, these statistics do not include the tens of thousands of students who attend private and religious schools, nor do they include the scores of students who may have serious problems with learning, but who may not meet the criteria established by school districts to receive special education services.

The most common learning disability is a difficulty with language and reading. Two-thirds of students with learning disabilities in high school are reading at least three grade levels behind. A recent National Institutes of Health study showed that 67 percent of young students identified as being at risk for reading difficulties were able to achieve average or above-average reading ability when they received help early.

All children learn in highly individual ways. Children with learning disabilities simply process information differently, but they are generally of normal or above-average INTELLIGENCE.

Sometimes overlooked as "hidden handicaps," learning disabilities are often not easily recognized, accepted, or considered serious once detected. The impact of the disability, which often runs in families, ranges from relatively mild to severe. Learning disabilities can be lifelong conditions that, in some cases, affect many parts of a person's life: school or work, daily routines, friendships, and family life. In some people, many overlapping learning disabilities may be apparent, while others may have a single, isolated learning problem that has little impact on other areas of their lives.

Learning disabilities are not the same as MENTAL RETARDATION, AUTISM, deafness, blindness, or behavioral disorders. Nor are learning disabilities caused by poverty, environmental factors, or cultural differences. Learning disabilities are not curable, but individuals can learn to compensate for and even overcome areas of weakness. ATTENTION DEFICITS and HYPERACTIVITY sometimes appear with learning disabilities, but not always.

Common learning disabilities include

- DYSLEXIA: a language-based disability in which a person has trouble understanding words, sentences, or paragraphs
- DYSCALCULIA: a mathematical disability in which a person has a very difficult time solving arithmetic problems and grasping math concepts
- DYSGRAPHIA: a writing disability in which a person finds it hard to form letters correctly or write within a defined space
- auditory and visual processing disabilities: a sensory disability in which a person has difficulty understanding language despite normal hearing and vision

Experts do not know exactly what causes learning disabilities, but they are assumed to be disorders of the central nervous system triggered by many different factors. These may include heredity, problems during pregnancy or birth, and incidents after birth.

The fact that learning disabilities tend to run in families indicates that there may be a genetic link. For example, children who lack some of the skills needed for reading, such as hearing the separate sounds of words, are likely to have a parent with a related problem. However, a parent's learning disability may take a slightly different form in the child. A parent who has a writing disorder may have a child with an expressive language disorder. For this reason, it seems unlikely that specific learning disorders are inherited directly. Instead, what is inherited might be a subtle brain dysfunction that can lead to a learning disability.

There may be an alternative explanation for why LD might seem to run in families. Some learning difficulties may actually stem from the family environment. For example, parents who have expressive language disorders might talk less to their children, or the language they use may be distorted. In such cases, the child lacks a good model for acquiring language and, therefore, may seem to be learning disabled.

LD problems also may be caused by illness or injury during or before birth, or by the use of drugs and ALCOHOL during pregnancy, untreated Rh incompatibility with the mother, premature or prolonged labor, or lack of oxygen or low weight at birth.

Throughout pregnancy, the fetal brain develops from a few cells into a complex organ made of billions of specialized, interconnected nerve cells called neurons. During this process, things can go wrong that may alter how the neurons form or interconnect.

In the early stages of pregnancy, the brain stem forms the part of the brain that controls basic functions such as breathing and digestion. Later, a deep ridge divides the cerebrum (the thinking part of the brain) into two halves, a right and left hemisphere. Finally, the areas involved with processing sight, sound, and other senses develop, as well as the areas associated with attention, thinking, and emotion.

As new cells form, they move into place to create various brain structures. Nerve cells rapidly grow to form networks with other parts of the brain. These networks allow information to be shared among various regions of the brain.

Throughout pregnancy, this brain development is vulnerable to disruptions. If the disruption occurs early, the fetus may die or the infant may be born with widespread disabilities and possibly mental retardation. If the disruption occurs later, when the cells are becoming specialized and moving into place, it may leave errors in the cell makeup, location, or connections. Some scientists believe that these errors may later show up as learning disorders.

Scientists have found that mothers who smoke during pregnancy may be more likely to bear smaller babies, who tend to be at risk for a variety of problems, including learning disorders. Alcohol also may be dangerous to the fetus's developing brain, distorting the developing neurons. Heavy alcohol use during pregnancy has been linked to FETAL ALCOHOL SYNDROME, a condition that can lead to low birth weight, intellectual impairment, hyperactivity, and certain physical defects. Any alcohol use during pregnancy may influence the child's development and lead to problems with learning, attention, memory, or problem solving. Drugs such as cocaine (especially crack cocaine) seem to affect the normal development of brain receptors that help to transmit incoming signals from skin, eyes, and ears. Because children with certain learning disabilities have trouble understanding speech sounds or letters, some researchers believe that learning disabilities (as well as ATTENTION DEFICIT HYPERACTIVITY DISORDER [ADHD]) may be related to faulty receptors. Current research points to drug abuse as a possible cause of receptor damage. Other research indicates that mothers exposed to toxins such as pesticides and even substances normally considered harmless (such as caffeine) can interfere with fetal development. Children born to these mothers have a higher frequency of learning problems. This area of research is highly controversial.

After birth, learning disabilities may be caused by head injuries, nutritional deprivation, poisonous substances, or child abuse. New brain cells and neural networks continue to be produced for a year or so after the child is born, and these cells are vulnerable to certain disruptions, too.

Some ENVIRONMENTAL TOXINS may lead to learning disabilities, possibly by disrupting childhood brain development or brain processes. Cadmium and LEAD, both prevalent in the environment, are becoming a leading focus of neurological research. Cadmium, used in making some steel products, can get into the soil, then into food. Lead was once common in paint and gasoline, and is still present in some water pipes. A study of animals sponsored by the National Institutes of Health showed a connection between exposure to lead and learning difficulties. In the study, rats exposed to lead experienced changes in their brain waves, slowing their ability to learn. The learning problems lasted for weeks, long after the rats were no longer exposed to lead.

In addition, there is growing evidence that learning problems may develop in children with cancer who had been treated with chemotherapy or radiation at an early age. This seems particularly true of children with brain tumors who received radiation to the skull.

Symptoms and Diagnostic Path

The earlier a learning disability is detected, the better chance a child will have of succeeding in school and in life. Parents are encouraged to understand the warning signs of a learning disability from as early as preschool, since the first years in school are especially crucial for a young child.

However, the very definition of *learning disability* hinders its identification with young children. The crucial element in identifying learning disabilities is their effect on academic performance, but the problems learning disabilities cause are not apparent until the child goes to school. How can a learning disability in reading be identified when a child is too young to be taught to read? With young children, the range of what is "normal" is so wide that it is extremely difficult in most cases, and impossible in others, to tell the difference between simple developmental immaturity and a learning disability.

There is no one indication of learning disabilities. Although most children have an occasional problem with learning or behavior, a consistent pattern of the following problems may suggest the need for further testing:

Preschool

If the child has problems

- learning the alphabet
- rhyming words
- connecting sounds and letters
- counting or learning numbers
- being understood when speaking to a stranger
- using scissors, crayons, or paint
- reacting too much or too little to touch
- using words or using phrases
- pronunciation
- walking up and down stairs
- talking (identified as a "late talker")
- remembering names of colors
- dressing

Elementary School

Does the child have trouble with

- learning new vocabulary
- speaking in full sentences
- understanding conversation rules
- retelling stories
- remembering information
- playing with peers
- moving from one activity to another
- expressing thoughts
- holding a pencil
- handwriting
- handling math problems
- following directions
- self-esteem
- remembering routines
- learning
- reading comprehension
- drawing or copying shapes
- deciding what information presented in class is important
- modulating voice

- neatness and organization
- meeting deadlines

Adulthood

Does the adult have trouble with

- remembering new information
- organization
- reading comprehension
- getting along with peers or coworkers
- finding or keeping a job
- sense of direction
- understanding subtle jokes
- making appropriate remarks
- self-expression
- following directions
- reading, writing, spelling, and math
- self-esteem
- using proper grammar
- meeting deadlines

Symptoms may appear in only one skill area, such as reading or writing, in many people with learning disabilities. The following is a brief outline of warning signs for possible learning disabilities in specific skill areas:

Attention

- has short attention span
- is impulsive
- has difficulty conforming to routines
- is easily distracted

Auditory

- does not respond to sounds of spoken language
- consistently misunderstands what is being said
- overly sensitive to sound
- has trouble differentiating simultaneous sounds

Language

- can explain things orally but not in writing
- has trouble telling or understanding jokes or stories

- misinterprets language
- does not understand what is said
- responds in an inappropriate manner, unrelated to what is said
- responds only partially to what is said

Math

- problems with arithmetic, math language, and math concepts
- reverses numbers
- problems with time, sequencing, or problem solving

Memory

- learns information presented one way but not another
- trouble memorizing information
- unable to repeat what has just been said

Movement

- performs similar tasks differently each day
- has trouble dialing phone numbers or holding a pencil
- has poor coordination, is clumsy
- is unaware of physical surroundings
- has a tendency to self-injury

Organization

- has trouble following a schedule
- is often late
- has trouble learning about time
- has difficulty organizing belongings

Reading

- poor reading ability or poor comprehension
- may misread information
- problems with syntax or grammar
- confuse or reverse similar letters or numbers
- problems reading addresses, small print, or columns

Social

- has trouble with social skills
- misinterprets nonverbal social cues
- experiences social isolation
- does not use appropriate eye contact

Thinking Skills

- acquires new skills slowly
- has trouble following directions
- confuses right/left, up/down, under/over, behind/between
- gets lost in large buildings
- seems unaware of time or sequence of events

Writing

- has problems writing down ideas
- has problems organizing thoughts on paper
- reverses or omits letters, words, or phrases when writing
- has problems with sentence structure, writing mechanics
- may spell the same word differently in a single paper
- may read well but not write well (or vice versa)

It is important to remember most people have one or more of the above warning signs and experts are not worried if a child has one or two of these symptoms. Experts get more concerned if a child has many of these symptoms, especially if the child is older or symptoms are severe.

It is also important to understand what is not included in the LD category. For example, although attention deficit disorder and attention deficit hyperactivity disorder (ADHD) are not learning disabilities themselves, there is a 20 percent probability that someone with attention deficit disorder or ADHD also has one or more learning disabilities. Other conditions that are not considered to be learning disabilities themselves include autism, blindness and deafness, emotional problems, hyperactivity, illiteracy, mental retardation, "slow learner," or physical disability.

LD is a broad term that covers a range of possible causes, symptoms, and treatments. Partly because learning disabilities can show up in so many forms, it is difficult to diagnose or to pinpoint the causes. And since a diagnosis depends on the classification used, (INDIVIDUALS WITH DISABILITIES EDUCATION IMPROVEMENT ACT [IDEIA] vs. *DIAGNOSTIC AND STATISTICAL MANUAL OF MENTAL DISORDERS*), a child may be identified as learning disabled under one system but not another.

Not all learning problems are necessarily learning disabilities; many children are simply slow to develop certain skills. Because children show natural differences in their rate of development, sometimes what seems to be a learning disability may simply be a delay in maturation or a difference in learning style. To be diagnosed as a learning disability, specific criteria must be met. These criteria appear in the *Diagnostic and Statistical Manual of Mental Disorders—Third Edition, Revised (DSM-III-R)* and IDEIA. *DSM-III-R* divides learning disorders into three broad categories: developmental speech and language disorders, academic skills disorders, and "other," a term that includes certain coordination disorders and learning handicaps not covered by the other terms. Each of these categories includes a number of more specific disorders.

IDEIA uses a slightly different classification system that specifies seven areas of learning disability

- basic reading skill
- reading comprehension
- mathematics calculation
- mathematics reasoning
- written expression
- oral expression
- listening comprehension

Under IDEIA, each area of learning disability is divided by the "severe discrepancy between potential and achievement" the law requires.

Developmental speech and language disorders Speech and language problems are often the earliest indicators of a learning disability. While not classified as learning disabilities themselves, they often accompany learning disabilities. People with developmental speech and language disorders have trouble producing speech sounds, using spoken language to communicate, or understanding what other people say. Depending on the problem, the specific diagnosis may be

- developmental articulation disorder
- developmental expressive language disorder
- developmental receptive language disorder

With a *developmental articulation disorder,* children may have trouble controlling their rate of speech, or they may lag behind their friends in learning to make speech sounds. These disorders are common, appearing in at least 10 percent of children younger than age eight. Fortunately, articulation disorders can often be outgrown or successfully treated with speech therapy.

Some children with *developmental expressive language disorder* have problems expressing themselves in speech, such as calling objects by the wrong names, speaking only in two-word phrases, or not being able to answer simple questions.

Some people have trouble understanding certain aspects of speech; this is *developmental receptive language disorder.* This explains the toddler who does not respond to his name or the worker who consistently cannot follow simple directions. While hearing is normal, these individuals cannot make sense of certain sounds, words, or sentences. Because using and understanding speech are strongly related, many people with receptive language disorders also have an expressive language disability.

Of course, some misuse of sounds, words, or grammar is a normal part of learning to speak. It is only when these problems persist that there is any cause for concern.

Academic skills disorders Students with academic skills disorders often lag far behind their classmates in developing reading, writing, or arithmetic skills. The diagnoses in this category include:

- developmental reading disorder
- developmental writing disorder
- developmental arithmetic disorder

Developmental reading disorder (also known as dyslexia) is quite widespread, affecting between 2 percent and 8 percent of elementary school children. The ability to read requires a rich, intact network of nerve cells that connect the brain's centers of vision, language, and memory. While a person can have problems in any of the tasks involved in reading, scientists have found that a significant number of people with dyslexia share an inability to distinguish or separate the sounds in spoken words. For example, a child might not be able to identify the word "cat" by sounding out the individual letters, c-a-t, or to play rhyming games. Fortunately, remedial reading specialists have developed techniques that can help many children with dyslexia acquire these skills. However, there is more to reading than recognizing words. If the brain cannot form images or relate new ideas to those stored in memory, the reader will not be able to understand or remember the new concepts. This is why other types of reading disabilities can appear in the upper grades when the focus of reading shifts from word identification to comprehension.

Writing, too, involves several brain areas and functions. The brain networks for vocabulary, grammar, hand movement, and memory must all work well if the child is to be able to write well. A *developmental writing disorder* may be caused by problems in any of these areas. A child with a writing disability, particularly an expressive language disorder, might be unable to compose complete, grammatical sentences.

Arithmetic involves recognizing numbers and symbols, memorizing facts such as the multiplication table, aligning numbers, and understanding abstract concepts like place value and fractions. Any of these may be difficult for children with *developmental arithmetic disorders*. Problems with numbers or basic concepts are likely to show up early, whereas problems that appear in the later grades are more often tied to problems in reasoning.

Many aspects of speaking, listening, reading, writing, and arithmetic overlap and build on the same brain capabilities. So it is not surprising that people can be diagnosed as having more than one area of learning disability. For example, the ability to understand language underlies the ability to learn to speak. Therefore, any disorder that interferes with the ability to understand language will also interfere with the development of speech, which in turn hinders learning to read and write. A single problem in the brain's operation can disrupt many types of activity.

"Other" Learning Disabilities There are additional categories of learning disabilities, such as "motor skills disorders" and "specific developmental disorders not otherwise specified." These diagnoses include delays in acquiring language, academic, and motor skills that can affect the ability to learn but do not meet the criteria for a specific learning disability. Also included are coordination disorders that can lead to poor penmanship, as well as certain spelling and memory disorders.

Attention disorders Nearly 4 million school-age children have learning disabilities; of these, at least 20 percent also have a type of disorder that leaves them unable to focus their attention. Some children and adults who have attention disorders are easily distracted or appear to daydream constantly. Children with this problem may have a number of learning difficulties.

In a large proportion of affected children (mostly boys) the attention deficit is accompanied by hyperactivity, running into traffic, or toppling desks. Hyperactive children cannot sit still: they blurt out answers, they interrupt, they cannot wait their turn. Because of their constant motion and explosive energy, hyperactive children often get into trouble with parents, teachers, and peers. By adolescence, physical hyperactivity usually subsides into fidgeting and restlessness, but the problems with attention and concentration often continue into adulthood.

At work, adults with ADHD often have trouble organizing tasks or completing their work. They do not seem to listen to or follow directions. Their work may be messy and appear careless.

Attention disorders (with or without hyperactivity) are not considered learning disabilities in themselves, but, because attention problems can seriously interfere with school performance, they often accompany academic skills disorders.

Treatment Options and Outlook

By law, a learning disability can be defined as a significant gap between a person's intelligence and the skills the person has achieved at each age. This means that a severely retarded 10-year-old who speaks like a six-year-old probably does not have a language or speech disability. He or she has mastered language up to the limits of intelligence. On the other hand, a fifth-grader with an IQ of 100 who cannot write a simple sentence probably does have a learning disability.

LEARNING DISORDERS may be informally flagged by observing significant delays in the child's skill development. Psychologists generally determine delays in the development of academic skills by comparing the statistical relationship between the IQ and achievement tests. If this statistical relationship is not known, psychologists must resort to less reliable ways of comparing potential and actual achievement. One alternative procedure is to simply compare IQ scores with the standard scores children obtain on achievement scales. The problem with this procedure is that directly comparing IQ and achievement test standard scores does not take into account how strongly the IQ and achievement test may be related. If a child's IQ is 85, for example, the predicted standard score in basic reading may be 90 on one test and 94 on another. Using a direct comparison of IQ and standard scores assumes that all IQ tests are related to all achievement tests to the same degree.

Parents and professionals should each gather information and discuss concerns about a child who is struggling with learning problems. The child's parents should arrange for a comprehensive psychoeducational evaluation, which can take place only with the parent's written consent. Evaluations can help identify the child's relative strengths and difficulties, and help determine whether the student is eligible for special assistance in school.

When parents and school staff agree, the public school system must provide an evaluation to determine if a student is entitled to special education services. Evaluations can be arranged for free through the school system, or through private clinics, private evaluators, hospital clinics, or university clinics. However, some school districts may not automatically accept test results from outside sources. Parents should check with their school district before seeking evaluation services from private facilities.

The actual diagnosis of learning disabilities is made using standardized tests that compare the child's level of ability to what is considered normal development for a person of that age and intelligence. Test outcomes depend not only on the child's actual abilities, but also on the reliability of the test and the child's ability to pay attention and understand the questions.

Each type of LD is diagnosed in slightly different ways. To diagnose speech and language disorders, a speech therapist tests the child's pronunciation, vocabulary, and grammar and compares them to the developmental abilities seen in most children that age. A psychologist tests the child's intelligence. A physician checks for any ear infections, and an audiologist may be consulted to rule out auditory problems. If the problem involves articulation, a doctor examines the child's vocal cords and throat. In the case of academic skills disorders, academic development in reading, writing, and math is evaluated using individually administered standardized tests. In addition, vision and hearing are tested to be sure the student can see words clearly and can hear adequately. The specialist also checks if the child has missed much school. It is important to rule out these other possible factors. After all, treatment for a learning disability is very different from the remedy for poor vision or missing school.

ADHD is diagnosed by checking for the long-term presence of specific behaviors, such as considerable fidgeting, losing things, interrupting, and talking excessively, and by ruling out medical factors that may sometimes cause the same behavioral symptoms. Other signs include an inability to remain seated, stay on task, or take turns. A diagnosis of ADHD is made only if the child shows such behaviors substantially more than other children of the same age.

If the school fails to notice a learning delay, parents can request an outside evaluation. Federal law requires school districts to maintain lists of sources for outside evaluations that can be obtained at public expense. Parents are also free to seek private evaluations by qualified individuals. By federal law, school districts must consider the results of any outside evaluation, although they may challenge the validity of those results, the qualifications of the examiner, or the appropriateness of the conclusions reached by the evaluator. After confirming the diagnosis, the public school is obligated to provide an appropriate educational program.

Parents should stay abreast of each step of the school's evaluation, and they may appeal the school's decision if they disagree with the findings of the diagnostic team. Parents always have the option of getting a second opinion. However, even when parents decide to obtain an outside evaluation, school districts must follow the same procedures required by federal law before they place a child in special education. For example, school districts must try to intervene with a child's learning problems for a reasonable period of time and document that their strategies for overcoming the problems are not working. An outside evaluator's recommendation for immediate placement cannot take precedence over such requirements. In addition, even if parents get an outside evaluation, the decision to classify or not classify a child as "learning disabled" rests with the placement team, to which the parents belong. Parents are free to appeal the decision to classify or to not classify and, if they lose, they may take court action. But contrary to the common perception, a private evaluator may not dictate classification and placement to the placement team.

Remediation   Although a diagnosis is important, even more important is creating a plan for getting the right help. Schools typically provide special education programs either in a separate all-day ("self-contained") classroom or as a special education class that the student attends for several hours each week ("resource classes"). Some parents hire trained tutors to work with their child after school. If the problems are severe, some parents choose to place their child in a special school for the learning disabled. However, a child's school district is not obligated to pay for this placement unless the district agrees to the placement, or they are directed to pay as the result of a due process hearing or court action. Parents cannot simply decide on their own to place their child into a facility and expect reimbursement from their local school district.

Planning a special education program begins with systematically identifying what the student can and cannot do. The specialist looks for patterns in the child's gaps, such as the failure to hear the separate sounds in words or other sound discrimination problems. Special education teachers also identify the types of tasks the child can do and the senses that function well. By using the senses that are intact and bypassing the disabilities, many children can develop needed skills. These strengths offer alternative ways in which the child can learn.

After assessing the child's strengths and weaknesses, the special education teacher designs an INDIVIDUALIZED EDUCATION PROGRAM (IEP). The IEP outlines the specific skills the child needs to develop as well as appropriate learning activities that build on the child's strengths. Many effective learning activities engage several skills and senses. For example, in learning to spell and recognize words, a student may be asked to see, say, write, and spell each new word. The student may also write the words in sand, which engages the sense of touch. Many experts believe that the more senses children use in learning a skill, the more likely they are to retain it.

An individualized, skill-based approach often succeeds in helping where regular classroom instruction fails. Therapy for speech and language disorders focuses on providing a stimulating but structured environment for hearing and practicing language patterns. For example, the therapist may help a child who has an articulation disorder to produce specific speech sounds. During an engaging activity, the therapist may talk about the toys, then encourage the child to use the same sounds or words. In addition, the child may watch the therapist make the sound, feel the vibration in the therapist's throat, then practice making the sounds before a mirror.

Assistive technology   Learning disabilities cannot be cured, but with the help of certain tools a child with a learning disability can work around difficulties with reading, writing, numbers, spelling, organization, or memory. Complex, high-tech tools and devices, called ASSISTIVE TECHNOLOGY, can help people work around specific deficits.

Tools for people with learning disabilities can be as simple as highlighters, color coding files or drawers, books on tape, tape recorders, calculators, or a different paper color or background color on a computer screen. Sometimes standard technologies (such as voice recognition systems) can be adapted or designed to help people with learning disabilities perform everyday tasks. Complex assistive technology includes talking computers that help people with reading and writing difficulties, speech recognition systems that translate oral language into written text, talking calculators that assist people with math difficulties, and software that suggests spelling for people with spelling difficulties.

Researchers are also investigating nonstandard teaching methods. Some create artificial learning conditions that may help the brain receive information in nonstandard ways. For example, in some language disorders, the brain seems abnormally slow to process verbal information. Scientists are testing whether computers that talk can help teach children to process spoken sounds more quickly. The computer starts slowly, pronouncing one sound at a time. As the child gets better at recognizing the sounds and hearing them as words, the sounds are gradually speeded up to a normal rate of speech.

History   Early in the 20th century, certain children had come to the attention of a British physician, eye surgeon James Hinshelwood, M.D., who tried to correlate his knowledge of patients who had received head injury from disease or trauma with the similar symptoms he saw in children with reading problems. In 1917 he published research in which he used "word blindness" to refer to dyslexia.

In the early 1930s, American psychiatrist SAMUEL ORTON, M.D., refused to accept the belief that emotional difficulties were behind learning problems. He noted, for example, that children with learning problems often displayed "mixed laterality," and suggested that the failure of one hemisphere of the brain to become dominant caused the disorder. Today, factors around hemispheric dominance are still considered important in the field of learning disabilities.

After World War I, an encephalitis epidemic left a number of cases of brain damage, which lead to the description of the disorganized and erratic behavior associated with hyperactivity. In 1947, German neurologist and psychiatrist Alfred Strauss described this syndrome in children, noting both perceptual and abstract reasoning problems. Although for a time hyperactivity was described as "Strauss syndrome," the terms *brain damaged* and *brain injured* became common.

In 1959, noting perceptual and learning similarities in patients with cerebral palsy and other neurological handicaps, researchers in the field proposed the term *cerebral dysfunction* to include cerebral palsy, mental retardation, and what was then called "hyperkinetic behavior disorder," characterized by irritability, short attention span, purposeless activity, and poor school work in reading, arithmetic, and handwriting.

In 1963, American experts began planning a series of task forces to investigate learning disabilities, in part because of parental pressure.

Certainly since 1968 the field of learning disabilities has been characterized by conflict and confusion, as the original focus and the term *learning disability* stretched to include all children who were underachieving for any reason. On the other hand, it is very possible that this "exclusion clause" has had the effect of excluding from appropriate programs children with learning disabilities who have come from disadvantaged backgrounds. Often the learning problems of such children would be diagnosed only in terms of their deprived environment, and not looked at in the real context of physiological causes. Thus, learning disabilities have tended to become a middle-class phenomenon—while the child of the middle class would be diagnosed as having a learning disability, a child of the slums would automatically be considered deprived. Unfortunate also has been the designation of learning disabilities as solely an educational problem and not a medical or health problem.

In 1981, a position paper on the definition was prepared by the National Joint Committee for Learning Disabilities (NJCLD), composed of five major and concerned organizations in the United States. The committee urged that the disorders represented by the collective term *learning disabilities* be understood as intrinsic to the individual, and that the basis of the disorders be presumed to be due to central nervous system dysfunction.

Controversy   The term *learning disability* was coined by psychologist Samuel A. Kirk in 1963 to describe children who experience difficulty acquiring academic skills despite normal intelligence. He proposed this term because of his discomfort with the widespread use in an educational setting of medically oriented terms such as *dyslexia, congenital word blindness, reading and math retardation,* and MINIMAL BRAIN DYSFUNCTION. Although the term has become widely accepted, there has been a great deal of controversy about the exact definition and methods of ASSESSMENT and identification of the condition.

The term has provided a focal point for legislation and advocacy that has resulted in far-reaching changes in the nature of public and postsecondary education in the United States. At the same time, the term *learning disabilities*, the range of potential learning problems that it includes, and the broad and rapidly changing field that it describes, continue to be controversial. In fact, there is still no consensus on the definition of learning disabilities or on what the category should include or exclude, and the coming years are likely to see continuing debate on the fundamental issues of definition, classification, diagnosis, and treatment.

According to the NJCLD, the term refers to a group of disorders marked by significant difficulties in listening, speaking, reading, writing, reasoning, or mathematical abilities. These disorders are presumed to be caused by central nervous system dysfunction, and may occur at any time. Although learning disabilities may appear at the same time as other handicapping conditions (such as deafness, blindness, mental retardation, or serious emotional disturbance), they are not caused by these conditions.

The primary legal definition of a learning disability, according to Public Law 94-142 (as amended by Public Law 101-76), indicates a disorder in one or more of the basic psychological processes involved in understanding or in using spoken or written language. This may include an imperfect ability to listen, think, speak, read, write, spell, or to do mathematical calculations. The term includes such conditions as perceptual handicaps, brain injury, minimal brain dysfunction, dyslexia, and developmental aphasia. The term does not include children who have problems primarily caused by visual, hearing, or motor disabilities, or by mental retardation, emotional disturbance, or by environmental, cultural, or economic disadvantage.

Most definitions suggest that learning disabilities are permanent, affect a range of language and mathematics functions, and are caused at least in part from problems within the central nervous system. In addition, definitions of LD have generally focused on two key identifying factors: discrepancy and exclusion.

Discrepancy means that a child with a learning disability exhibits a significant gap between aptitude and performance. In many states, a diagnosis of a learning disability depends on a very strict statistical measurement of this discrepancy between achievement and aptitude.

Unfortunately, Congress has never provided any guidance as to what it meant by the requirement of "a severe discrepancy between potential and achievement," which has led to widely differing practices for making such a determination.

Exclusion means that a learning disability is not caused by some other handicapping condition, such as physical impairment or social status. A child who struggles to learn because she cannot see, or because he comes from a background of poverty and disadvantage, is not considered to have a learning disability if these are the primary factors in the learning problems.

Both the discrepancy formulation for learning disabilities, and the role that exclusion of other conditions plays, have become subjects for increasing debate in recent years. Many researchers have proposed redefining the concept of learning disabilities to focus on specific language and thought processing problems that may be identified by appropriate testing, without necessarily involving the question of aptitude or intellectual potential.

Some experts have argued that the exclusionary element in definitions of LD has led to the underidentification or misdiagnosis of individuals who come from poverty or from minority cultural, racial, or ethnic backgrounds. They argue that the difficulties such children have in learning are more likely to be caused by their backgrounds and upbringing than to a potential learning disability, and that approaches to diagnosis that depend on aptitude/achievement discrepancies are also likely to underrepresent such individuals.

A third major area of controversy has to do with excluding social and behavioral disabilities from standard definitions of learning disabilities, and to excluding ADHD from this general category. This debate is highlighted by the difference between the NJCLD definition quoted above and the following definition from the National Institute of Mental Health:

Learning Disabilities (LD) is a disorder that affects people's ability to either interpret what they see and hear or to link information from different parts of the brain. These limitations can show up in many ways—as specific difficulties with spoken and written language, coordination, self-control, or attention. Such difficulties extend to school-work and can impede learning to read or write, or to do math.

Learning disabilities can be lifelong conditions that, in some cases, affect many parts of a person's life: school or work, daily routines, family life, and sometimes even friendships and play. In some people, many overlapping learning disabilities may be apparent. Other people may have a single, isolated learning problem that has little impact on other areas of their lives.

The continuing controversy and debate that surrounds the concept of learning disabilities is complicated by different disciplines and theoretical perspectives, as well as the advocacy of parents, economic pressures on school districts, and political and legal developments. These controversies are likely to continue in the years to come.

Treatment for learning disabilities is extremely important if the child is to be successful. In fact, 35 percent of students with untreated learning disabilities do not finish high school, and drop out before they receive transitional vocational services to help them get a job. Most students with learning disabilities were not fully employed one year after graduating from high school. Adolescents with untreated learning disabilities are at higher risk for drug and alcohol abuse. One study showed that up to 60 percent of adolescents in treatment for substance abuse had learning disabilities.

Even though learning disabilities cannot be cured, there is still cause for hope. Because certain learning problems reflect delayed development, many children do eventually catch up.

Of the speech and language disorders, children who have an articulation or an expressive language disorder are the least likely to have long-term problems. Despite initial delays, most children do learn to speak. For people with dyslexia, the outlook is mixed. But an appropriate remedial reading program can help learners make great strides. With age, and appropriate help from parents and clinicians, children with ADHD become better able to suppress their hyperactivity and to channel it into more socially acceptable behaviors.

Federal Protection As of 1981, people with learning disabilities were included under the pro-
tection of laws originally designed to protect the rights of people with mobility handicaps. More recent federal laws specifically guarantee equal opportunity and raise the level of services to people with disabilities. Once a learning disability is identified, children are guaranteed a free public education specifically designed around their individual needs. Adolescents with disabilities can receive practical assistance and extra training to help make the transition to jobs and independent living. Adults have access to job training and technology that open new doors of opportunity.

The INDIVIDUALS WITH DISABILITIES EDUCATION IMPROVEMENT ACT of 1990 assures a public education to school-age children with diagnosed learning disabilities. Under this act, public schools are required to design and implement an individualized education program tailored to each child's specific needs. The 1991 IDEIA extended services to developmentally delayed children as young as five. This law makes it possible for young children to receive help even before they begin school.

IDEIA was updated December 3, 2004. The signing marked the end of a three-year reauthorization process and represented the first update to the nation's special education law in seven years. At the foundation of the new law are the findings of the 2002 President's Commission on Excellence in Special Education, which recommended special education reforms based on academic results for students, early intervention, parental choice, and paperwork reduction.

The revision is an attempt to update and improve the criteria for identifying a specific learning disability by eliminating the requirement that students must exhibit a severe discrepancy between ability and achievement in order to be found eligible for services under IDEIA (regardless of age). This requirement had been part of IDEIA federal regulations since 1977 and, according to a 2000 survey conducted by the National Association of State Directors of Special Education (NASDSE), all 50 states have required a severe discrepancy between ability and achievement for purposes of LD special education eligibility. There is widespread agreement that such policies require students to experience failure for several years in order to show the requisite degree of discrepancy. Despite the fact that clinical judgment, curriculum-based assessments, discrepant results on achievement assessments, parental information and other factors might all point to the presence of a learning disability, before the IDEIA revision, a student could not have been found eligible under the specific learning disability category if this severe discrepancy did not exist. This new language represents the first change in how states may determine the existence of a specific learning disability since the law was passed nearly 30 years ago. The change in the evaluation procedures section of the law will grant greater flexibility to local and state education agencies as they begin to implement new models for identification, and will inflate the incidence of learning disabilities, according to some experts.

The 2004 revisions to IDEIA maintain the definition of specific learning disabilities that is contained in the current IDEIA, including the disorders that are not included under this definition, such as a learning problem that is primarily the result of visual, hearing, or motor disabilities, of mental retardation, of emotional disturbance, or of environmental, cultural, or economic disadvantage.

The AMERICANS WITH DISABILITIES ACT of 1990 guarantees equal employment opportunity for people with learning disabilities and protects disabled workers against job discrimination. Employers may not consider the learning disability when selecting among job applicants, and must make "reasonable accommodations" to help workers who have handicaps do their job. Such ACCOMMODATIONS may include shifting job responsibilities, modifying equipment, or adjusting work schedules.

By law, public colleges and universities must remove barriers that keep out disabled students. As a result, many colleges now recruit students with learning disabilities. Depending on the student's areas of difficulty, the school may offer help including recorded books and lectures, providing an isolated area to take tests, or allowing a student to tape rather than write reports. Students with learning disabilities can arrange to take college entrance exams orally or in isolated rooms free from distraction. Many colleges are creating special programs to specifically accommodate these students.

Local school districts can help parents identify the requirements and the process for getting special education services for their child. If parents do not get the answers here, they can contact their state department of public instruction. Other agencies serve disabled infants and preschool children, while still others offer mental health and counseling services. The National Information Center for Children and Youth can provide referrals to appropriate local resources and state agencies.

Counselors at each state department of vocational rehabilitation serve the employment needs of adolescents and adults with learning disabilities. They can refer adults to free or subsidized health care, counseling, and high school equivalence (GED) programs. They can assist in arranging for job training that sidesteps the disability. State departments of vocational rehabilitation can also assist in finding special equipment that can make it possible for disabled individuals to receive training, retain a job, or live on their own.

Finally, state-run protection and advocacy agencies and client assistance programs serve to protect these rights. As experts on the laws, they offer legal assistance, as well as information about local health, housing, and social services. School districts must maintain lists of agencies and organizations that parents can contact for help in obtaining services for a child suspected of having a handicap.

Consequences People with learning disabilities who have not been diagnosed or properly treated, experience serious, lifelong negative consequences including low SELF-ESTEEM, delinquency, and ILLITERACY. Thirty-five percent of students identified with learning disabilities drop out of high school (this does not include students who drop out without being identified as having learning disabilities). Fifty to 80 percent of adults with severe literacy problems have undetected or untreated learning disabilities. Fifty percent of young criminal offenders tested were found to have previously undetected learning disabilities; when offered educational services that addressed their learning disability, the recidivism rates of these young offenders dropped to below 2 percent.

learning disorder A more specific term than LEARNING DISABILITY, but without the same legal weight. A learning disorder may include any of a broad spectrum of dysfunctions in the ability to learn, including some syndromes and difficulties that are not generally grouped under the category of learning disabilities.

Learning disorders refer to the specific mental processes involved in learning problems. For example, the inability to remember information that the student hears in a specific order (referred to as a disorder in auditory-sequential memory) would be referred to as a learning disorder.

learning modalities   The way in which information is received and expressed, such as visual, tactile, auditory, or kinesthetic. Generally, individuals have strengths in a certain modality and learn better when information is presented through that channel. For example, an individual whose strongest learning modality is visual will have difficulty learning information given by lecture alone, with no visual aids such as notes on the board.

Research shows that since people have different learning strengths, it is better to design lessons that use more than one modality, such as a combination of visual and auditory. This allows all learners, including those with learning disabilities, to access information using their strongest learning modality.

learning strategies   The idea that *how* an individual learns is more important than *what* he or she learns. This is an especially useful approach with individuals who have a LEARNING DISABILITY and who may not learn efficiently.

Learning strategies include the cognitive (thinking) aspect of learning as well as the behavioral (actions) aspect of learning to help individuals in planning, executing, and evaluating a learning task. Components of teaching learning strategies would include teaching individuals to be active participants in their learning, encouraging collaborative learning, and utilizing questioning to aid in comprehension.

learning style   An individual's behavior, temperament, and attitude in a learning situation. Some of the best-known learning styles are visual, auditory, or kinesthetic. Some experts argue that it is important to match an individual's learning style with the style of instruction to make learning easier. For example, an individual with a strong visual learning style should be taught to read with an emphasis on the shapes of words.

There are many different learning styles, but none are either "right" or "wrong." Although a student may prefer one style over another, preferences develop like muscles: the more they are used, the stronger they become. Successful students have flexible and integrated learning styles. No one uses one of the styles exclusively, and there is usually significant overlap in learning styles.

Visual learners relate most effectively to written information, notes, diagrams, and pictures. Typically they will be unhappy with a presentation where they cannot take detailed notes. To a degree, information does not exist for a visual learner unless it has been seen written down. This is why some visual learners take notes even when they have printed notes in front of them. Visual learners will tend to be most effective in written communication. They make up about 65 percent of the population.

Auditory learners relate most effectively to the spoken word. They tend to listen to a lecture and then take notes afterward, or rely on printed notes. Because written information will often have little meaning until it is heard, it may help auditory learners to read written information out loud. Auditory learners may be sophisticated speakers, and may specialize in subjects like law or politics. Auditory learners make up about 30 percent of the population.

Kinesthetic learners learn best through touch, movement, and space, and learn skills by imitation and practice. Kinesthetic learners can appear slow, because information is usually not presented in a style that suits their learning methods. Kinesthetic learners make up around 5 percent of the population.

learning style inventory   A test or questionnaire that tries to assess the way a person learns (LEARNING STYLE). Understanding a person's learning style can help a teacher develop appropriate ways to teach.

There are many learning style inventories available, such as the Myers-Briggs Personality Type Indicator, based on Carl Jung's theories of conscious functioning, or the Grasha-Riechmann Student Learning Style Scales, developed by Anthony Grasha and Sheryl Riechmann, who designed a test to assess adolescent differences by focusing on how students interact with teachers and colleagues with respect to their learning processes.

Interest in learning style inventories has increased since the growth in popularity of a multiple intelligences perspective to learning.

least restrictive environment   The setting where a pupil with a disability can be educated with no more segregation than is absolutely necessary. Students with disabilities should have the opportunity to participate as fully as possible in school and school activities with classmates who are not disabled.

The concept of "least restrictive environment" is one of the most confusing and controversial in education for children with disabilities. As originally formulated in Public Law 94-142, children with disabilities were to be guaranteed a "free appropriate public education" in the "least restrictive environment," but it was not clear what that meant.

The concept was more fully described in the INDIVIDUALS WITH DISABILITIES EDUCATION IMPROVEMENT ACT, which required that learning disabled students be placed, when appropriate, in settings with regular (non-special education) students to provide maximum opportunities to learn in the least restrictive environment.

Generally, there is a presumption that a child with a disability should be served in the regular classroom with as much interaction with non-handicapped classmates as possible, although some disagree. According to current federal law, a child with a disability may be removed from the regular classroom only when the nature or severity of the disability is such that the education in regular classes cannot be achieved satisfactorily, even with the use of supplementary aids and services.

However, for specific areas of intensive training or if a child's handicap makes him disruptive to others, it is appropriate to remove a child from the regular classroom. For example, a child with a reading disability may appropriately be educated in most academic areas in the regular classroom with assistance in note taking and test taking, but it may be necessary to remove the child from the classroom to work in a small group or one-on-one,

specifically in the area of reading. The child's placement and services depend on the child's individual needs, not on administrative convenience.

Before a student's least restrictive environment is determined, the student's educational needs must be identified. This is the job of the CHILD STUDY COMMITTEE, made up of the student's parents, teacher, school administrator, and others who know the student. After the team determines the student's educational strengths and needs, it develops annual program goals and objectives, which are part of the INDIVIDUALIZED EDUCATION PROGRAM (IEP). Only after the IEP is developed does the team consider the placement options. In fact, the IEP drives all aspects of the child's educational program.

There must be compelling educational reasons, based on the individual student's educational needs, for removing the student from the regular classroom. Those reasons must be listed on the IEP.

legally blind   A legal term that is used to determine eligibility for services. Many individuals who are legally blind are not totally blind, but have—and use—some vision.

legal rights/protection   See INDIVIDUALS WITH DISABILITIES EDUCATION IMPROVEMENT ACT; REHABILITATION ACT OF 1973.

legislation related to learning disabilities   A number of federal laws have been passed to ensure that children with LEARNING DISABILITIES (LD) are given a free and appropriate education. These include the recently revised INDIVIDUALS WITH DISABILITIES EDUCATION IMPROVEMENT ACT (once known as the Education for All Handicapped Children Act of 1975), and the REHABILITATION ACT OF 1973.

Individuals with Disabilities Education Improvement Act (IDEIA)   IDEIA is a federally mandated program that assures a free and appropriate public education for children with diagnosed educational deficits. It was revised in 2004 in an attempt to update and improve the criteria for identifying a specific learning disability by eliminating the requirement that students must exhibit a severe discrepancy between ability and achievement in order to be found eligible for services under the IDEIA (regardless of age). This requirement had been part of the IDEIA federal regulations since

1977 and, according to a 2000 survey conducted by the National Association of State Directors of Special Education (NASDSE), all 50 states have required a severe discrepancy between ability and achievement for purposes of LD special education eligibility. There is widespread agreement that such policies require students to experience failure for several years in order to show the requisite degree of discrepancy. Despite the fact that clinical judgment, curriculum-based assessments, discrepant results on achievement assessments, parental information, and other factors might all point to the presence of learning disability, before the IDEIA revision, a student could not have been found eligible if this severe discrepancy did not exist.

A child under age three with special needs should be eligible for an early intervention program available in every state, provided by qualified workers in the child's home or place familiar to the child. This might include a physical activity to help develop coordination and body awareness, such as stringing beads or working on a puzzle. Social interaction is encouraged, and children learn by doing with positive reinforcement.

Rehabilitation Act [RA] of 1973 This major law requires that schools must not discriminate against children with a list of specific disabilities (including learning disabilities) and that they must provide children with reasonable ACCOMMODATIONS. While the IDEIA focuses on free appropriate public education for children with disabilities, section 504 of the Rehabilitation Act is intended to prohibit discrimination against individuals with handicaps in programs receiving federal money. This law is more general, with a broader definition of "disabled" rather than the "handicapped" definition in IDEIA.

Unlike IDEIA, which applies mostly to public elementary and high school children with disabilities, the RA also applies to postsecondary institutions that receive federal money. Eligibility for this law is based on the existence of an identified physical or mental condition that substantially limits a major life activity, such as learning. Children diagnosed with ATTENTION DEFICIT HYPERACTIVITY DISORDER (ADHD) are therefore entitled to protection of section 504 if the disability substantially limits their ability to learn. Children who are not eligible for SPECIAL EDUCATION services may still be guaranteed access to related services if they meet the section 504 eligibility criteria.

letter recognition The ability to recognize all letters in the alphabet, the building blocks of words and sentences. Early readers and individuals with learning disabilities may confuse visually similar letters such as "b" and "d" or "m" and "n." Letter recognition is an important pre-reading skill that leads to word recognition in the decoding process. It is generally introduced in preschool or kindergarten.

As young children master the alphabet song and recite their ABCs, they also must learn to identify the shapes that represent those sounds. Children are often quick to recognize the letters in their names, but other letters may be less familiar.

lifetime education A philosophy of education that suggests learning need not be restricted to a certain early period of a person's life, but should engage in learning activities throughout their lives.

limbic system A combination of neural structures folded around the top of the brainstem that is linked to the development of LEARNING DISABILITIES. The limbic system is involved in the production of emotional responses connected to fear and aggression and is also associated with interest in food, drink, and sex. It includes the hippocampus, the amygdala, and the hypothalamus.

lindane A solid organochloride pesticide that evaporates quickly into the air and that does not occur naturally in the environment. Its primary use is to kill head lice, body lice, and scabies, and it was used for 50 years in agriculture to kill bugs on fruits and vegetables. As a toxic chemical, it was used as a chemical weapon during World War I, and it is also used for medical research to induce seizures in rats. The Agency for Toxic Substances and Disease Registry has prioritized lindane as 33rd on its list of 275 most hazardous substances.

Although there has been little study on human exposure to lindane during pregnancy, some research suggests there is a possibility that lindane can damage the central nervous system of an unborn child, leading to developmental, behavioral, and LEARNING DISABILITIES. Traces of lindane have been found in human breast milk all over the world. In 2003, the U.S. Food and Drug Administration (FDA) repackaged lindane and included a detailed and restrictive "black box" warning. The FDA classifies lindane as a second choice treatment to more efficient and less toxic alternatives and states that children, the elderly, and pregnant women should not use this product due to its toxicity.

Lindane is found in the air near factories that produce it and locally after it has been applied. It can remain in the air for up to 17 weeks, traveling quite far. It takes rain or snow to remove it from the air, bringing it down to earth, and into the water.

Lindane is being phased out of production and use in the United States but is still widely used in other countries that export products here.

The most serious exposure occurs through direct skin contact such as lice or scabies treatment, especially for children. Other points of contact come from eating contaminated food such as meats, fruits, vegetables, and milk. Breathing it in the air near factories that produce it is hazardous as well is drinking contaminated water.

linguistic approach   A method of teaching reading and spelling that uses similar word patterns (word families). The linguistic approach emphasizes the predictability and regularity of English word patterns by incorporating them in sentences and stories such as "The fat cat sat on the big mat."

linguistics   The formal study of language, including the sound system, development, and function of human languages. Linguistic theory and the understanding of natural language processing provided by linguistics are essential to understanding how language processing may differ for individuals with language-based LEARNING DISABILITIES.

listening comprehension level   The highest grade level of material that can be understood well when it is read aloud to a student. Listening comprehension level, measured by reading successively more difficult passages to a student, is useful in estimating the student's potential silent reading level.

Although the suggested criteria vary, better than 75 percent comprehension is often used as a standard in judging whether a student understands material at this level.

listening vocabulary   The number of words a person understands when they are heard in speech; also, hearing vocabulary, sometimes called "receptive vocabulary."

literacy   The ability to read and write in a person's native language. The development of literacy is fairly recent in terms of human history; the first literate cultures appeared about 5,000 years ago. The development of literacy made possible the transmission of culture and scientific knowledge, historical chronicles, and stories and poetry, across generations in a relatively stable form. Many of the advances of global civilization are indebted in major ways to the role of literacy.

Before the rise of literacy, the transmission of culture was by word of mouth. Many famous texts such as the Homeric epics and the Bible first existed and were transmitted in oral form before they were written down. Until the most recent century, literacy was primarily limited to those within the socioeconomic elite of various cultures. Even today, the illiteracy rate is very high in many developing countries and among disadvantaged individuals in industrialized nations.

The rise of universal public education in Western industrial nations during the 1800s set the stage for a much broader literacy within the general population. It is not surprising that it was during this period that reading problems among some schoolchildren were first described. These early investigations were the first steps toward understanding the nature of DYSLEXIA and LEARNING DISABILITIES.

Illiteracy continues to be a major social problem in the United States, and is the focus of many contemporary movements toward reform in public school systems. However, the causes of illiteracy are complex, relating to social, economic, and cultural factors that schools are not capable of addressing independently. The role that undiagnosed learning disabilities play in the rate of illiteracy is most likely significant.

Local Education Agency   A formal term for a designated school district, as differentiated from the state education agency.

locus of control   A motivational term related to that source to which people attribute their successes or failures. People with an internal locus of control believe they are responsible for their own successes and failures, whereas people with an external locus of control would most often blame (or thank) fate, destiny, luck, society, or some other force beyond their control. Locus of control has great influence on a person's motivation, expectations, SELF-ESTEEM, risk-taking behavior, and even on the actual outcome of actions. Determining a person's locus of control is important in helping to address the individual's problems.

Children's motivation at school is linked to their belief in whether they have control over personal successes and failures. Children will not try hard if they believe they have no control over the outcome of the situation.

That influence extends to students with high ability as well as to students with low ability. For example, students with high ability but with an external locus of control attribute their early successes in school to fixed inborn ability. These students come to believe that they can coast on their inborn ability and that they will never make low grades because of that inborn ability. These students sometimes begin to earn drastically lower grades in middle school and high school than they did in elementary school because middle and high school grades are more performance-based, and because they do not feel any obligation to put forth strong effort.

Many children will fall between these two extremes of internal and external locus of control, and possess characteristics of each type. A child's locus of control tells a lot about behavior, actions, and motivations. An internalizer will do much better at school and in life than an externalizer, while an externalizer will think mistakes at school are caused by work that is too hard. Believing nothing can be done, this child will not try hard. Externalizers develop lower expectations, choose easier challenges, and give up quickly. These feelings of helplessness will extend to other situations and influence the child's outlook, attitudes, and motivation toward all activities.

Without a feeling of control or influence on what other people think, these children will not contact new people or try to repair friendships when problems occur.

An internalizer will expect to do well as a result of hard work, and will easily initiate conversations and play with other children. Internalizers will take the lead in solving problems and learning to share, reciprocate, and get along with others. An internalizer will excel at school and do better than other children of equal intelligence who are not internalizers.

Whether a child is an internalizer or externalizer is partly due to the parents' attitudes. A child's locus of control begins to develop at infancy, when they start to learn if they have control over the world around them. The more a child's crying is ignored during the first years, the more likely a child will feel powerless. As the child grows, parents should continue to nurture the child's locus of control. Encouraging independence will go a long way toward making a child an internalizer. Children who are allowed to make decisions, go places, and are given time to solve everyday problems tend to become internalizers. Children who are not granted these privileges usually become externalizers.

Externalizers will often have a dominating mother and father who make all the necessary decisions for them.

long-term memory   The long-range storage of information in MEMORY on a relatively permanent basis. A person can store an indefinite number of chunks of information in long-term memory in interconnected semantic networks.

What a person chooses to store in long-term memory is probably closely tied to the emotions. In fact, the LIMBIC SYSTEM, which mediates emotion in the brain, is highly involved in memory function. Because humans generally seek pleasure and shun pain, they tend to repeat something that is rewarding (remember it) and avoid what is painful (forget it).

Researchers divide long-term memory into three types: procedural, semantic, and episodic.

Procedural memory is the ability to remember how to do something (such as ride a horse or write a letter). Semantic memory involves remembering factual information, such as the capital of Oregon or the multiplication tables. It has no connection to where or when a person learned the information. Episodic memory involves remembering personal events, such as a first kiss or where one learned to ride a bike.

Long-term memory differs from short-term memory in more than the length of time that a memory is able to be retrieved. The nerve changes involved in long-term memory may be different; the process is not easily disrupted and its capacity is virtually unlimited. Retrieval from short-term memory is virtually automatic, but retrieval in long-term memory is not easy or always automatic.

M

mainstreaming The placement of disabled students in the regular education classroom, or in activities such as sports, field trips, or school programs, with nonhandicapped students. Mainstreaming was introduced in the 1970s as a result of PUBLIC LAW 94-142, which mandated that special needs children be placed in the LEAST RESTRICTIVE ENVIRONMENT. Until the approval of PL 94-142 in 1975, most special needs children (from mildly to severely disabled) were educated in self-contained settings.

The philosophy of mainstreaming disabled children into the regular classroom comes from the idea that, since most individuals will be "mainstreamed" into society, the integration of regular and special needs students should begin at an early age. It was also believed that school resources could be used more efficiently if special needs students were placed in the regular classroom. Mainstreaming also required regular educators to share the responsibility for disabled students with special educators. Conversely, mainstreaming benefits regular education students by increasing their understanding and tolerance of students with differences.

Longitudinal studies of mainstreaming over the past two decades indicate that mainstreaming is defined differently depending on the school and school district. In most school systems, mainstreaming involves placing a special needs student in the regular classroom setting for one subject area or a portion of the day depending on what is best for the student. According to research, mainstreaming can be a valid alternative to self-contained classrooms, but it is not an appropriate practice for all special needs students. A delicate balance must be struck among the student's need, teacher training, attitudes toward mainstreaming, and cost factors.

Most students with LEARNING DISABILITIES are educated in the regular classroom while receiving support services. Although parents sometimes worry that their children's needs will not be met in a regular classroom setting, mainstreaming does not mean that SPECIAL-EDUCATION students are "dumped" into classes indiscriminately. Rather, students are placed in a regular classroom with support services so they can perform adequately. The concept of mainstreaming is a response to the fact that students can benefit from regular classroom placement if they get additional assistance at the same time. Forms of assistance might be an aide, modification of instruction, more instruction time, and communication with the regular classroom teacher.

Parents of nondisabled children often complain that the disabled child might disrupt the class or take up too much of the teacher's time. Both are legitimate concerns, and if any child is so disruptive he interferes with the functioning of the class, then intervention is necessary. In fact, recent court decisions have established the school's right to remove disruptive students to more restrictive settings if they are preventing others from learning.

Considerable time, energy, and planning go into every successful mainstreaming experience. Parents must be advocates for their children and provide input about the type and amount of mainstreaming that takes place, and they need to forge positive relationships with school personnel. This should be done during the development and implementation of the INDIVIDUALIZED EDUCATION PROGRAM (IEP).

Mainstreaming works when

- parents and teachers work together
- specific mainstreaming experiences are recorded in the child's INDIVIDUALIZED EDUCATION PROGRAM (IEP)

- special education teachers meet with regular classroom teachers in the mainstreamed setting

- mainstream teachers get information on the special education student's strengths, needs, and techniques considered helpful for the student's particular learning disability

- mainstream teachers have time to consult with special education teachers to discuss student progress

- regular students are given information to better understand students with special needs

manic depression   See BIPOLAR DISORDER.

mapping   In educational terms, a strategy for displaying related ideas in a visual format. Mapping may refer to flow charts, diagrams, or using color-coding to draw connections and help recall information. One important example of mapping is "mind-mapping" (also called clustering), which is used in the process of writing to generate and organize ideas and information that can eventually be translated into a linear outline.

A mind map might consist of a core topic at the center of the page, with major subtopics spreading outward from it, and relevant details attached to each subtopic. Such an approach may be especially helpful for individuals who have difficulty with sequencing information but are strong in the area of visual-spatial reasoning.

Likewise, a GRAPHIC ORGANIZER for representing information may help a student who has trouble with reading comprehension because of problems organizing and identifying key information and relationships between concepts and supporting evidence.

margin notes   Notes placed in the margins of texts in order to paraphrase main ideas or important details in the reader's words. Margin noting is an effective way to become an active reader. By condensing information in the reader's own words, margin notes serve to enhance comprehension, boost recall, and simplify reviewing.

mastery   Learning a skill to the point where an individual uses the skill automatically, consistently,

and without cuing, in a variety of contexts. Mastery of a specific skill can be measured in a number of ways. One such measurement may be a mastery test, which is designed to assess the application of a specific skill.

In order to master material, children need to be appropriately placed and given adequate instruction. The following four criteria should be used to place children appropriately in an instructional setting:

1. A child should understand material taught with 70 percent correctness.

2. A child should score 90 percent on material previously taught and reviewed.

3. Children should complete material in a "lesson" in the anticipated amount of time and shouldn't need more practice.

4. Children should completely understand material presented at the end of each lesson.

These criteria are rarely met in a school setting in which classes are heterogeneous, with children of varying abilities, and when individual instruction time may be limited. Proponents of DIRECT INSTRUCTION suggest that rote drill and practice is required for mastery of basic skills. Nonetheless, children often are moved from one grade level to the next without mastering skills or course content.

mathematics disorder   A disorder in which mathematical ability, as measured by individually administered standardized tests, is substantially below what is expected given the child's chronological age, intelligence, and education level. The disorder significantly interferes with academic achievement and with activities of daily living that require mathematical ability.

math facts   Basic addition, subtraction, and multiplication, the automatic recall of which helps speed up computation.

math manipulatives   Objects such as blocks, coins, or buttons that students can use to help them learn math.

math phobia   A fear or anxiety about learning mathematics.

math skills Mathematics is a core academic curriculum, which typically is taught sequentially through each grade level. The sequence of math skills starts from simple and concrete (counting and classification in kindergarten) to more complex and abstract skills (scientific notation in middle school).

Sound math instruction should include teaching concepts, skills, and problem solving rather than an accumulation of computation skills. Math skill development requires opportunities for practice and review, learning to generalize skills to a variety of situations, and understanding math vocabulary.

To master arithmetic, children must understand numbers (that is, the quantity that each number represents), counting, the conceptual (such as understanding the base-10 number system) and procedural (such as borrowing from one column to the next) features involved in solving simple and complex arithmetic problems.

Just when and how children acquire these skills is fairly theoretical, although most current research supports psychologist JEAN PIAGET's theory that youngsters develop math concepts in four stages. Although recent research has revised Piaget's time line, the sequence remains the same. Piaget's stages included

1. sensorimotor: birth to two years (manipulates objects, uses trial and error, thinks through solutions mentally)

2. preoperational: two to four years (uses reason, but not logic)

3. concrete operational: seven to 11 years (solves concrete problems, can reverse thought process, develops classification skills, learns to sort by category, understands serial order)

4. formal operations: 11 to 15 years and up (uses abstract reasoning, applies logic, solves verbal problems and problems dealing with the future, develops capacity to think scientifically

A LEARNING DISABILITY in math can result from problems in learning any one or any combination of these more basic skills. To complicate matters further, it is possible that different children can have different patterns of strength and weakness when it comes to understanding and learning these basic skills.

maturation Developmental growth based on chronological aging. Theories based on maturation and development generally suggest that individuals will perform in certain ways at certain stages of development. However, if interpreted or applied too narrowly, such approaches may fail to recognize the wide range in individual development over time.

maturation lag A delay in normal development exists as a core feature of many learning disorders. In general, maturation lag refers to any developmental difficulty in which an element of an individual's intellectual, cognitive, social, or behavioral functioning lags behind that predicted by normal development.

meaning-based instruction Instruction that is directed toward purposeful reading and writing with an emphasis on comprehension and composition.

mean score The average score in a grouping of scores. To identify the mean, all scores in a group are added together and then divided by the number of individual scores. For example, a grouping of scores includes the following: 10, 16, 13, 12, 3, 6. These scores are added together for a sum of 60. This sum is then divided by the total number of test scores (in this case, six). The mean in this case would be 10.

megavitamins and ADHD The use of very high doses of vitamins and minerals to treat ATTENTION DEFICIT HYPERACTIVITY DISORDER is based on the theory that some people have a genetic abnormality that requires higher levels of vitamins and minerals.

However, there is a complete lack of supporting scientific evidence for megavitamin treatment for learning disabilities, and there are no well-controlled studies supporting these claims. Both the American Psychiatric Association and the American Academy of Pediatrics have concluded that the use of megavitamins to treat behavioral and learning problems is not justified.

memory A general term that covers a wide range of cognitive functions related to taking in, processing, storing, and retrieving information. Memory is closely tied to attention, and may also be profoundly influenced by linguistic, auditory, or visual-spatial processing abilities.

In general, types of memory can be categorized in two fashions: first, by the stage in the sequence of processes involved in taking in, storing, and recalling information; and second, by the sensory modality involved in the initial stage of memory input (such as auditory, visual, kinesthetic, and so on).

In terms of stages or types of the cognitive processes involved in memory, present theory identifies three major types of memory: short-term memory, active working memory, and long-term memory. Short-term memory involves immediate storage and processing of information, as a prelude to direct response or manipulating the information in some fashion, or to moving the information into long-term memory, or to shifting attention and forgetting the information. Short-term memory may be auditory or visual in form depending on the nature of the input, or may involve other perceptual systems as well. The capacity of short-term memory is very limited, and the duration in which information is held in short-term memory is brief and measured in seconds.

Active working memory refers to the capacity to hold information in mind, either temporarily storing it while referring to more immediate tasks or information, or focusing on it in reflection, consideration, or some other form of mental manipulation. Active working memory has to do with concentration or focus, and is closely linked to attention. Information sustained and processed in working memory may be verbal or nonverbal in nature. The role of active working memory in a broad range of academic, social, and personal domains is extremely important. It is a fundamental component in the process of writing or reading, for example, and it is active working memory that enables reflection on past behavior or helps us note the passing of time. Current theories regarding attention disorders see the impact that deficits in impulse control have on working memory as a core factor in the symptoms of ATTENTION DEFICIT HYPERACTIVITY DISORDER (ADHD).

Long-term memory refers to storage of information in memory on a relatively permanent basis, operating over an extended period of time. In academic settings, success in many areas depends on the ability to recognize and remember salient information, and to transfer this information into long-term memory in a fashion that will enable effective recall on demand, as in a testing situation. In general, long-term memory is not affected directly by learning disabilities or attention disorders. However, the dual ability to move information from short-term memory into long-term memory—and to retrieve information stored in long-term memory—may be significantly affected by a wide range of LEARNING DISORDERS.

memory, active working A type of short-term MEMORY that enables a person to hold information in mind while manipulating or using it. For example, when adding several numbers together, a person might hold the amount "carried" in active working memory while adding a new row of numbers. When learning this skill, children typically are taught to write the "carried" amount above the next number, because they will not yet be able to perform this operation mentally.

Research suggests that remembering gets easier with age because using these processes becomes more automatic after extended use and practice. Active working memory also allows a person to return to earlier steps in a problem-solving sequence so the process can be integrated. Because it has a limited capacity, this kind of memory is linked to ATTENTION.

Active working memory is critical to success at school, at home, and in personal relationships, and it is a fundamental component in the process of reading and writing. It enables reflection on past events and helps monitor the passing of time. Individuals who have ATTENTION DEFICIT HYPERACTIVITY DISORDER (ADHD) or a LEARNING DISABILITY that includes difficulties with IMPULSIVITY and attention may find it difficult to use active working memory effectively.

mental age A score that equates performance on an INTELLIGENCE TEST with the expected mental development for individuals at a specific age. In other words, the individual receives the same number of correct answers on a standardized IQ test as the average person of that age in the sample population.

Saying that an older person with MENTAL RETARDATION is like a person of a younger age, or that a 30-year-old person with mental retardation "has the mental age of a 6-year-old," is not a correct usage of "mental age."

The mental age refers only to the intelligence test score. It does not describe the level and nature of the person's experience and functioning in aspects of community life.

Most intelligence tests have questions that become increasingly challenging and are rated for a specific age. When a child achieves a mental age score of 12, he or she is said to be performing at the level of 12 years of age for the skills measured by the specific test, regardless of actual chronological age.

mental retardation This is defined as below-average intelligence (IQ below 70–75), significant limitations in two or more ADAPTIVE SKILL areas; and the condition present from childhood.

An estimated 7.5 million Americans have mental retardation, which is 10 times more common than CEREBRAL PALSY and 28 times more prevalent than neural tube defects such as spina bifida. Mental retardation cuts across the lines of racial, ethnic, educational, social, and economic backgrounds; one out of 10 American families is directly affected by mental retardation. According to the World Health Organization, about 156 million people—about 3 percent of the Earth's population—have mental retardation.

INTELLIGENCE TESTING alone is only one measure of functioning ability. A person with limits in intellectual functioning who does not have limits in adaptive skill areas may not be diagnosed as having mental retardation. "Adaptive skill areas" are those living skills a person needs to live, work, and play independently. They include communication, self-care, home living, social skills, leisure, health and safety, self-direction; reading, writing, basic math; community use, and work. Adaptive skills are assessed in the person's typical environment, by interviewing people who know the client. For example, parents, caregivers, house supervisors,

and others rate the individual on the VINELAND SOCIAL MATURITY SCALES. The Vineland asks many questions regarding the client's abilities in communication, socialization, daily living skills, and (for children five and below) motor function.

Many individuals have been diagnosed with mental retardation, particularly at a young age, who are later diagnosed with profound LEARNING DISABILITIES but with average or above-average intelligence. This was much more common before states and federal agencies began to require that the evaluations to identify individuals as mentally retarded use multiple measures, including not only IQ testing but assessment of adaptive behavior.

Mental retardation can be caused by anything that affects development of the brain before birth, during birth, or during childhood. Several hundred causes have been discovered, but about a third of the time, the cause remains unknown. The three major known causes of mental retardation are DOWN SYNDROME, FETAL ALCOHOL SYNDROME, and FRAGILE X SYNDROME.

Genetic conditions   Mental retardation can be caused by abnormal genes, or from other disorders of the genes caused during pregnancy by infections, overexposure to X-rays, and other factors. More than 500 genetic diseases are associated with mental retardation, including

- PKU (PHENYLKETONURIA): a single gene disorder caused by a defective enzyme
- Down syndrome: a sporadic chromosomal disorder caused by too many or too few chromosomes, or by a change in structure of a chromosome
- fragile X syndrome: a single-gene disorder located on the X chromosome

Problems during pregnancy   ALCOHOL, drugs, or smoking during pregnancy can cause mental retardation. Other problems include malnutrition, certain environmental contaminants, and illnesses of the mother during pregnancy, such as toxoplasmosis, cytomegalovirus, rubella, and syphilis. Pregnant women who are infected with HIV may pass the virus to their child, leading to future neurological damage.

Problems at birth   Although any unusual stress during birth may injure the infant's brain, prematurity and low birth weight are more likely to predict serious problems than any other condition.

Problems after birth Brain damage can be caused by whooping cough, chickenpox, measles, and Hib disease (which may lead to meningitis and encephalitis). Accidents such as a blow to the head, near drowning, or lead, MERCURY, and other environmental toxins can cause irreparable damage to the brain and nervous system.

Poverty and cultural deprivation Low-income children may become mentally retarded as a result of malnutrition, disease, inadequate medical care, and environmental health hazards. Children in disadvantaged areas also may be deprived of common cultural enriching experiences, resulting in irreversible damage.

Symptoms and Diagnostic Path

The effects of mental retardation vary considerably among people, just as the range of abilities varies considerably among people who do not have mental retardation. About 87 percent will be mildly affected and will be only a little slower than average in learning new information and skills. As children, their mental retardation is not easy to see, and may not be identified until school age. As adults, many individuals with mental retardation will be able to lead independent lives in the community.

The remaining 13 percent of people with mental retardation (those with IQs under 50) will have serious limits in function. However, with early intervention, a good education, and appropriate supports as an adult, all can lead satisfying lives in the community.

People with mental retardation may have trouble communicating, interacting with others, and being independent. There may also be concerns with regard to understanding health and safety issues. Not all skills are necessarily impaired, and individuals with mental retardation may learn to function independently in many areas. However, education programs, providing skilled assistance and ongoing support, are necessary for determining appropriate living and work environments.

While the term *mental retardation* still exists as a clinical diagnosis, contemporary usage is moving toward terms such as *developmental disabilities*, which some believe do not carry the same negative connotations or misuse. In the past, those who were retarded were traditionally divided by IQ scores into *educable, trainable*, and *custodial;* today, the more commonly used terms include *mild, moderate, severe,* or *profound* categories, based on the level of functioning and IQ. Individuals with mental retardation are not a homogenous group, but have widely differing levels of functioning.

Mild retardation This classification is used to specify an individual whose IQ test scores lie between 55 and 68 or 69, and correspond to an educators' label of "educable retarded." The individual is capable of learning basic academic subjects. Many people with mild retardation are able to live and work independently.

Moderate retardation This classification is used to specify an individual whose IQ test scores are between 40 and 55; it corresponds to the earlier label of trainable retarded. These individuals can usually learn functional academics and vocational skills. They often achieve coached employment goals and live with limited assistance.

Severe and profound mental retardation This classification applies to individuals with IQ scores below 25. These are the most seriously impaired of the mentally retarded, often characterized by physical and sensory impairment as well as mental retardation. They can sometimes achieve supported employment goals; more typically they can function at the level of sheltered employment. They generally require significant assistance with daily living skills.

Mental retardation is diagnosed primarily on the basis of intelligence testing, but affected individuals often demonstrate other brain problems such as attention deficits, movement problems, and perceptual difficulties. Dexterity and coordination may also be limited.

The first step is to administer standardized intelligence tests and a standardized adaptive skills scale. Next, an expert should describe the person's strengths and weaknesses in intellectual and adaptive behavior skills, emotions, physical health, and environment. These skills can be assessed by formal testing, observations, interviews, and interacting with the person in daily life.

Risk Factors and Preventive Measures

It is possible to prevent some forms of mental retardation. For example, every year in the United

States, about 250 cases of mental retardation due to PKU are prevented by newborn screening and dietary treatment. Newborn screening and thyroid hormone replacement therapy prevent 1,000 cases of mental retardation a year due to congenital hypothyroidism; and more than 1,000 cases of mental retardation from Rh disease and severe jaundice are prevented by using anti-Rh immune globulin to prevent Rh disease. The Hib vaccine prevents another 5,000 cases of mental retardation caused by Hib diseases, and 4,000 cases of mental retardation due to measles encephalitis can be prevented because of the measles vaccine. Countless numbers of cases of mental retardation caused by rubella during pregnancy are prevented thanks to the rubella vaccine.

Removing lead from the environment can reduce brain damage in children, and child safety seats and bicycle helmets reduce head trauma. Early intervention programs with high-risk infants and children have shown remarkable results in reducing the predicted incidence of subnormal intellectual functioning.

Early prenatal care and preventive measures before and during pregnancy increase a woman's chances of preventing mental retardation; dietary supplementation with folic acid reduces the risk of neural tube defects. Research continues on new ways to prevent mental retardation, including research on the development and function of the nervous system, a wide variety of fetal treatments, and gene therapy to correct the abnormality produced by defective genes.

mercury   A naturally occurring metal characterized by its "quicksilver" properties. At room temperature, mercury is a shiny, silvery liquid that beads up and rolls around. Mercury is very dense and can be absorbed into the skin and lungs. It is emitted into the environment naturally by volcanic eruptions and unnaturally by industrial coal burning. Mercury has been linked to the development of MENTAL RETARDATION, developmental disabilities, brain damage, and organ damage. It is suspected to cause cancer but has not yet been proven to do so.

Mercury is found in the ground and in oceans, lakes, rivers, and streams. It is found in high levels in seafood, mostly tuna, shellfish, shark, tilefish, and king mackerel. There are some uses for mercury such as in dental fillings, fluorescent lights, batteries, and thermometers; some cosmetic creams contain other forms of mercury called methylmercury.

Mercury also can pass from mother to child through the placenta and breast milk. In newborns, it causes mental retardation, brain damage, lack of coordination, blindness, seizures, and the inability to speak. As a result, it has been recommended that women who are pregnant or who may become so eat no more than two cans of tuna per week and limit their intake of other possibly tainted fish.

metacognition   The awareness and knowledge of an individual's own mental processes; the ability to think about thinking. Metacognition refers to one's understanding of what strategies are available for learning and what strategies are best used in which situations. It involves the ability to select and manage cognitive strategies effectively. Ordinarily these abilities develop in childhood; children learn that mental activities go along with decision making. They know when they know something and when they do not.

Metacognition skills are directly related to reading, writing, problem solving, and any process that requires error monitoring. Students must be able to examine how they learn best and what resources they can draw upon in order to set and achieve academic goals.

One of the reasons individuals with LEARNING DISABILITIES tend to have academic difficulties is a lack of skills in selecting and managing task-appropriate strategies. Many theorists and educators believe that these skills can be intentionally taught and developed.

metacognitive awareness   In reading, when a child knows that what he or she is reading makes sense, by monitoring and controlling one's own COMPREHENSION.

metacognitive learning   Knowledge of strategies to enhance an individual's learning. Metacognitive learners know their strengths and weaknesses and can direct their learning accordingly.

Individuals with LEARNING DISABILITIES often lack metacognitive skills, but can greatly benefit from being explicitly taught such skills. Metacognitive learning skills would include the ability to classify, self-monitor, evaluate, and predict their own learning.

Beyond monitoring progress, evaluating how well a person has performed is a metacognitive skill. Because metacognitive learners are aware of their limitations, they can also predict their learning.

Metropolitan Achievement Test   A national commercial, norm-referenced achievement group test created to rank test takers. Norm-referenced tests provide a quick snapshot of some of the things most people expect students to learn. They are relatively cheap and easy to administer. Published by Harcourt Assessment, Inc., the test is designed to provide ASSESSMENT of students' achievement in reading, mathematics, language, arts, science, and social studies at appropriate levels.

See also NORM-REFERENCED TEST.

methylphenidate (Ritalin)   A medication prescribed for individuals (usually children) who have an abnormally high level of activity, or ATTENTION DEFICIT HYPERACTIVITY DISORDER (ADHD). About 3 to 5 percent of the general population has the disorder, which is characterized by agitated behavior and an inability to focus on tasks.

This central nervous system stimulant has effects similar to, but more potent than, caffeine—but weaker than amphetamines. It has a notably calming effect on hyperactive children and a "focusing" effect on those with ADHD.

Scientists think ADHD occurs in part because certain receptors in the brain involved in focusing attention and reining in impulsiveness fail to respond to DOPAMINE and norepinephrine, the brain's natural neurotransmitters. It is the interaction between these chemicals and the brain's receptors that helps most people stick with tedious chores, or rein in inappropriate impulses. Researchers think that drugs like Ritalin boost the level of these brain chemicals and stimulate the inhibitory receptors—which is why a stimulant drug can increase INHIBITION. The drugs enter the body quickly, curing nothing but helping a child focus on the important work of learning.

Although the drug clearly reduces the symptoms of ADHD, and many students have been taking the drug for years, no studies have continued long enough to see if it has a lasting effect on academic performance or social behavior. Moreover, a positive response to Ritalin does not automatically mean a child suffers from ADHD. Stimulants can temporarily sharpen almost anyone's focus. Ritalin has become one of the more widely sought-after drugs on the black market because of its attention-focusing effects. Many college students buy black market Ritalin to enhance their study skills.

However, while most experts agree that medication can help, it is not the only solution—parents and teachers need to learn new ways (such as rewards and consequences) in which to teach their children how to focus and sit still.

Extensive research suggests a combination of stimulants and behavior management is the best way to treat ADHD. First introduced in the 1940s, Ritalin is usually prescribed as a part of a treatment plan that includes educational and psychosocial interventions for children with behavior characterized by

- moderate-to-severe distractibility
- short attention span
- hyperactivity
- emotional liability
- impulsivity

The widespread use of Ritalin in children is not without controversy. Some experts are vehemently opposed to medicating children who are deemed too inattentive or active for a "normal" classroom. However, there is no specific evidence that clearly establishes the mechanism by which Ritalin produces its mental and behavioral effects in children. Because a diagnosis of ADHD itself is not always straightforward, and because some doctors prescribe it after a brief conversation with concerned parents, without obtaining the proper diagnostic information, critics argue that far too many children who are simply extremely energetic are given a diagnosis of ADHD and medicated.

A doctor should prescribe Ritalin only after medical, psychological, behavioral, and educational assessments. The doctor or therapist should talk both to parents and the child, and get information from teachers before prescribing stimulants. Pediatric neurologists and developmental pediatricians warn that ADHD symptoms are often caused by other symptoms. The diagnosis should only be made after these conditions are ruled out.

Dosage Closely monitored treatment with stimulants (Ritalin is one of four commonly prescribed, and its use has increased 700 percent in one decade) can erase enough symptoms of ADHD to eliminate the diagnosis for 82 to 85 percent of children. While most parents give their children a typical twice-daily dose, one recent government study suggests that three times a day works better, with a nighttime dose about half the size of the first two.

It may take up to one month for the medication to achieve its maximum effect in children, and 30 minutes to take effect in adults. Medications like Ritalin are usually taken for as long as it is helpful or necessary. While there has been an increase in the number of stimulant prescriptions for children under age five, there is no evidence that these drugs are safe or effective when used on young children.

Risk of abuse Because of its stimulant properties, however, there have been reports of Ritalin abuse by adults who turn to the drug for its stimulant effects: appetite suppression, wakefulness, increased focus and attentiveness, and euphoria. When abused, the tablets are either taken orally or crushed, and snorted or smoked. Some abusers dissolve the tablets in water and inject the mixture, although this can cause problems if insoluble fillers in the tablets block small blood vessels.

Because stimulant medicines such as Ritalin have the potential for abuse, the U.S. Drug Enforcement Administration (DEA) has placed stringent, Schedule II controls on their manufacture, distribution, and prescription. For example, DEA requires special licenses for these activities, and prescription refills are not allowed. States may impose further regulations, such as limiting the number of dosage units per prescription.

Side effects Common side effects include decrease or loss of appetite, nervousness, sleep problems, weight loss, or dizziness. There is also evidence that brain growth slows in children who take Ritalin and other stimulants. However, once these children stop taking Ritalin, there is usually a substantial growth rebound, although the extent of the rebound varies.

Contraindications Ritalin should not be used in children with ANXIETY, tension, agitation, irregular heart rhythms, severe angina pectoris, or glaucoma, or in anyone with motor tics or a family history or diagnosis of TOURETTE'S SYNDROME. Although a relationship has not been established, suppression of growth (such as weight gain and/or height) has been reported with the long-term use of stimulants in children. Therefore, patients who need long-term therapy should be carefully monitored; it may be a good idea to withhold the drug on weekends and during school holidays.

See also STIMULANT MEDICATION.

micro-uniting Breaking a large task into smaller steps. For many learners, especially learning-disabled learners, completing assignments or projects on time can be a challenge. Micro-uniting assignments can make an overwhelming project become manageable by outlining the subtasks necessary and creating a timeline to complete each task.

mild mental retardation MENTAL RETARDATION in which the IQ level is between 50 and 70. Adults with mild mental retardation typically achieve functional LITERACY and are able to live independently (or with minimal assistance) in the community.

Millon Clinical Multiaxial Inventory A personality test that was recently updated, this assessment was written by Theodore Millon to assess personality disorders, as opposed to the MINNESOTA MULTIPHASIC PERSONALITY INVENTORY, which screens for a broad range of psychological problems. A teen version of this test also exists.

minimal brain dysfunction (MBD) A general term used to describe a young child who shows behavioral, cognitive, and affective signs of brain injury. The term is usually used for cases in which the pattern of thought and action would typically be caused by organic abnormality, but none is apparent.

Historically, MBD was the term used to define and classify learning and behavioral difficulties now classified under the category of ATTENTION

DEFICIT HYPERACTIVITY DISORDER. It generally includes HYPERACTIVITY, IMPULSIVITY, various neurological soft signs, and any of a number of learning and LANGUAGE DISABILITIES such as DYSLEXIA and DYSCALCULIA.

The term is often used as though there were an identifiable MBD syndrome, a collection of fairly specific disorders that could be taken as hallmarks of some underlying neurological cause. Although the issue is far from settled, the evidence to support a single MBD syndrome is largely unconvincing.

minimum competency testing An ASSESSMENT that tries to establish the minimum level of achievement. At least 36 states now require some type of minimum competency, which may be tied in with the ability to graduate.

There is a great deal of controversy about minimum competency tests. Critics worry that the blame for a poor school program may be shifted to the students. While the goal of minimum competency testing is to improve overall achievement, critics worry that the tests will in fact depress some students' achievement levels. There is also concern about the impact of such tests on minority achievement.

Students with an identified LEARNING DISABILITY can waive the tests, although some schools suggest that these students take the tests anyway in the freshman year. If the student fails the entire test, he or she could then take it again with modifications as stipulated in one's INDIVIDUALIZED EDUCATION PROGRAM. A student with learning disabilities as a senior can sometimes waive the tests.

Minnesota Multiphasic Personality Inventory (MMPI) The oldest personality test, this true-false ASSESSMENT is used by psychologists in a wide variety of settings to help diagnose the possible existence of mental disorders. The MMPI was first published in 1943 and was restandardized in 1989 as the MMPI-2. It can be used to identify social and personal maladjustment, identify good candidates for high-risk public safety jobs, help in the criminal justice system, and help design effective treatment strategies. There is also a widely used adolescent form.

miscue analysis A type of reading ASSESSMENT in which the errors (miscues) that students make in reading provide a diagnostic window into the underlying language processes that caused the mistakes. Miscue analysis focuses on the differences between a student's oral reading performance and the printed text.

Miscue analysis does not look at problems solely with single sounds and their written symbols. It also focuses closely on the ways in which patterns and structures in a student's underlying language differ from those of the text.

mixed dominance See CROSS DOMINANCE.

mixed receptive-expressive language disorder A LANGUAGE DISABILITY causing problems in both understanding and expressing language. The condition was formerly called "developmental receptive language disorder." Today, it is generally understood that receptive language deficits do not occur all by themselves, but appear together with problems expressing language.

Three percent to 5 percent of all children have both receptive and expressive language disorder. The cause of this disorder is unknown, but problems with receptive skills begin before the age of four. Difficulty understanding and using language can cause problems with social interaction, and make it difficult to function independently as an adult.

Symptoms and Diagnostic Path
There are a number of symptoms that indicate this condition, including problems in

- language comprehension
- language expression
- articulation
- recalling early visual or auditory memories

Parents who are concerned about their child's acquisition of language should have the child tested, since early intervention offers the best possible outcome. Standardized receptive and expressive language tests can be given to any child suspected of having this disorder. An audiogram should also be given to rule out the possibility of deafness.

Treatment Options and Outlook

Speech and language therapy are the best way to treat this type of language disorder. Psychotherapy is also recommended for children because of the possibility of emotional or behavioral problems.

See also EXPRESSIVE LANGUAGE DISORDERS; COMMUNICATION DISORDER.

mnemonic devices   MEMORY aids devised to help an individual remember information. Mnemonic strategies include rhymes, nonsense words or sentences, anagrams, and images.

A common mnemonic for remembering the colors of the rainbow is *Roy G. Biv* in which each letter represents the colors in order: Red, Orange, Yellow, Green, Blue, Indigo, and Violet. The well-known poem that starts "Thirty days hath September . . ." is often the only way in which adults can remember how many days are in a particular month.

Most mnemonic strategies do not have any inherent connection with the material to be learned, but they impose meaning on material that is otherwise disorganized. In general, these strategies usually involve adding something to the material to be learned to make it easier to remember.

Individuals with LEARNING DISABILITY who have trouble remembering information often find using mnemonic strategies helpful. Mnemonics can be especially useful in remembering unrelated information that is not connected to anything meaningful.

modality   The CHANNEL or mode through which information is taken in and processed. The most common examples are visual (sight), auditory (hearing), tactile (touch), and kinesthetic (movement).

modified self-contained classroom   A self-contained program in which students receive instruction from a regular education teacher for some part of the school day.

mold, toxic black   Molds are fungi that grow in damp, dark places; although most are harmless, toxic black mold can be detrimental to people's health. Children who are exposed to mold at school may exhibit symptoms similar to LEARNING DISABILITIES. They may not be able to focus or remember things very well. They may be tired, fatigued, have headaches or stomachaches. The toxic effect from molds comes from their spores, which grow on the surface of a mold and can be blown into the air.

Molds are found everywhere in the environment, but they grow quickly in moist places and on porous materials such as wood, paper, cardboard, and ceiling tiles. They also can grow well in drywall, upholstery, carpets, and wallpaper. Humans breathe air and dust that contain mold spores. Poor ventilation in buildings increases the likelihood of growth and therefore exposure.

morpheme   The smallest unit of meaning in a language. There are two types of morpheme, "free" and "bound." Morphemes that stand alone and have a meaning by themselves are called "free morphemes"; these include words such as *house, create, talk.* "Bound" morphemes are the prefixes and suffixes that do not have meaning as independent words. Individuals with LEARNING DISABILITIES can enhance their vocabularies by improving their awareness of the smallest unit of meaning in a language through explicit training in prefixes, roots, and suffixes.

For example, psychology can be broken into two morphemes: *psych,* meaning "mind," and *ology,* meaning "the study of." When an individual becomes aware of meaningful word parts such as *psych,* dozens of other words (such as psychedelic, psychometric, psychic) become understandable.

morphological awareness   An explicit awareness that words are composed of base forms, roots, prefixes, and suffixes and that those parts affect the word's meaning. For example, an individual who has acquired morphological awareness can see how the following words are similar: unforgivable, forgave, forgiving, and give.

Research has shown that morphological awareness has a significant impact on spelling, vocabulary development, and READING COMPREHENSION. The more skilled in morphological awareness individuals are, the better they are at spelling. Individuals with LEARNING DISABILITIES do not perform as well as their normal peers with spelling words that change phonologically (such as run/ran or diving/dove).

Vocabulary development is also related to morphological awareness. Children who are taught about parts of words tend to have more developed vocabularies than children without such instruction. Young children with language difficulties in particular benefit from explicit instruction on how words work.

Reading comprehension also improves with an awareness of how words are put together. Research has shown that teaching morphological awareness before learning to read can predict how well a student comprehends by grade two. Explicit instruction in elementary grades on prefixes, roots, and suffixes provides morphological awareness. Older students benefit from learning the origins of words for vocabulary and spelling enrichment. Teaching vocabulary using word families helps individuals with learning difficulties negotiate between spelling and phonological shifts (such as democracy/democrat/hypocrisy/technocrat).

morphology The study of how words are constructed. For individuals with a LEARNING DISABILITY, studying how words are composed is an important way to boost language competence.

See also MORPHEME; MORPHOLOGICAL AWARENESS.

motivation The internal process that causes an individual to move toward the completion of a goal or to back away from a negative situation or stimulus. Motivation is frequently discussed in relation to learners. Various theories exist that attempt to explain what motivates individuals to act or to strive to complete difficult tasks.

See also LEARNED HELPLESSNESS; LOCUS OF CONTROL.

Motor Free Visual Perception Test A test of VISUAL PERCEPTION designed for children aged four through eight years, 11 months that should be used in combination with a copying measure such as the BENDER VISUAL-MOTOR GESTALT TEST or the developmental test of visual-motor integration.

In this test, the child selects the correct figure during tasks involving spatial relationships, VISUAL DISCRIMINATION, figure-ground relationships, visual closure, and visual memory.

motor planning Thinking about a desired result and judging what motor activities or strategies will produce that result. For example, motor planning would be involved in determining how hard to throw a ball in order to reach another person.

motor sequencing Determining an appropriate sequence of movements to fulfill a task or produce a desired outcome. Movements are ordered both in terms of what is done first and next (temporal sequence), and what movements are performed simultaneously.

For example, in cutting with scissors, the hand holding the scissors alternates in temporal sequence opening and closing the hand; when the hand holding the scissors is in open position, the forearm concurrently moves the hand forward, so that the cutting advances. In describing the sequencing involved in an activity process, in addition to observing what is the sequence, it is possible to note whether the sequencing is simple, moderate, or complex. Many different movements would result in complex motor sequencing.

motor skills A wide range of capabilities involved in movement, such as the use and regulation of muscles and muscle groups with appropriate timing and sequencing, the ability to recall through motor memory the muscular steps used to perform a task in the past, and the use of ongoing sensory feedback to regulate muscular responses and activities.

motor tics Movements that a person cannot control. Motor tics can include eye blinking, rolling the eyes, grimacing, or shrugging the shoulders.

multicategorical classroom A classroom that mixes together children with a variety of disabilities or handicapping conditions, under the instruction of a single SPECIAL EDUCATION teacher.

multicultural assessment ASSESSMENT that takes into account the specific environmental and sociocultural factors that may be involved in determining ability and potential.

See also SOCIOCULTURAL PERSPECTIVE.

multidisciplinary team   A group of specialists who work together to meet students' needs. This type of team combines members' varied expertise to gather information and make decisions about students' eligibility for special services. Members of the team may include a LEARNING DISABILITY specialist, school nurse, teacher, social worker, school psychologist, speech and language pathologist, and parents. Amendments to the INDIVIDUALS WITH DISABILITIES EDUCATION IMPROVEMENT ACT in 1997 included general teachers on the multidisciplinary team.

multifactored evaluation   An ASSESSMENT of more than one area of a child's functioning so that no one factor may contribute to a misdiagnosis.

multimodal   See LEARNING MODALITIES.

multiple disabilities   A child with a combination of two or more disabilities, such as deafness, blindness, MENTAL RETARDATION, or speech and language problems. Children with multiple disabilities usually have many problems with socialization, communication, and adaptation. Placement in a program designed for just one of the disabilities may not be effective, so children are usually placed in a program designed to handle all their problems.

ATTENTION DEFICIT HYPERACTIVITY DISORDER (ADHD) often appears in children with multiple disabilities, but it is not always diagnosed. Because these problems are often complex, it can be quite challenging to identify the primary obstacle to learning.

multiple intelligences   Advances in cognitive science, developmental psychology, and neuroscience suggest that each person's level of INTELLIGENCE, as it has been traditionally considered, is actually made up of a number of faculties that can work individually or together with other abilities. Harvard professor Howard Gardner originally identified eight such types of intelligences, including verbal/linguistic, logical/mathematic, visual/spatial, musical/rhythmic, body/kinesthetic, interpersonal, intrapersonal, and naturalistic. Each of these eight types represents abilities within a specific area of human functioning.

Gardner believed that the forms of intelligence that are measured by most INTELLIGENCE TESTS correspond to verbal/linguistic, logical/mathematic, and visual/spatial intelligences, meaning that traditional measures of intelligence overlook or fail to recognize abilities and gifts in other areas.

Although not based on or validated by research Gardner's theories have become increasingly influential. However, standard measures of intelligence continue to focus on verbal and nonverbal reasoning measures that depend heavily on linguistic, logical, and visual-spatial abilities, and the common understanding of intelligence continues to be mostly closely linked to verbal capabilities.

Many school curricula narrowly emphasize linguistic and mathematical intelligences, which can be the weakest areas for learning-disabled students. Often individuals with LEARNING DISABILITIES have talents that are not valued in academic settings. The theory of multiple intelligences emphasizes the need to acknowledge and cultivate different kinds of thinking and different abilities.

Musical intelligence   Child prodigies such as Menuhin, Mozart, Saint-Saens, Boulez, and others experience music "naturally." The ability to perform and compose music has been scientifically pinpointed in certain areas of the brain. Indeed, cases of autistic and other impaired children who can perform brilliantly but are unable to talk or interact with others illustrate this.

Each individual has a different musical ability, and there are even people who are totally amusical, yet continue to have very normal and successful lives. Although musical intelligence may not seem as obvious a form of intellect as mathematical or logical ability, from a neurological point of view the ability to perform and comprehend musically appears to work independently from other forms of intelligence.

Body/Kinesthetic   One of the most controversial of Gardner's intelligences is the idea of body-kinesthetic intelligence. In Gardner's theory, each person possesses a certain control of movements, balance, agility, and grace. For some extraordinary individuals, such as Michael Jordan or Jackie Joyner Kersey, strength in body-kinesthetic intelligence appeared even before they began formal training. Super athletes all seem to have a natural sense of how their body should act and react in a demanding physical situation. It is also long known that each hemisphere of the brain controls the opposite side of the body's movements; in APRAXIA or other conditions, some people lack the ability to voluntarily control muscles, though they continue to move involuntarily.

Some people, however, argue that physical control does not constitute a designation as a form of intelligence. But Gardner and other multiple intelligences researchers maintain that body-kinesthetic ability does indeed deserve such a recognition.

Logical/Mathematic The most easily understood cognitive faculty is logical-mathematic intelligence—the ability to mentally process logical problems and equations—the type most often found on multiple-choice standardized tests. Logical-mathematic intelligence often does not require verbal articulation. Individuals who have good logical-mathematic abilities are able to process logical questions at an unusually rapid rate.

Before the advent of the theory of multiple intelligences, logical-mathematic intelligence was considered a pseudonym for intelligence itself, the "raw intellect" that Western culture revered. Although the theory of multiple intelligences agrees that logical-mathematic intelligence is indeed a key section of the intellect, it is by no means the only one that should be developed.

Linguistic Everyone possesses the ability to use language; although some can master only basic levels of communication, others can speak many languages with grace and ease. For years, researchers have recognized the connection between language and the brain. Damage to one portion of the brain (BROCA'S AREA) will affect the ability to express clear grammatical sentences, although a person's understanding of vocabulary and syntax remains intact. As Howard Gardner notes, even young children and deaf individuals will begin to develop their own unique language if they are not offered an alternative. A person's ability to construct and comprehend language may vary, but as a cognitive trait it is still universal.

Spatial Spatial intelligence involves the ability to comprehend shapes and images in three dimensions. Whether trying to put together a puzzle or create a sculpture, we use spatial intelligence to interpret what we may or may not physically see. Advances in neuroscience have now provided researchers with clear-cut proof of the role of spatial intelligence in the right hemisphere of the brain.

In rare instances, for example, certain brain injuries can cause people to lose the ability to recognize their closest relatives. Though they may see the other person perfectly well, they are unable to comprehend who they see.

And yet a blind person may feel a shape and identify it with ease, although he or she is unable to see it. Because most people use spatial intelligence in conjunction with sight, its existence as an autonomous cognitive attribute may not seem obvious, but recent research suggests that it is an independent portion of the intellect.

Interpersonal Humans are social animals who thrive when involved with others. This ability to interact with others, understand them, and interpret their behavior is called interpersonal intelligence. According to Gardner, individuals' interpersonal intelligence allows them to notice the moods, temperaments, motivations, and intentions of others.

From a psychological and neurological point of view, the connection between interpersonal intelligence and the brain has been explored for generations; if the frontal lobe is damaged, that person's personality and ability to interact well with others is destroyed. Interpersonal intelligence allows us to affect others by understanding others; without it, an individual loses the ability to exist socially.

Intrapersonal Related to interpersonal intelligence, intrapersonal intelligence is the cognitive ability to understand and sense the "self." Intrapersonal intelligence allows individuals to tap into internal feelings and thoughts. A strong intrapersonal intelligence can lead to SELF-ESTEEM, self-enhancement, and a strength of character that can be used to solve internal problems.

On the other hand, a weak intrapersonal intelligence (such as with autistic children) prevents a person from recognizing the self as separate from the surrounding environment.

Intrapersonal intelligence often is not recognized from the outside unless it is expressed in some form, such as rage or joy.

Naturalistic   Recently added to the original list of seven multiple intelligences, naturalistic intelligence is a person's ability to identify and classify patterns in nature. During prehistory, hunter-gatherers would rely on naturalistic intelligence to identify what plants or animals were edible and which were not. Today, naturalistic intelligence may be seen in the way we relate to our surroundings. People who are sensitive to changes in weather patterns or are adept at distinguishing nuances among large numbers of similar objects may be expressing naturalistic intelligence abilities.

Impact on Schools   If the theory of multiple intelligences is true, it means that the most common form of assessment in the United States may not be the best. This type of assessment involves multiple-choice or fill-in-the-blank questions that have been developed from a given set of information that has been deemed worthy of being "necessary knowledge." Correct answers on this type of test do little to help students understand the subject. Though some can demonstrate their knowledge of the "facts," many cannot truly explain the context of the knowledge and the ramification of the facts. Limited response assessment gives educators and politicians an efficient means of ranking students as successful or not, but does very little for the student in terms of understanding the subject.

multisensory   Learning that involves more than one sense, including visual, auditory, kinesthetic, and tactile, to help reinforce learning.

See also LEARNING MODALITIES; VAKT.

near-point copying The ability to copy when text or other visual information is close at hand.

near-point deficits The ability to see material close at hand is an essential factor in reading well. It has to do with the ability to see forms and letters clearly at a distance of about 16 inches, the standard distance used in reading.

An individual with near-point deficits has a problem with vision itself rather than with the visual-perceptual system, and may require corrective lenses or other treatment.

needs assessment A broad-based appraisal of educational objectives and conditions in an attempt to relate goals to existing strengths and weaknesses. A needs assessment may examine the goals and assets of a particular school system and may lead to specific recommendations for improvement.

negative reinforcement Unpleasant reinforcement that is used to increase a certain behavior. Contrary to popular belief, it is not the same as punishment, which is used to decrease a certain behavior. For example, in the classroom a child may be sent to time-out (negative experience) for an inappropriate behavior, but once the child has maintained appropriate behavior, she may return from time-out, encouraging better behavior in the future.

neurobiology The biological makeup of the brain, including brain structure and functions, as well as biochemical processes.

neurological assessment Testing based on a NEUROLOGICAL EXAMINATION, providing information about the ways in which dysfunctions or differ-

ences in brain function may affect function of movement, thought, or social, emotional, psychological, or behavioral activities.

neurological disorders A spectrum of potential effects on human development, performance, and behavior ranging from profound disorders that may affect every aspect of human functioning, to minimal dysfunctions that create little impairment in the ability to learn and perform effectively. In all cases, neurological disorders or dysfunctions involve impairments in neurological functioning that are based in the biochemistry and structure of the brain.

neurological examination A test that may typically include a conventional ASSESSMENT of brain function, and an examination of "soft" (subtle) neurological signs.

A conventional assessment will include a family and medical history, as well as physical examination of specific neurological functions, such as cranial nerves, reflexes, and other motor functions. In some cases, a neurological examination also may involve more specialized procedures such as an electroencephalogram to measure electrical activity in the brain, X-rays, brain-imaging techniques, or biochemical, endocrinologic, or genetic studies.

Examination of subtle neurological signs may include a variety of tasks designed to identify more subtle gross-motor, visual-motor, or fine-motor difficulties. Such tasks are relatively informal, involving activities such as copying forms, hopping or standing on one foot, or testing finger dexterity.

neurological impress method An approach to reading instruction for students with significant reading disabilities. With this method, the teacher and student read the same material aloud, rapidly and at the same time, as the teacher directs his voice into the ear of the student at close range. The theory behind this system is that the auditory feedback will help the student develop reading fluency.

neurologist   A physician specializing in brain function who can assess and treat with medication a variety of neurological conditions and disorders.

A neurologist can perform detailed examinations of all the neurological structures in the body, including the nerves of the head and neck, muscular strength and movement, sensation, balance, and reflex testing. In some cases, detailed questions about MEMORY, speech and language, and other cognitive functions are part of the examination. Neurologists also use other common tests, including a variety of brain imaging scans, to provide detailed pictures of the brain, spinal structures, and blood vessels. A neurologist also can perform a lumbar puncture (spinal tap) to obtain a patient's cerebrospinal fluid for analysis. Some neurologists interpret EEG (electroencephalography) for the evaluation of seizure disorders or perform other tests to diagnose nerve and muscle problems.

In addition, neurologists use many types of drugs to treat problems involving the nervous system. A neurologist may send a patient for a surgical evaluation but does not perform surgery.

A neurologist must complete a four-year premedical university degree and four years of medical school. This is followed by at least three years of specialty training in an accredited neurology residency program. After residency training, neurologists may choose to enroll in a one- or two-year fellowship program, which offers the opportunity to focus on a subspecialty of neurology such as stroke, dementia, or movement disorders.

After completing the educational requirements, neurologists may seek certification from the American Board of Psychiatry and Neurology (ABPN). To be eligible for certification, an applicant must be a licensed physician with the required years of residency who has passed both a written and oral exam administered by the ABPN.

neurology   The branch of medicine that focuses on the study of diseases and disorders of the nervous system.

neuropsychological examination   Testing that explores a number of broad areas in brain and behavioral functioning, including intellectual functioning, ATTENTION, language, sensorimotor functions, executive functions, and social and emotional functions. They also measure specific skills, such as MEMORY, CONCENTRATION, PROBLEM SOLVING, and learning.

A neuropsychological examination typically involves administration of a complex battery of tests designed to identify levels of functioning within specific areas and to compare abilities and problems in all areas.

Also called "information processing tests," this type of testing reveals how the brain and nervous system interact. A complete neuropsychological evaluation begins with information about a child's education and physical, social, and psychological development. Then tests are used to measure a wide range of areas, including focus and attention, motor skills, sensory acuity, working memory, learning, intelligence, language, arithmetic skills, problem solving, judgment, abstract thinking, mood, temperament, the ability to interpret and apply meaning to visual information, and other skills.

A neuropsychological examination might be recommended if a child has experienced a medical condition or injury that could affect brain health, a sudden or unexpected change in thinking, failure to improve with therapy or SPECIAL EDUCATION help, or complex learning and behavior patterns that other evaluations have not identified.

neuropsychologist   A psychologist who focuses on the relationship between behavior and neurological functions. Neuropsychologists are trained to think about the link between brain function and behavior and would therefore typically be called to assess a child with LEARNING DISABILITIES if the child's abilities are complicated or difficult to assess, if there are thinking problems or behavior patterns that might be closely linked to disrupted brain function, or if the child might have some kind of brain damage.

Clinical neuropsychologists have a doctoral degree (Ph.D., Psy.D., or Ed.D.) from a university or professional school, usually with the same kind of experience that a clinical psychologist needs but sometimes in different areas of psychology such as "school" or "counseling." They also have specialized education in neuropsychology and neuroscience, including at least two years of postdoctoral training in a clinical setting, and often have passed a national board certification exam. Those holding an ABCN/ABPP Diploma in Clinical Neuropsychology have the clearest evidence of competence as a clinical neuropsychologist.

See also NEUROPSYCHOLOGY.

neuropsychology   The study of the relationship between brain function and behavior. This field includes NEUROPSYCHOLOGISTS who work in experimental and clinical settings; experimental neuropsychologists who work with both human and animal models; and clinical neuropsychologists, who look for procedures that will help people with neurologically based disorders by studying brain and behavior relationships.

neurotransmitter   A chemical messenger in the brain that is released from the ends of a brain cell to carry information across the gap between cells, where it arrives at specific sites on a receiving cell. Examples of neurotransmitters include acetylcholine, DOPAMINE, epinephrine, serotonin, and various neuropeptides.

Treatment for ATTENTION disorders involving medications focuses primarily on regulating the action of neurotransmitters.

See also ATTENTION DEFICIT HYPERACTIVITY DISORDER.

noncategorical   An approach to grouping children in a classroom without reference to any diagnostic label or category.

nonfluent aphasia   A language disorder characterized by pauses and hesitancy, with little speech and poor articulation in which a person uses primarily nouns and verbs. Automatic phrases, such as "yes" and "no," prevail. This condition is also called BROCA'S APHASIA. A person with severe nonfluent aphasia may use only single words and may experience these same deficits in writing and read-

ing. People with nonfluent aphasia typically can understand speech.

Treatment Options and Outlook
Speech-language therapy can help patients with aphasia recover some language skills, use the remaining skills they still have, and learn other ways to communicate. There is no guarantee of a cure.

Risk Factors and Preventive Measures
There is no specific way to prevent the onset of aphasia after a stroke or head injury, but seeking early medical treatment when a stroke occurs may lessen injury to the brain and improve recovery.

nonphonetic word   A word whose pronunciation may not be accurately predicted from its spelling.

nonsense words   See PSEUDOWORD DECODING.

nonverbal learning disabilities (NLD)   A form of LEARNING DISABILITY that primarily affects social functioning in areas such as interpersonal skills, social perception, and interaction. Also called "right-hemisphere learning disorders," "right hemisphere processing deficit" and "nonverbal processing deficit," this problem often goes unrecognized. Since abnormalities of the right hemisphere interfere with understanding and adaptive learning, experts believe that nonverbal learning disabilities are more debilitating than verbal disabilities.

Experts suspect that nonverbal learning disabilities are caused by a problem in the right hemisphere of the brain, either from brain injury or damage before birth. The damage primarily affects visual-spatial perception, processing, and reasoning. Individuals with NLD often display significant strengths in verbal areas and may develop reading and speaking skills earlier than their peers; consequently, their nonverbal learning difficulties may be overlooked. Both parents and teachers will often suspect that something is wrong early on, but they cannot quite figure out what it is.

Nonverbal learning disorders remain predominantly misunderstood and largely unrecognized. The discovery of this pattern of problems began in the 1970s, when researchers began to notice children who had much weaker performance IQ (putting block patterns or puzzles together) than verbal IQ (defining vocabulary words or explaining answers to commonsense questions). But even today education professionals are largely unfamiliar with nonverbal learning disorders. Typically, parents are assured that everything is fine and that their child is "just a perfectionist," or is immature, bored, or a bit clumsy. Rarely are a parent or teacher's concerns accepted until the child reaches a point in school where he is no longer able to function. These children are often labeled "behavior problems" or "emotionally disturbed" because of their frequent inappropriate and unexpected conduct, despite the fact that NLD has a neurological rather than an emotional origin.

It is especially important to identify children with nonverbal learning disorders because overestimates of the child's abilities and unrealistic demands made by parents and teachers can lead to ongoing emotional problems. Unfortunately, there are few resources available for the child with NLD syndrome through schools or private agencies, and it is hard to find a professional who understands nonverbal learning disabilities.

Nonverbal learning disorders are much less common than language-based learning disorders (affecting only between .1 percent to 1 percent of the general population). Unlike language-based learning disabilities, the NLD syndrome affects girls as often as boys. Although there are not many people with NLD, experts suspect that as school ASSESSMENT procedures improve, a higher proportion of children will be identified with NLD.

Language-based learning disorders are believed to be inherited, but a specific genetic problem has not yet been discovered. Nonverbal learning disabilities involve the performance processes that originate in the right cerebral hemisphere of the brain, which specializes in nonverbal processing. Brain scans of individuals with NLD often reveal mild abnormalities of the right cerebral hemisphere. A number of children suffering from NLD have at some time early in their development

- sustained a moderate to severe head injury
- received repeated radiation treatments on or near their heads over a prolonged period of time

- had a congenital absence of the CORPUS CALLOSUM
- been treated for hydrocephalus
- had brain tissue removed from the right hemisphere

All of this damage listed above would involve significant destruction of white matter connections in the right hemisphere. Current evidence suggests that a contributing cause of the NLD syndrome involves early damage of the right cerebral hemisphere, or white matter disease that forces the left hemisphere system to function on its own.

Symptoms and Diagnostic Path
Individuals with NLD may experience significant difficulties in perceiving and understanding the subtle visual cues important to nonverbal communication that form the basis of social interaction and interpersonal relations. They may misread overt signals of impatience, annoyance, or the desire to end an interaction, and consequently may respond in ways that are perceived by others as inappropriate.

A person with NLD syndrome may have trouble adapting to new situations, or accurately reading nonverbal signals and cues. Although these students make progress in school, they have trouble "producing" in situations where speed and adaptability are required.

There are three categories of dysfunction

- lack of coordination, severe balance problems, or difficulties with fine motor skills
- poor visual recall, faulty spatial perceptions, or difficulties with spatial relations
- lack of ability to comprehend nonverbal communication, trouble adjusting to new situations, or significant problems with social judgment and social interaction

Children with nonverbal learning disorders commonly appear awkward and uncoordinated in both fine and GROSS MOTOR SKILLS. They may have had extreme difficulty learning to ride a bike or to kick a soccer ball. FINE MOTOR SKILLS, such as cutting with scissors or tying shoe laces, seem to be impossible for them. Young children with NLD are less likely to explore their environment because they cannot rely on their own perceptions. These children do not learn much from experience or repetition and cannot generalize information.

In the early years, children may appear confused much of the time despite a high intelligence and high scores on receptive and expressive language measures. Closer observation will reveal a social ineptness due to misinterpretations of body language and tone of voice. These children do not perceive subtle cues in their environment, such as the idea of personal space, the facial expressions of others, or nonverbal displays of pleasure or displeasure. These are all social skills that are normally grasped intuitively through observation, not directly taught.

Instead, these children cope by relying on language as their principal means of social relating, gathering information, and relieving anxiety. They often develop an exceptional memory for rote material. Since the nonverbal processing area of the brain is not giving automatic feedback, they rely solely on MEMORY of past experiences, each of which they labeled verbally to guide them in future situations. This, of course, is less effective and less reliable than being able to sense and interpret another person's social cues. Normal conversational "give and take" seems impossible for these children.

It is hard for these children to change from one activity to another or to move from one place to another. A child with NLD needs to concentrate merely to get through a room. Owing to the inability to handle such information processing demands, these children will instinctively avoid any kind of novelty.

Problems with NLD grow more apparent and more profound during the latter stages of childhood development and into adolescence and adulthood, as pressures on social interaction increase and the requirements for appropriate social performance become more subtle and complex.

Testing for NLD must cover all the potential areas of strength and weakness. Diagnosis usually begins with standard IQ and achievement tests, followed by assessment of other information processing areas such as fine motor, touch, attention, conceptual reasoning, and memory.

All too often, children with NLD are never diagnosed, in part because the early verbal skills are a source of pride to parents and teachers. Verbally precocious kids with NLD can even be considered gifted in their early school careers and are often able to read at a very early age. As they move on to late elementary and then middle school, however, nonverbal and conceptual reasoning problems become more obvious. Despite the early verbal ability, they can begin to have trouble organizing written work and begin to hand in written homework assignments late (if at all). By the time teachers and parents notice that this child is not continuing to progress, the child may already have begun to give up or become bogged down in academic failure. The child may still be able to memorize well, but memorization may not be enough to meet the demands of high school.

A child with NLD is especially prone to developing DEPRESSION and ANXIETY problems if untreated or unrecognized, especially if he or she is often told just "not working up to ability" or "not working hard enough," so a sensitive evaluation of emotional status through interviewing and observation is needed in addition to testing.

Treatment Options and Outlook

Parents and the school should not underestimate the gravity of this disability. The main problem in the painstaking approach to teaching the child is the caregiver's faulty impression that the child is much more adept than he is. Everyone tends to overestimate the intelligence of NLD adolescents. The child should be shielded from teasing, persecution, and other sources of anxiety.

Intervention should involve a combination of extra instruction and compensation (such as keyboard training to sidestep bad handwriting)—the earlier the better. When considering treatment, it is important to remember that NLD is different from a language-based learning disability. Academic help is typically different from what would be done in more common reading and language disorders. Academic subjects that many children with NLD need help with include math, some aspects of written language, READING COMPREHENSION, and complex visual tasks such as understanding and creating maps, charts, and graphs.

A comprehensive INDIVIDUALIZED EDUCATION PROGRAM (IEP) should outline what help will be given in speech and language therapy to improve social communication, as well as occupational therapy to address visual perception and fine motor skills. On the other hand, since NLD as an underlying pattern is not itself one of the 13 categories of SPECIAL EDUCATION or one of the seven specific types under the category of learning disability in the federal law, the school should look closely for any way to qualify a child under one of these existing categories. Particular attention should be paid to deficits in math computation, math reasoning, reading comprehension, and written expression.

During class, the child's teacher should be careful to speak clearly and outline expectations without ambiguity. Copying text from the board or another paper is not usually helpful and should be avoided, but simplifying tests will help. Whenever possible, timed tests should be reduced or eliminated.

Independence should be introduced gradually, in controlled, nonthreatening situations. The more completely the strengths and weaknesses of the child are understood, the better prepared the care providers will be to promote the child's independence. These children should never be left to their own devices in new activities or situations that lack sufficient structure. Goals and expectations must be attainable.

OCCUPATIONAL THERAPY is a good idea for the younger child. Use of a computer word processor can help, since the spatial and fine motor skills needed for typing are not as complicated as those involved in handwriting. Tasks requiring folding, cutting with scissors, or arranging material (maps, graphs, mobiles) will require considerable help. Timed assignments will need to be modified or eliminated.

Adults need to check often that the child understands, and that information is presented clearly. All expectations need to be direct and explicit, and the student's schedule needs to be as predictable as possible. He or she should be prepared in advance for changes in routine, such as: assemblies, field trips, minimum days, vacation days, finals, and so on.

This type of child needs to be assigned to one case manager at school who will oversee progress and can make sure all of the school staff are making the necessary ACCOMMODATIONS and modifications. In-service training and orientation for all school staff that promotes tolerance and accept-

ance is a vital part of the overall plan for success, as everyone must be familiar with and supportive of the child's academic and social needs.

This child needs to be in a learning environment that provides daily, nonthreatening contact with nondisabled peers—not a "special" or alternative program—in order to boost social development. This child will benefit from cooperative learning situations when grouped with good role models.

Transitions will always be difficult for this child, so he will need time during the school day to collect thoughts before "switching gears."

Teachers will need to present strategies for conversation skills, how and when to change the subject, tone and expression of voice, and nonverbal body language (facial expressions, correct social distance).

Isolation, deprivation, and punishment are not effective methods to change the behavior of a child who is already trying his or her best to conform, but who misinterprets nonverbal cues. If inappropriate behavior causes problems at school, a behavioral intervention plan detailing a course of action may need to be a part of this child's IEP or 504 plan.

How well these children progress seems to depend on early identification and accommodation. Typically, the NLD child is regularly punished for circumstances he or she cannot help, without ever really understanding why, and is often left with little hope that the situation will ever improve. As a result, these children tend to have depression, anxiety, and suicidal thoughts.

nonverbal memory   MEMORY for figures, spatial relationships, and so on. Nonverbal memory is assumed to be based in the deep structures of the right temporal lobe.

normalization   The procedure of placing handicapped individuals in situations as close to normal ones as possible, such as placing a mentally retarded person in a group home rather than in an institution.

norm-referenced test   An ASSESSMENT that compares a person's score with the typical scores of a sample of people who have already taken the same exam, called the "norm group." The norm defined by this group represents the distribution of test scores

norm-referenced test 167

among them. An example of a norm group might be a nationwide sample of ninth graders, or a sample identified by gender, age, and ethnic background. Most standardized achievement tests are norm-referenced. Norm-referenced testing is different from criterion-referenced testing, and does not serve the same purposes or share the same characteristics.

Commercial, national, norm-referenced achievement tests include the CALIFORNIA ACHIEVEMENT TEST (CAT); Comprehensive Test of Basic Skills (CTBS) (which includes the Terra Nova), Iowa Test of Basic Skills (ITBS), and Tests of Academic Proficiency (TAP); METROPOLITAN ACHIEVEMENT TEST (MAT); and STANFORD ACHIEVEMENT TEST (SAT, not to be confused with the college admissions SAT). IQ, cognitive ability, school readiness, and developmental screening tests are also NRTs.

NRTs are designed to compare students' scores. A commercial norm-referenced test does not compare all the students who take the test in a given year; instead; test makers select a sample from the target student population (say, ninth graders). The test is "normed" on this sample, which is supposed to fairly represent the entire target population (all ninth graders in the nation). Students' scores are then reported in relation to the scores of this norm group.

To make comparing easier, test makers create exams in which the results are designed to resemble a bell-shaped curve: most students will score near the middle, and only a few will score low or high.

Scores are usually reported as percentile ranks. The scores range from 1st to 99th percentile, with the average student score set at the 50th percentile. If Jake scored at the 83rd percentile, it means he scored higher than 83 percent of the test takers in the norm group. Scores also can be reported as "grade equivalents," "stanines," and "normal curve equivalents."

One more question right or wrong can cause a big change in a student's score. In fact, having one more correct answer can sometimes cause a student's percentile score to jump more than 10 points.

In making an NRT, it is often more important to choose questions that sort people along the curve than it is to make sure that the content covered by the test is adequate; thus, tests sometimes emphasize small and meaningless differences among test takers. Since the tests are made to sort students, most of the things everyone knows are not tested. Questions may be obscure or tricky, in order to help rank the test takers.

In addition, tests can be biased, favoring one kind of student or another for reasons that have nothing to do with the subject area being tested. For example, knowledge that is more commonly learned by middle- or upper-class children outside of school is often included in tests. To help make the bell curve, test makers usually eliminate questions that students with low overall scores might get right, but those with high overall scores get wrong. Thus, most questions that favor minority groups are eliminated.

NRTs usually have to be completed in a time limit. Some students do not finish, even if they know the material. This can be especially unfair to students with a LEARNING DISABILITY or whose first language is not English. This is another way in which test makers sort people out.

No test is perfectly reliable, and all tests have a "measurement error." A score that appears as an absolute number—say, Jake's 83—really is an estimate. For example, Jake's real score is probably between 76 and 90, but it could be even further off; therefore, results may be reported in "score bands," which indicate the range within which the true score probably lies. Subscores on tests are even less precise, usually because there are often very few items on this portion. A score band for Sally's math subtest might show that her score is between the 45th and 99th percentile because only a handful of questions were asked.

Measurement error may be due to the fact that a student may not feel well, and test-taking conditions are not the same from place to place. Moreover, scores for young children are much less reliable because their moods and attention are more varied. Also, young children develop quickly and unevenly, so a score that is accurate today could be completely wrong next month.

If a child or a school's score goes up on a norm-referenced test, that may or may not mean the child knows more or the school has improved. Schools cannot teach everything. They teach some facts, some procedures, some concepts, some skills—but not others. Often, schools focus most on what is tested and stop teaching many things that are not tested. When scores go up, it does not mean the students know more, it means they know more of what is on that test.

"Teaching to the test" explains why scores usually go down when a new test is used. A district usually uses an NRT for five to 10 years. Each year, the score goes up as teachers become familiar with what is on the test, but when a new test is introduced, the scores suddenly drop. The students do not know less; it is just that different things are now being tested.

It is often easier to use a norm-referenced test to compare students because they were created to rank test takers. These tests provide a quick snapshot of some of the things most people expect students to learn. They are relatively cheap and easy to administer.

Unfortunately, politicians often call for all students to score above the national average. Since NRTs are constructed so that half the population is always below the midpoint, it is impossible to have all students score above the 50th percentile.

If these tests were used only as one additional piece of information and not much importance was placed on them, this would not be much of a problem. Many mistakes can be made by relying on test scores to make educational decisions. Every major maker of NRTs tells schools not to use them as the basis for making decisions about retention, graduation, or placement. The test makers know that their tests are not designed to be used that way. According to the Standards for Educational and Psychological Measurement, in elementary or secondary education, a decision or characterization that will have a major impact on a test taker should not automatically be made on the basis of a single test score.

Any one test can measure only a limited part of a subject area or a limited range of important human abilities. A reading test may measure only some particular reading skills, not a full range of the ability to understand and use texts. Multiple-choice math tests can measure skill in computation or solving routine problems, but they are not good for testing whether students can reason mathematically and apply their knowledge to real-world problems.

Most NRTs focus too heavily on memorization and routine procedures. Multiple-choice and short-answer questions do not measure most knowledge that students need to do well in college, qualify for good jobs, or be active and informed citizens. Tests like these cannot show whether a student can write a research paper, understand current events or the impact of science on society, or debate important issues. They do not test problem solving, decision-making, judgment, or social skills.

Tests often force teachers to overemphasize memorization over thinking and knowledge application. Since the tests are very limited, teaching just what is on the test weakens a curriculum. Defining "improvement" in a school district as a rise in test scores often leads to test coaching. Linking teacher raises to test scores is almost a guarantee that test coaching will occur.

Norm-referenced tests also can lower academic expectations. NRTs support the idea that learning or intelligence fits a bell curve. If educators believe it, they are more likely to have low expectations of students who score below average.

Norm-referenced tests are the opposite of CRITERION-REFERENCED TESTS, which determine whether each student has achieved specific skills or concepts. Unlike NRTs, CRTs are used to find out how much students know before instruction begins and after it has finished. They measure specific skills that make up a designated curriculum and compare each individual with a preset standard for acceptable achievement. The performance of others is irrelevant.

norms The typical distribution of scores on a given test among a specific norm group.

objective left-right discrimination A higher level of discrimination in which an individual can consistently and accurately be aware of the relation of left and right sides of the body on another person as well as himself. The client can imitate in a mirror fashion the movements of another; later he can reverse the sides, imitating the action of another so that his right hand is truly performing what another person's right hand is doing. Naming the sides of the self and in other objects and in pictures is a conceptual skill and might be considered at the lower level of cognitive function.

obsessive-compulsive disorder (OCD) An ANXI-ETY disorder characterized by severe obsessions and/or compulsions. People with obsessive-compulsive disorder suffer intensely from recurrent, unwanted thoughts (obsessions) or rituals (compulsions), which they feel they cannot control. Rituals such as handwashing, counting, checking, or cleaning are often performed as a way of preventing obsessive thoughts or making them go away. Performing these rituals, however, provides only temporary relief, and not performing them markedly increases anxiety. Left untreated, obsessions and the need to perform rituals can take over a person's life. OCD is often a chronic, relapsing illness.

OCD is often linked with other anxiety disorders, major DEPRESSION, and TOURETTE'S SYNDROME. While OCD can coexist with ATTENTION DEFICIT HYPERACTIVITY DISORDER, it is not yet clear how that link occurs.

OCD strikes men and women equally, affecting about one in 50 people. It can appear in childhood, adolescence, or adulthood, but usually first appears in the teens or early adulthood. One-third of adults with OCD experienced their first symptoms as children.

There is growing evidence that OCD is caused by a physical problem in the brain, related in part to genetics, brain chemicals, and problems in communication between different parts of the brain. Brain cells use a chemical called serotonin to communicate with one another and some experts believe that low levels of serotonin are linked to OCD. Symptoms improve when the person with OCD is given drugs that increase the brain concentration of serotonin (such as certain antidepressants, such as Prozac). Brain scans also show that the brain cell circuits involved in OCD become normal after the person takes a serotonin-boosting medication or receives cognitive-behavioral psychotherapy.

Although experts have not yet identified any specific genes for OCD, research does suggest that heredity may play a role in some cases. Childhood-onset OCD tends to run in families (sometimes along with tic disorders). If a parent has OCD, there is a slightly higher risk that the child will develop the condition, although the risk is still low.

OCD is not caused by the person's home environment or by attitudes learned in childhood (such as an emphasis on cleanliness or a belief that certain thoughts are dangerous or unacceptable).

Symptoms and Diagnostic Path
Many healthy people have some of the symptoms of OCD, such as checking the stove several times before leaving the house. But the disorder is diagnosed only when such activities consume at least an hour a day, are very distressing, and interfere with daily life. Most adults with this condition know that what they are doing is senseless, but they cannot stop. However, children with OCD may not realize that their behavior is unusual.

The symptoms may come and go, may get better over time, or may grow progressively worse.

Often, people with OCD may avoid situations in which they might have to confront their obsessions, or they may try unsuccessfully to use ALCOHOL or drugs to calm themselves. Severe OCD can keep someone from working or from carrying out normal responsibilities at home, but more often it does not develop to those extremes.

Brain scans using positron emission tomography (PET) have found that people with OCD have different patterns of brain activity than those people with other mental illnesses, or people with no mental illness at all.

In addition, PET scans show that in patients with OCD, both behavioral therapy and medication produce changes in a part of the brain called the caudate nucleus. This is graphic evidence that both psychotherapy and medication affect the brain.

Treatment Options and Outlook

A combination of medication and psychotherapy is often helpful for most patients; some individuals respond best to one therapy, some to another. A number of medications that were originally approved for treatment of depression have been found to be effective for anxiety disorders, including citalopram (Celexa), escitalopram (Lexapro), fluoxetine (Prozac), fluvoxamine (Luvox), paroxetine (Paxil), and sertraline (Zoloft).

Behavioral therapy (specifically "exposure and response prevention") is also helpful in treating OCD. This type of therapy involves exposing the person to whatever triggers the problem and then helping the person avoid the usual ritual. This might involve having the patient touch something dirty and then not wash his hands. This therapy is often successful in patients who complete a behavioral therapy program, although results have been less favorable in some people who have both OCD and depression.

Cognitive therapy is another therapy favored by many specialists. Cognitive therapists treat what they consider to be unproductive self-statements (such as "If I do not wash my hands, it will be horrible") that they believe are responsible for the discomfort that people with OCD experience.

The most popular type of cognitive therapy is rational-emotive therapy (RET) developed by psychologist Albert Ellis. In RET, the therapist emphasizes replacing unproductive self-statements such as, "If I do not wash may hands I will die," with more productive self-statements such as "If I do not wash my hands, I may be uncomfortable, and I may feel an urge to wash my hands, but I will not die." Through extensive practice in rephrasing self-statements, RET therapists believe, the person eventually overcomes the discomfort they have experienced and are able to change the rituals and obsessions that have made them (and the people around them) miserable.

occipital lobe One of four major pairs of lobes of the cerebral cortex that include the center of the visual perception system. Although protected from injury because of the location at the back of the brain, any significant trauma could produce subtle changes to the visual-perceptual system, such as visual field defects.

The occipital lobe is involved in visual-spatial processing, discrimination of movement, and color discrimination. Damage to one side of the occipital lobe causes loss of vision. Disorders of the occipital lobe can cause visual hallucinations and illusions. Lesions in the parietal-temporal-occipital association area can cause word blindness, ALEXIA, and AGRAPHIA.

occupational therapists Professionals who work directly with individuals with impaired physical or motor functions caused by disease, injury, or surgical or other medical interventions. They work with individuals who have conditions that are mentally, physically, developmentally, or emotionally disabling, and help them to develop, recover, or maintain daily living and work skills. They help clients not only to improve basic motor functions and reasoning abilities, but also to compensate for permanent loss of function. Their goal is to help clients have independent, productive, and satisfying lives.

Occupational therapists may work exclusively with individuals in a particular age group, or with particular disabilities. In schools, for example, they evaluate children's abilities, recommend and provide therapy, modify classroom equipment, and in general, help children participate as fully as possible in school programs and activities.

Occupational therapists help clients perform activities of all types, such as using a computer.

Physical exercises may be used to increase strength and dexterity, while paper and pencil exercises may be chosen to improve visual acuity and the ability to discern patterns. A client with short-term memory loss, for instance, might be encouraged to make lists to aid recall. One with coordination problems might be assigned exercises to improve hand-eye coordination. Occupational therapists also use computer programs to help clients improve decision making, abstract reasoning, PROBLEM SOLVING, and perceptual skills, as well as memory, sequencing, and coordination—all of which are important for independent living.

In mental health settings, they may treat mentally retarded individuals, choosing activities that help people learn to cope with daily life, such as time management skills, budgeting, shopping, homemaking, and use of public transportation. They may also work with individuals who are dealing with alcoholism, drug abuse, DEPRESSION, eating disorders, or stress-related disorders.

Occupational therapists must have at least a bachelor's degree in occupational therapy, and the profession is regulated in all states. To obtain a license, applicants must graduate from an accredited educational program and pass a national certification examination. Those who pass the test are called "registered occupational therapists." Occupational therapy coursework includes physical, biological, and behavioral sciences, and the application of occupational therapy theory and skills. Completion of six months of supervised fieldwork is also required.

Office for Civil Rights The government office that ensures equal access to education and promotes educational excellence throughout the nation through vigorous enforcement of civil rights.

Part of the Department of Education, this office is responsible for monitoring the scope of laws and regulations regarding civil rights in educational contexts.

The Office for Civil Rights enforces five federal laws that prohibit discrimination in education programs and activities that receive federal financial assistance. Discrimination on the basis of race, color, and national origin is prohibited by Title VI of the Civil Rights Act of 1964: sex discrimination is prohibited by Title IX of the Education Amendments of 1972; discrimination on the basis of disability is prohibited by Section 504 of the REHABILITATION ACT OF 1973; and age discrimination is prohibited by the Age Discrimination Act of 1975. The Department of Justice also has delegated OCR responsibility for enforcing Title II of the AMERICANS WITH DISABILITIES ACT of 1990.

The civil rights laws enforced by OCR include all state education agencies, elementary and secondary school systems, colleges and universities, vocational school, proprietary schools, state vocational rehabilitation agencies, libraries, and museums that receive U.S. Department of Education funds.

A complaint of discrimination can be filed by anyone who believes that a school that receives federal financial assistance has discriminated against someone on the basis of race, color, national origin, sex, disability, or age. The person or organization filing the complaint need not be a victim, but may complain on behalf of another person.

Most of OCR's activities are conducted by its 12 enforcement offices throughout the country involved in preventing, identifying, ending, and remedying discrimination against America's students.

Office of Special Education Programs A component of the Office of Special Education and Rehabilitative Services, which is one of the principal components of the U.S. Department of Education. The office's mission and organization focus on the free appropriate public education of children and youth with disabilities from birth through age 21.

They are the primary administrative agency for the implementation of the INDIVIDUALS WITH DISABILITIES EDUCATION IMPROVEMENT ACT (IDEIA). While many matters relating to IDEIA legislation are typically handled at the state level, the Office of Special Education Programs has the authority to investigate complaints, withhold funds, and review individual state plans pertaining to compliance.

oppositional behavior Behavior that is negative, hostile, and defiant in nature. Some degree of oppositional behavior is normal in childhood and adolescence, and represents one method by which a child separates from parental or social expectations in order to define individual identity.

In some cases, an unusual degree of oppositional behavior may accompany an ATTENTION DISORDER or SELF-ESTEEM or self-concept difficulties arising from learning problems in school.

A significant and ongoing pattern of oppositional behavior may indicate the presence of OPPOSITIONAL DEFIANT DISORDER, a condition that may occur together with attention disorders.

See also CONDUCT DISORDER.

oppositional defiant disorder (ODD) A psychological disorder characterized by angry, hostile, and impulsive behavior in opposition to authority figures. This antisocial disorder of early to middle childhood may evolve into a CONDUCT DISORDER, usually diagnosed before the age of 12.

There are probably many different causes for ODD, but biological, genetic, and environmental factors all may play a role. Some parents report that their child with ODD was more rigid and demanding than their other youngsters at an early age, which could suggest that a difficult temperament might predispose a child to ODD. Some experts believe ODD may be linked to how a child was disciplined.

Authoritarian child-rearing practices are often associated with the development of ODD characteristics. ODD is considered less severe than conduct disorder and may involve behaviors that include overt resistance to rules and instructions, lying, and violations of other social norms.

This is the most common psychiatric problem in children, which affects more than 5 percent of all youngsters. In younger children it is more common in boys than in girls, but as they grow older, the rate is the same in both.

ODD can occur together with ATTENTION DEFICIT HYPERACTIVITY DISORDER (ADHD). Indeed, many behavioral problems associated with ADHD may in fact be symptoms of ODD.

It is extremely rare for a physician to see a child with only ODD; usually, the child has another psychiatric disorder—often ADHD. A child with ADHD has a 30 percent to 40 percent risk of also having ODD.

Symptoms and Diagnostic Path

ODD is characterized by aggressiveness, but not impulsiveness. In ODD, individuals annoy others on purpose, while this behavior is usually not so purposeful in ADHD. ODD signs and symptoms are much more difficult to live with than ADHD. ADHD sometimes goes away, but ODD rarely does. Unlike ADHD, ODD is not characterized by poor social skills, and children with ODD can sit still.

Children and adolescents with ADHD alone are impulsive, but they are not necessarily aggressive. A child with ADHD may impulsively push someone too hard on a swing or knock a child down, but he or she would probably be sorry afterward. A child with ODD plus ADHD might push the child out of the swing and then deny it, bragging about it to friends later. Children with ADHD and ODD often get in a lot of trouble as their impulsiveness and hyperactivity often lead to fights, rough play, and huge temper tantrums.

Children with ODD develop signs of mood disorders or anxiety as they get older; by the time these children reach the end of elementary school, about 25 percent will have disabling mood or anxiety problems. When ODD is present with ADHD, DEPRESSION, TOURETTE'S SYNDROME, anxiety disorders, or other disorders, it makes life with that child far more difficult.

The criteria for diagnosing ODD include a pattern of negative, hostile, defiant behavior lasting at least six months. The disturbance in behavior causes significant problems with social, school, or job functioning. At least four of the following symptoms must be present. The individual often

- loses his or her temper
- argues with adults
- actively defies or refuses to comply with adults' requests or rules
- deliberately annoys people
- blames others for mistakes or misbehavior
- is touchy or easily annoyed by others
- is angry and resentful
- is spiteful and vindictive

All of the criteria above include the word *often*—this may mean different things to different people. After all, these behaviors occur to a varying degree in all normal children. Researchers have found that "often" is best solved by the following criteria:

At least four times a week the child is angry and resentful and deliberately annoys people.

At least twice a week the child is touchy or easily annoyed by others, loses his or her temper, argues with adults, and actively defies or refuses to comply with adults' requests or rules.

In the last three months, the child is spiteful and vindictive and blames others for his or her mistakes or misbehavior.

The problems usually begin between ages one and three, and appears to run in families. If a parent is alcoholic and has been in trouble with the law, their children are almost three times as likely to have ODD.

Treatment Options and Outlook

Unfortunately, children with ODD only sometimes respond well to treatment. Children with oppositional and defiant behavior along with attention problems typically benefit from some form of structured behavior-management program at home and school; interventions based on improved parenting may be effective.

Anyone working with children with ODD should use clear, specific commands and work on reinforcing positive behaviors. Consistent negative consequences delivered in a neutral way in response to inappropriate behaviors is also effective, but more positive incentives than reprimands should be tried.

oral language   Speaking and listening. Development of good oral language in young children is important for the development of good reading and writing skills later. Difficulties in early oral language development in sounds, word meanings, and sentence structure can be a warning sign for possible LANGUAGE DISORDER.

Language includes four dimensions, which are developed in children in the following order: listening, speaking, reading, and writing. Thus, oral language plays an important role in the normal development of reading and writing.

oral reading   Reading out loud. Oral reading is used to measure an individual's reading skills, which are usually recorded as "grade level." For example, a child's oral reading rate of 3.4 means he is reading material at a third grade, fourth month level.

Recording an individual's oral reading errors can be used to diagnose reading problems. By looking for reading patterns, it is possible to design a remediation program accordingly.

organicity   A term used to refer to unusual or abnormal behavior that is likely to have a biological basis.

organizational strategies   Individuals with a LEARNING DISABILITY often have trouble with a lack of organization and can benefit from learning to use strategies to help them manage their time, materials, and information.

For school-age students, teachers can provide clear routines and structures in the classroom. Students can be taught to prepare a notebook for each class and keep materials neat. Keeping a daily planner can help map out assignment due dates, appointments, and daily schedules. Teaching strategies such as active reading and note-taking skills are also useful for organizing information, which can often be overwhelming for learning-disabled individuals.

orthographic awareness   An individual's command of the sound-letter relationship. As children learn to write, their approaches to spelling change as they become more aware of sounds and letters. In the beginning, children often spell very simply (such as "bt" for "boat"). As they get older they may apply conventions of spelling but still misspell ("bote" for "boat").

With more exposure to written language, as they become more proficient readers and learn specific spelling patterns, young writers begin to apply more sophisticated spelling patterns ("boat" for "boat"). Individuals with LEARNING DISABILITIES who have underdeveloped orthographic awareness often have problems with spelling.

orthography   The formal name for spelling—the system of representing spoken language in written form. The spelling of English can be difficult to learn due to many irregular spelling patterns. For example, "do," "due," and "dew" are all pronounced the same way. English has 44 sounds, but it has only 26 letters.

The letter-sound correspondence is essential for reading, as is the sound-letter correspondence for correct spelling. Difficulties in these relationships can result in language disabilities.

Orton, Samuel Torrey (1879–1948)   A neuropsychiatrist and pathologist who was a pioneer in reading failure and related language processing difficulties; he also was the first to identify DYSLEXIA.

Orton first called dyslexia *strephosymbolia* (twisted symbols), after noting the letter reversals that some dyslexics demonstrate in their writing. Although transposing letters also occurs in the writing of most young children, and reversals are not necessary for a diagnosis of dyslexia or reading disability, it remains as a common stereotype of the disorder.

A professor of neuropsychiatry and neuropathology at the Neurological Institute of Columbia University, Orton was a pioneer in focusing attention on language differences by bringing together neuropsychiatric information and principals of remediation. As early as 1925 he had identified the syndrome of developmental reading disability, separated it from mental defect and brain damage, and offered a physiological explanation with a favorable prognosis.

As early as the 1920s, Orton had extensively studied children with the kind of language processing difficulties now commonly associated with dyslexia and had formulated a set of teaching principles and practices for such children. During his lifetime, Orton directed many research projects dealing with developmental reading disabilities.

It was during one of these projects that he met Anna Gillingham (1878–1963), a teacher and psychologist in the field of language disabilities. Together, they developed procedures and comprehensive materials for early identification and remediation of dyslexic children. Their program is known today as the ORTON-GILLINGHAM APPROACH to reading instruction. Their manual, published first in 1936, is now in its seventh edition.

Modern research has continued to confirm Orton's theories about the physiological differences experienced by dyslexics. Although early remediation is most effective, these methods have been successfully adapted for use with older students and adults.

See also GILLINGHAM, ANNA.

Orton-Gillingham approach   A multisensory approach to reading, writing, and spelling born of a theory of reading disabilities devised by Samuel Orton, Anna Gillingham, and Bessie Stillman in the 1930s. Their approach was based on the idea that the brain stores information in both hemispheres; when the connection between the two hemispheres is not fully developed, individuals may read words in reverse.

People with DYSLEXIA have the potential to be accomplished readers and adequate spellers. The ability to achieve this potential depends on two variables: the instructional approach and the amount of practice. The Orton-Gillingham approach to reading and spelling ensures success by developing multisensory techniques for memory and retrieval. This practical teaching technique emphasizes the reading-decoding process.

The teacher introduces the elements of the language systematically, and students are taught letter-sound relationships using all senses: seeing the letter (visual), saying the letter (auditory), and writing the letter (kinesthetic). In this respect. Orton-Gillingham differs from traditional PHONICS instruction. Once letters are mastered, letters are grouped into blends, and short, structured passages are used for reading and dictation. Infinitely flexible, it is a philosophy rather than a system. The student learns the elements of language-consonants, digraphs, blends, and diphthongs in an orderly fashion.

As students learn new material, they continue to review old material until it becomes automatic. The teacher addresses vocabulary, sentence structure, composition, and reading comprehension in a similar structured, sequential, and cumulative manner.

At best, the teacher tries to understand how an individual learns and to devise appropriate teaching strategies. In every lesson, the student experiences success and gains confidence as well as skill. Learning becomes a happy experience. The Orton-Gillingham approach is appropriate for teaching individuals, small groups, and classrooms. It is appropriate for teaching in the primary, elementary, and intermediate grades, and at the secondary and college level, as well as for adults.

An Orton-Gillingham approach, while not the only program available, is probably the best known for helping children with dyslexia learn to read. The fundamental principles on which it is based, including developing phonemic awareness, and using a multisensory approach, are considered essential components in reading instruction today.

The Orton-Gillingham approach has proven successful with students who have struggled in learning to read and spell through traditional classroom methods, despite normal intelligence, hearing, and vision. It is the program most recommended by experts in the field of dyslexia.

Modern research has continued to confirm Dr. Orton's theories about the physiological differences experienced by people with dyslexia. Early remediation is most effective; however, these methods have been successfully adapted for use with older students and adults. The result is the development of lifelong language skills and the wonderful feeling of success in the world of written language.

See also GILLINGHAM, ANNA; ORTON, SAMUEL TORREY.

outcomes assessment The ASSESSMENT of student attainment or mastery of specific learning objectives. While the term may be used in relation to assessment of an individual student's program and performance, it is more commonly used in the context of overall institutional research and evaluation. This allows a school to see whether student performance meets the educational goals defined by the school, and helps the school evaluate the effectiveness of those goals.

The nature and focus of outcomes assessment varies according to the nature of a school and its mission. For example, outcomes assessment for a high school might focus on the percentage of students in specific grades who meet established standards for competence in reading, writing, and critical skills.

While outcomes assessment typically focuses on academic accomplishments, it may also take into account social and emotional development. In the past decade, outcomes assessment has become an increasingly important activity for educational institutions, both public and private, as a primary means of demonstrating institutional effectiveness and justifying their use of federal, state, and local funds.

parapnasias Use of incorrect words or word combinations.

parenting skills training A type of behavioral therapy that can be helpful in dealing with children with a LEARNING DISABILITY. Rearing children under the best of circumstances is challenging, but when one or children have a learning disability, special discipline techniques may be necessary to help modify behavior. For instance, many therapists recommend consistent use of "time outs" when a child loses control. Other techniques include rewards and penalties or stress-reduction methods, such as meditation. Parents are further encouraged to spend "quality time" each day with the child; read a book together, toss a football, or play a board game, for example. Since children with learning disabilities tend to receive more than an average share of negative feedback, parents can balance that out by praising good behavior and good deeds, large and small, and pointing out the child's strengths and abilities.

parietal lobes One of four major pairs of lobes of the CEREBRAL CORTEX. It is an located at the upper middle part of the head above the temporal lobes, and includes the sensory cortex and the association areas involved in processing information about body sensation, touch, and spatial organization. The association areas in the parietal lobes are also involved in secondary language and visual processing.

Lesions in association areas in the parietal lobe can cause difficulties in learning tasks that require an understanding of spatial perception and the body's position in space. GERSTMANN'S SYNDROME is associated with damage to these areas; this syndrome may include left to right confusion, difficulty naming fingers when specific fingers are touched (FINGER AGNOSIA), problems in writing (dysgraphia), and problems with mathematics (DYSCALCULIA).

pattern recognition The ability to remember and recognize patterns is a key component of learning. Pattern recognition is an important element in reading development, in which an effective reader will increasingly come to recognize that certain patterns (such as specific consonant clusters like *th* or *st*) represent stable sounds, or that certain prefixes and suffixes (such as *re-* or *-ing*) convey specific meanings.

The ability to recognize and remember patterns is essential in developing mathematical and writing abilities, and also plays an essential role in developing higher order cognitive abilities such as critical thinking, analysis, and problem solving.

Pattern recognition may be a significant difficulty for individuals with a LEARNING DISABILITY or attention disorders.

Peabody Picture Vocabulary Test–Third Edition (PPVT-III) A developmental test of language ASSESSMENT that measures receptive vocabulary (that is, vocabulary a person understands when he hears it used by someone else) by having a student point to the correct picture that depicts a dictated word from among a group of four pictures. Children who have poor visual comprehension of pictures, or who tend to respond impulsively, may have a low score on the PPVT-III, even though they have adequate language skills.

Because this test assesses only one aspect of language development, it should be used together with other tests that measure other aspects of language ability, such as oral communication skills and comprehension of grammatical structures.

Receptive vocabulary is only a small subset of COGNITIVE ABILITY and should never be confused with INTELLIGENCE.

pedagogy   The study of teaching methods, including the educational goals and objectives and the means of achieving such goals. Pedagogy encompasses educational psychology and theories of learning.

pemoline (Cylert)   A stimulant medication that had been used for 30 years to treat ATTENTION DEFICIT HYPERACTIVITY DISORDER (ADHD) but that was discontinued in spring 2005 by its manufacturer. The drug caused very rare reported cases of serious liver damage in patients, but the manufacturer said it was removing the drug from the market because of declining sales. Cylert earned less than $1 million in 2004.

The nonprofit group Public Citizen had petitioned the U.S. Food and Drug Administration in early 2005 to remove Cylert and all its generic versions, citing an increased risk of serious liver problems and death from liver failure. Pemoline had been approved in 1975, but since that time, other drugs have become available to treat ADHD. The petition noted that as of May 1996, Cylert had caused 13 cases of acute liver failure, resulting in death or liver transplantation in 11 cases. The petition also said that from 1975 to 1996, there were 193 adverse drug reactions involving the liver in patients younger than 20 years old. It also has been banned in Canada and England.

percentile   A value on a scale of 100 that indicates the percent of a distribution that is equal to or below it. It is the point on a distribution of NORMS in a STANDARDIZED TEST below which a certain percentage of the scores fall. For example, if 50 percent of the scores fall below a raw score of 80 on a test, then the score of 80 is the 50th percentile.

perception   The process by which sensory information (hearing, sight, touch, movement, taste, smell) is recognized and interpreted.

Perception involves both the intake of information through the senses, and processing and making sense of that information within cognition. While sensory experience itself is largely automatic for humans, perception also involves learned behavior and intellectual capacity.

perceptual disorder   A disorder involving the perception of stimuli from one or more of the senses. Unlike visual or hearing problems, perceptual disorders involve the processing of information received through a sense, either in perception or understanding.

A number of distinct brain problems are caused by defects in visual, sensory, and hearing perception that represent fundamental defects in perception rather than complex problems of MEMORY, reasoning, or motor function. They usually involve only parts of the brain.

perceptual handicap   See PERCEPTUAL DISORDER.

perceptual learning disabilities   See PERCEPTUAL DISORDER.

perceptual-motor skills   In everything children do, they look, listen, and touch, and then make a perceptual judgment about the things they see, hear, and feel. It is this perceptual judgment that dictates the way they react to their world (what is seen, what is heard, and what is felt). When perceptions are well developed, then reactions are more likely to be appropriate for each given situation.

There are six perceptual systems that take in information from the environment: visual (sight), auditory (sound), tactile (touch), kinesthetic (muscle feeling), olfactory (smell), and gustatory (taste). Perceptual-motor skills or behavior generally will involve perceptual input through more than one of these systems, and a complex sequence of motor activities.

Motor learning is an important part of childhood development. There is a natural developmental sequence of perceptual motor skill development, beginning very early with skills such as rolling over and sitting up, and proceeding to activities such as crawling, standing, walking, running, and jumping. As development progresses, the requirements for integration of perceptual systems and motor behavior grow steadily more subtle and complex.

Delays in the development of age-appropriate perceptual-motor skills may have significant and sometimes pervasive effects on school and social performance.

perceptual processing   The systems and processes by which raw data from the surrounding environment is taken in through the perceptual system and interpreted by the brain. In general, visual processing and auditory processing are the most commonly referred to areas of perceptual processing, when addressing issues of learning and learning problems in clinical or educational settings.

perfectionism   A set of self-defeating thoughts and behaviors aimed at reaching excessively high and unrealistic goals. Many people who have trouble with writing or finishing school projects have problems with perfectionism, which may be closely related to anxiety or to OBSESSIVE-COMPULSIVE DISORDER. Individuals diagnosed with ATTENTION DEFICIT HYPERACTIVITY DISORDER (ADHD) frequently have perfectionist tendencies, particularly in areas they feel are important. One key factor in perfectionism that is often characteristic of both learning-disabled students and those with ADHD is the inability to differentiate between important and unimportant information. For example, a perfectionistic student may spend hours on a homework assignment because he or she repeatedly crumples up his or her paper and tosses it in the trash when some of the letters are not the same size as others, or because he or she keeps changing pencils to obtain a certain color of lead. In such cases, perfectionism is another manifestation of the social imperception that so often characterizes students with learning disabilities and ADHD.

The issue of perfectionism may seem to be linked to a failure to understand the nature of a task's requirements. However, it appears equally likely that perfectionist behavior may arise from deeper underlying factors, and may best be addressed through a combination of behavioral and cognitive treatments.

Perfectionism is often mistakenly seen as desirable or even necessary for success. However, recent studies have shown that perfectionistic attitudes actually interfere with success. The desire to be perfect can both deprive an individual of a sense of personal satisfaction and cause that person to fail to achieve as much as those with more realistic goals.

Most perfectionists learned early in life that they were valued because of how much they achieved. As a result, they learned to value themselves only on the basis of other people's approval, so that self-esteem came to be based primarily on external standards. This can leave people vulnerable and excessively sensitive to the opinions and criticism of others. In attempting to protect themselves from criticism, these individuals may decide that being perfect is their only defense.

A number of negative feelings, thoughts, and beliefs may be associated with perfectionism, including

- fear of failure: perfectionists often equate failure to achieve their goals with a lack of personal worth or value

- fear of making mistakes: perfectionists often equate mistakes with failure. In orienting their lives around avoiding mistakes, perfectionists miss opportunities to learn and grow

- fear of disapproval: if they let others see their flaws, perfectionists often fear that they will not be accepted. Trying to be perfect is a way of trying to protect themselves from criticism, rejection, and disapproval

- all-or-nothing thinking: perfectionists often think they are worthless if their accomplishments are not perfect, and they have trouble putting things in perspective. For example, a straight-A student who gets a "B" might think he or she is "a total failure"

- the "shoulds": the lives of perfectionists are often structured by an endless list of rigid rules about how their lives must be led. With such an overemphasis on shoulds, perfectionists rarely take into account their own desires

- others' success: perfectionists tend to perceive others as achieving success with a minimum of effort, few errors, little emotional stress, and maximum self-confidence, whereas their own efforts are inadequate

Perfectionists are often trapped in a vicious cycle in which they set unreachable goals and then fail to meet them because the goals were impossible to begin with. Failure was thus inevitable. The constant pressure to achieve perfection and the inevitable chronic failure lessen productivity and effectiveness. As perfectionists become more self-critical, their SELF-ESTEEM suffers, which may also lead to ANXIETY and DEPRESSION. At this point perfectionists may give up completely on their goals and set different unrealistic goals, but this thinking sets the entire cycle in motion again.

Perfectionists need to understand that perfectionism is undesirable, and they must challenge the self-defeating thoughts and behaviors that fuel perfectionism. Cognitive therapy is often helpful in achieving this.

perseveration   Persistent repetition of a behavior or activity regardless of the result, or having trouble switching from one activity to another. Extreme examples of perseveration may be seen in individuals with a DEVELOPMENTAL DISABILITY or AUTISM, for whom repetitive hand motions, rocking, or other movements are common characteristics. More typical examples in childhood might involve singing a song from a video again and again.

In a school setting, perseveration can be used to describe the fixation on a specific element in a broader task, such as spending all of the time of an exam on a single essay question. Psychologists often encounter perseveration in students they evaluate for LEARNING DISABILITIES. For example, if a student is told to copy six small circles in a straight row, the student may make the circles all the way across the width of the page, drawing 30 or more. Teachers and parents often report perseverative behaviors among students with learning disabilities and ADHD. For example, if they ask the student to hop four times on the left foot, the student may hop 20 or more times or until he or she loses balance.

This type of behavior may be caused by inflexible strategies and problems in shifting from one task to another.

personality test   A type of test that is meant to assess a broad range of personality traits and char-

acteristics, and provide a spectrum of potential information, from indications of personal styles or patterns to evidence of significant personality disorders or other psychological difficulties. Personality tests are often administered as part of a comprehensive ASSESSMENT battery in order to assure an accurate diagnosis of complex symptoms.

The oldest, most-studied personality test is the MINNESOTA MULTIPHASIC PERSONALITY INVENTORY (MMPI), a true/false test with 567 questions. It is used by psychologists in hospitals, clinics, and in private practice, to help diagnose the possible existence of mental disorders. The MMPI was first published in 1943, and was restandardized with updated language in 1989 as the MMPI-2. An adolescent version of the MMPI-2 (the MMPI-A) is also available.

The MILLON CLINICAL MULTIAXIAL INVENTORY (MCMI) is another personality test recently updated as the MCMI-III. It was written by Dr. Theodore Millon (founding editor of the *Journal of Personality Disorders*) to specifically assess personality disorders, as opposed to the MMPI, which screens for a broad range of psychological problems. An adolescent version of this test also exists.

A third widely used personality test is called the SIXTEEN PRIMARY FACTOR INVENTORY (also known as the 16PF or the Cattell 16PF), which is a more positive test that evaluates personality traits and identifies the test taker's strengths. Developed by Raymond Cattell, it is used primarily for job seekers and to assess relationship strengths and weaknesses. A children's version of the 16PF (the Children's Personality Questionnaire, or CPQ) and an adolescent version (the High School Personality Questionnaire) are also available.

pervasive development disorder—not otherwise specified (PDD-NOS)   A type of PERVASIVE DEVELOPMENT DISORDER characterized by significantly impaired social interactions or stereotyped behaviors without all of the features of AUTISM or ASPERGER'S SYNDROME. Children with Asperger's syndrome or PDD-NOS tend to function at a higher level than children with autism and may be able to function independently.

pervasive developmental disorders (PDD)   An older term for a category of neurological disorders now called AUTISM SPECTRUM DISORDERS, characterized by severe and pervasive impairment in several areas of development, including social interaction, imaginative activity, a limited number of repetitive activities or interests, and verbal and nonverbal communications skills.

The five disorders typically included under the PDD umbrella include autistic disorder (AUTISM), ASPERGER'S SYNDROME, CHILDHOOD DISINTEGRATIVE DISORDER (CDD), RETT SYNDROME, and PERVASIVE DEVELOPMENT DISORDER—NOT OTHERWISE SPECIFIED (PDD-NOS). Each of these disorders has specific diagnostic criteria as outlined by the *DIAGNOSTIC & STATISTICAL MANUAL OF MENTAL DISORDERS—FOURTH EDITION, Text Revision (DSM-IV-TR)*. Autism is the most common of the five PDDs, affecting an estimated 1 in 250 births, according to the U.S. Centers for Disease Control and Prevention. Rett syndrome is the least common, and recently, many experts tend to exclude it from the autism spectrum disorders.

The term *pervasive developmental disorders* was first used in the 1980s to describe a group of disorders that shared symptoms or characteristics. Unfortunately, the term occasionally causes confusion, since one of the disorders included under PDD has a very similar name—PDD-NOS. As a result, PDD and PDD-NOS are sometimes used interchangeably.

Pervasive Developmental Disorders Screening Test-II (PDDST-II) An easily administered ASSESSMENT tool designed to screen children as young as 18 months for several AUTISTIC SPECTRUM DISORDERS, including AUTISM, pervasive developmental delay, and ASPERGER'S SYNDROME. Designed to be a parent-report screening measure, the test helps to identify children with these problems in early childhood so that intervention can begin as soon as possible.

phenylketonuria (PKU) An inherited metabolic disease (one of the inborn errors of metabolism) that leads to MENTAL RETARDATION and other developmental disabilities if untreated in infancy. In this condition, an amino acid called phenylalanine builds up in the bloodstream, causing brain damage. Infants with untreated PKU appear to develop typically for the first few months of life, but by 12 months of age most babies will have a significant

developmental delay and will be diagnosed with mental retardation.

PKU is inherited as a single-gene disorder, which is a condition caused by a mutant or abnormal gene. It is an autosomal recessive disorder, which means that each parent of a child with PKU carries one defective gene for the disorder and one normal gene. In a recessive condition, an individual must have two defective genes in order to have the disorder. Individuals with only one copy of a defective gene are called "carriers," show no symptoms of having the disease, and usually remain unaware of their status until they have an affected child. In order for a child to inherit PKU, both parents must be PKU carriers. When this occurs, there is a one in four chance of their producing an affected child with each pregnancy. Boys and girls are equally at risk of inheriting this disorder.

Symptoms and Diagnostic Path
Before the 1960s, most infants born with PKU developed mental retardation and cerebral palsy. Although treatment for PKU using a low phenylalanine diet was first described in the 1950s, the inability to detect PKU early in the child's life limited effective treatment.

The first newborn screening test was developed by Dr. Robert Guthrie in 1959 specifically to test for PKU. This simple yet effective and economical test was developed to screen newborn infants for PKU before leaving the hospital. Today, all states routinely screen newborns for this condition. The American Academy of Pediatrics recommends that infants receiving the test during the first 24 hours of life be retested at two to three weeks of age during their first postnatal pediatric visit.

To test for PKU, a few drops of blood are taken from the infant's heel, and then tested in a state laboratory for abnormal amounts of phenylalanine. The normal phenylalanine level is less than 2 milligrams per deciliter (mg/dl). Those with phenylalanine levels of 20.0 mg/dl or higher are considered likely to have "classical" PKU. Infants with these high levels are further tested to confirm the diagnosis before treatment is started.

Some infants with slightly higher levels of phenylalanine have "mild hyperphenylalanemia." Today many clinicians believe that any child with a phenylalanine level greater than 6 or 8 mg/dl should be treated with a modified phenylalanine-restricted diet.

Treatment Options and Outlook

Although PKU is not preventable, its symptoms can often be treated successfully through the use of a carefully regimented diet with a restricted phenylalanine content. Babies are given a special formula that contains very low phenylalanine levels; then they gradually progress to eating certain vegetables and other foods that are low in phenylalanine. Affected children must have their blood tested regularly to ensure the presence of the correct level of phenylalanine. Foods recommended for those affected by PKU contain small amounts of protein, such as fruits and vegetables, limited amounts of cereal and grain products, and special low-protein products.

High-protein foods such as meat, fish, eggs, poultry, dairy products, nuts, peanut butter, legumes, soy products, and products containing Nutrasweet should be avoided. The food program used to treat those with PKU is quite expensive, typically costing up to $10,000 a year or more. Although health departments may pay for the formula in some states and mandated insurance coverage may cover the cost in other states, most insurance companies do not cover the cost of treatment for those with PKU because it is considered nutritional rather than medical therapy.

While phenylalanine-restricted diets have proven to be highly effective in preventing mental retardation, it is now recognized that subtle cognitive deficits may still occur. Usually the individual has a normal IQ, but the incidence of ATTENTION DEFICIT HYPERACTIVITY DISORDER (ADHD) and LEARNING DISABILITIES is higher compared to those children who do not have PKU.

Recent studies have found that children with PKU who stopped the diet in early childhood did not develop as rapidly as children who remained on the diet, and had more LEARNING DISABILITIES, behavioral problems, and other neurological problems. Thus, until research provides alternative treatments, everyone with PKU should remain on a restricted diet indefinitely in order to maintain a safe level of phenylalanine (believed to be in the range of 2-6 mg/dl).

Pregnancy and PKU Pregnant women with PKU who are not receiving dietary therapy will have high levels of phenylalanine that can damage their unborn child, causing mental retardation and other congenital defects in the baby. High levels of phenylalanine are extremely toxic to the brain of a fetus. Although the child does not have PKU, there will be brain damage from the toxic effects of phenylalanine in the womb. This is known as maternal PKU.

More than 90 percent of infants born to women with PKU who are not on a specialized diet will have mental retardation, and may also have small head size, heart defects, and low birth weight. These infants cannot be treated with a special diet since they do not have PKU.

Therefore, women who have PKU should follow a phenylalanine-restricted diet at least one year before getting pregnant, and should stay on the diet while breast-feeding to increase the chance of having a healthy child.

phoneme A single sound. English has 44 phonemes, which are represented by 26 letters (GRAPHEMES).

phonemic awareness The awareness of the sounds (PHONEMES) that make up whole words. A person who has weak phonemic awareness will have trouble judging sounds within words. This causes students to omit, substitute, or reverse sounds and letters within words, and can make learning a second language quite difficult. Individuals with weak phonological processing cannot judge whether what they say matches what they see. Although phonemic awareness is not necessary for understanding spoken language, the ability to break apart and manipulate the sounds in a written word is a crucial skill when learning to read and write.

For example, when an individual hears the word *sat*, the ear hears one continuous sound. When children develop phonemic awareness, they can break the word into three phonemes—/s/-/a/-/t/—making it possible to read and spell correctly. When children have developed phonological awareness, they can isolate sounds, rhyme, blend sounds, and manipulate the sounds of language.

Research indicates phonemic awareness is often underdeveloped for individuals with a LEARNING DISABILITY. Brain scans identify that the brains of learning-disabled individuals cannot segment words and syllables into phonemes nor can they blend sounds into words.

Since poor phonemic awareness is known to be a core deficit in learning-disabled individuals, explicit and systematic instruction in a PHONICS approach has significant benefits to children with reading problems from kindergarten to sixth grade.

The benefits of explicit phonics instructions, which improve phonemic awareness, are overwhelmingly supported by research done by the National Institute of Child Health and Human Development, which endorses this method for regular classroom reading instruction.

Many children have trouble judging sounds within words. Although they see letters correctly, they cannot detect and correct their errors in reading and spelling. This causes problems with decoding, spelling, and pronunciation. A child with this problem might read "secp" for "sleep," spell words like "girl" as "gril," and mispronounce common words.

Individuals who do not develop phonemic awareness in preschool often have trouble learning to read and spell. Therefore, it is important to measure phonemic awareness as children enter first grade. There are informal and formal means of assessing phonemic awareness. Some informal tests would include the following:

- asking an individual to add, delete, or change the sounds in a word
- matching rhyming words
- matching initial, middle, or final sounds of words
- asking an individual to tap on the table for each sound they hear in a given word

When children have trouble with such tasks, more formal assessment of phonemic awareness may be required. There are many formal tests available to assess phonemic awareness, such as the Lindamood Auditory Conceptualization Test or the Test of Phonological Awareness.

phonics   An approach to teaching reading and spelling that emphasizes symbol-sound relationships; used especially in beginning or remedial instruction. Being able to discriminate sounds is an essential element in reading and communicating well.

Phonics programs published by major educational publishers have been used to teach reading for decades. These programs offer books, workbooks, computer software, and other teaching materials that introduce letter and word patterns in a systematic and structured way.

There are two phonics approaches: synthetic and analytic. *Synthetic phonics* is a method where individuals are taught single letters and their sounds. Once the letters are mastered, individuals are taught to synthesize the letters into whole words. *Analytic phonics* teaches whole word families (cat, fat, mat, hat) and then teaches individuals to analyze the phonemic elements of the words. Traditionally, reading was taught in U.S. schools using phonics instruction, with its emphasis on developing word-recognition skills.

However, the phonics approach to learning was criticized in the 1980s when many schools changed direction and embraced the WHOLE LANGUAGE APPROACH, a more holistic and content-driven approach to teaching reading. This method attempts to get students to read right away, using high-quality children's literature, and emphasizes using contextual cues to aid comprehension.

As national reading scores declined, the movement toward whole language began to change again. Studies comparing whole language and phonics showed that children who are explicitly taught phonics in a direct and systematic way achieve higher scores on reading tests.

Today, most schools use a combination of both approaches. A growing body of research suggests that contextual cues cannot replace word recognition. Good readers do not skip words or rely on context but read virtually every word and see all letters. In fact, studies demonstrate that only poor readers rely on contextual cues for word identification. Teaching children to guess the meaning of words by context actually decreases the odds that they will learn to read well.

Children who do not understand what they read usually have poor word-recognition skills.

Because these children have to devote so much attention to slowly and carefully figuring out the words, they focus less attention on what the text means. Children who recognize words more readily can focus more attention on meaning.

Many experts in education today agree that word-recognition skills as taught in phonics are the critical building blocks for reading success. Still, research also demonstrates that phonics alone is less effective than phonics combined with whole language. An average child needs to read a word four to eight times before word-recognition becomes automatic.

Therefore, the process of reading strengthens the child's ability to perceive sounds in both verbal and written language. Moreover, for practice to be most effective, children need to read stories that are at their reading level; in other words, they should be able to recognize most of the words.

While the trends of teaching reading shift from year to year in general education, the field of learning disabilities has consistently found a phonics approach most effective to teach children with LEARNING DISABILITIES.

phonological processing   The ability to hear speech sounds (PHONEMES) and words and identify different sound segments.

See also PHONICS.

phonology   The sound system of a language. PHONICS comes from this word. A PHONEME (sound) is the smallest unit of language; different languages and dialects use different phonemes.

Piaget, Jean (1896–1980)   A pioneering Swiss developmental PSYCHOLOGIST whose lifelong studies in developmental psychology centered on figuring out how children acquire and develop knowledge. He believed that knowledge is a progressive construction of logically embedded structures. To him, this meant that children's logic and way of thinking are at first quite different from those of adults. By the end of his remarkable career, Piaget had developed several new fields of science, including developmental psychology, cognitive theory, and genetic epistemology. Modern educators laud Piaget for being the first to take children's thinking seriously.

His pervasive influence on education is based on the fact that he realized that children do not simply have empty minds to be filled with knowledge but that they are actively building knowledge, constantly creating and testing their own theories of the world. He believed that to understand children, one must understand how they evolve, grow, and learn.

He described four stages of childhood development: sensorimotor, preoperational, concrete operational, and formal operational, yet he never thought of himself as a child psychologist. Instead, his real interest was epistemology (the theory of knowledge). Piaget accepted that there are multiple ways of knowing, which he examined nonjudgmentally but rigorously. He believed that by looking carefully at how knowledge develops in children, it would be possible to understand the nature of knowledge in general.

In the late 1990s, experts challenged Piaget's ideas, stating that knowledge is an intrinsic property of the brain, bolstered by experiments showing that newborns already know some information that Piaget believed children constructed.

Piaget earned a Ph.D. in natural sciences at the University of Neuchâtel, and published two philosophical essays during this time. After a semester at the University of Zurich, where he developed an interest for psychoanalysis, he left Switzerland for France, where he worked for a year at a boys' institution created by Alfred Binet and then directed by Théodore Simon, who had developed an IQ test with Binet. At this school, Piaget performed his first experimental studies of the growing mind.

In 1923, he and Valentine Châtenay were married; Piaget studied their three children's intellectual development from infancy to language acquisition. Piaget occupied several chairs in psychology, sociology, and the history of science at Neuchâtel from 1925 to 1929; history of scientific thinking at Geneva from 1929 to 1939; the International Bureau of Education from 1929 to 1967; psychology and sociology at Lausanne from 1938 to 1951; sociology at Geneva from 1939 to 1952, then genetic and experimental psychology from 1940 to 1971. In 1955, he created and directed until his death the International Center for Genetic Epistemology.

PKU   See PHENYLKETONURIA.

PL 94-142   See EDUCATION FOR ALL HANDICAPPED CHILDREN ACT OF 1975.

portfolio assessment   A representative collection of a student's work that was completed over a period of time. Sometimes referred to as authentic assessment, the collection is used to assess progress and achievement in writing, art, reading, or mathematics. Portfolio assessment is a much more useful means of checking the progress of students with a LEARNING DISABILITY than traditional paper/pencil tests, which often are not true reflections of the student's progress.

However, ASSESSMENT of portfolios can present problems due to their subjective nature. Many educators have developed effective ways to identify progress in specific skill areas. Materials collected in portfolios may include writing samples, science projects, spelling tests, behavioral checklists, teacher observation notes, videotapes of performances, and/or math projects.

positive reinforcement   A method of promoting certain behavior by providing a positive stimulus. When the desired behavior is produced, the stimulus is presented. For example, teachers frequently use stickers or gold stars (positive stimulus) when a child has completed an assignment correctly (desired behavior). As the positive reinforcement is repeated, the desired behavior is reinforced.

See also NEGATIVE REINFORCEMENT.

Prader-Willi syndrome   A complex genetic disorder that causes short stature, MENTAL RETARDATION or a LEARNING DISABILITY, incomplete sexual development, characteristic behavior problems, low muscle tone, and an involuntary urge to eat constantly. This, coupled with a reduced need for calories, leads to obesity.

PWS is found in people of both sexes and all races—about one in 14,000 people in the United States. Prader-Willi syndrome is one of the 10 most common conditions seen in genetics clinics and is the most common genetic cause of obesity that has been identified.

IQs are usually in the 70s but vary from as low as 40 to as high as 100. However, normal IQs—even in the 90–100 range—are accompanied by learning disabilities. Almost all children with Prader-Willi require some form of SPECIAL EDUCATION.

Although PWS is associated with an abnormality of chromosome 15, it is generally considered not to be an inherited condition, but rather a spontaneous genetic birth defect that occurs at or near the time of conception. The faulty chromosome affects functioning of the hypothalamus.

Symptoms and Diagnostic Path
Newborns with PWS have poor muscle tone, and cannot suck well enough to get sufficient nutrients. Often they must be fed through a tube for several months after birth until muscle control improves. Sometime in the following years, usually by preschool age, children with PWS develop an increased interest in food and quickly gain excessive weight if calories are not restricted.

In addition to sometimes extreme attempts to obtain food, people with PWS are prone to temper outbursts, stubbornness, rigidity, argumentativeness, and repetitive thoughts and behaviors. Strategies to deal with these problems usually include structuring the person's environment, implementing behavioral management techniques, and, occasionally, drug therapy.

People with PWS can attend school, enjoy community activities, get jobs, and even move away from home, although they need a lot of help. Schoolchildren with PWS are likely to need special education and related services, such as speech and occupational therapy. In community, work, and residential settings, adolescents and adults often need special assistance to learn and carry out responsibilities and to get along with others.

Always, people with PWS need around-the-clock food supervision. As adults, most affected individuals do best in a special group home for people with PWS, where food access can be restricted without interfering with those who do not need such restriction. Although in the past many patients died in adolescence or young adulthood, preventing obesity will allow a person with PWS to live a normal lifespan.

Early diagnosis of Prader-Willi syndrome gives parents an opportunity to manage their child's diet and avoid obesity and its related problems from the start. Since infants and young children with PWS typically have developmental delays in all areas, diagnosis may facilitate a family's access to critical early intervention services and help identify areas of need or risk. Diagnosis also makes it possible for families to get information and support from professionals and other families who are dealing with the syndrome.

Many doctors will refer a suspected patient to a medical geneticist who specializes in diagnosing and testing for genetic conditions such as PWS. After taking a history and doing a physical examination, the diagnostician will arrange for specialized genetic testing to be done on a blood sample to evaluate for the genetic abnormality found in people with PWS.

Treatment Options and Outlook

Although there is no cure for Prader-Willi, advances in the use of psychotropic medications can improve behavior and mood, and growth hormone can improve short stature and lean body mass. It is also imperative that the person's insatiable appetite be controlled; otherwise, it can result in life-threatening obesity. This appetite, accompanied by easy weight gain and behavioral problems such as stubbornness and temper tantrums are major problems associated with Prader-Willi syndrome.

Although Prader-Willi is a lifelong condition, most children learn to feed themselves, are toilet-trained, walk, talk, swim, play, go to school, work, and enjoy life.

pragmatic language Verbal and nonverbal language that includes tone of voice, posture, gestures, and facial expression used in social interaction.

pragmatic skills The social element of language usage. Pragmatic skills include taking turns in conversation, asking relevant questions, staying on topic, and engaging in active listening. Individuals with LEARNING DISABILITY often have problems in processing or responding to pragmatic cues; this can cause poor social skills and problems in communication.

praxia Knowing or recognizing objects; this is dependent on intact PARIETAL LOBES.

praxis Also known as motor planning, this is the ability to integrate input from the senses and to formulate and execute a sequence of unfamiliar actions.

prefrontal lobes A part of the brain also known as the prefrontal cortex that is the center for EXECUTIVE FUNCTIONS and higher order thinking, and supports self-control, sequencing behaviors, planning, and the ability to modulate motor responses. The prefrontal lobes also are thought to be involved in the monitoring of internal emotional states. It is one of the largest cortical sub-regions of the brain and plays an important role in human problem solving.

preoperational stage The second of four stages in psychologist JEAN PIAGET's theory of cognitive development, which he believed occurred from about age two to six. During this period of time, the child learns to use language but lacks logic, relying instead on immediate experience. However, recent research has suggested that children reach cognitive milestones, such as the ability to sequence and categorize, at ages younger than Piaget estimated.

The most important advancement during this stage is the ability to use language and symbols. Children of this age have the ability to pretend, and they get great joy from pretending. They can pretend that sticks are boats and swords, and in their play they take on roles in complicated games. They pretend to be heroes and villains, mothers and fathers, and characters from the stories they hear.

Children tend to be egocentric during this stage, unable to see things from any perspective but their own. During this period, they reason by moving from particular to particular—for example, children might explain that the car goes because the radio is on or that it gets dark at night because they go to sleep. They do not understand the idea that objects remain the same in terms of mass or number when shape or arrangement changes.

See also PIAGET, JEAN.

pre-referral process Strategies a teacher uses when a student is obviously having trouble in class but has not yet been officially referred for a multidisciplinary team evaluation. In the pre-referral stage, a teacher informally collects data concerning the area of difficulty.

There are several pre-referral models of intervention used to avoid the lengthy and involved process of referral. In the consultation model, the teacher brings data to a child study team or identified school consultant. Another popular model is peer collaboration, in which a teacher meets with a colleague to share data.

In all pre-referral models the teacher develops a statement of the concern, shares data, and brainstorms interventions with colleagues. The pre-referral process is important because intervention on an informal level may effectively address the child's difficulty. If intervention strategies fail, the student will most likely be formally referred to the school's child study committee or team.

pretest   A test given in a specific skill area before instruction or remediation has taken place. Typically it is followed by a post-test given after instruction to measure progress.

print disabilities   A range of visual, perceptual, or physical impairments that may prevent a person from reading standard print. Examples of print disabilities include blindness, visual impairment, DYSLEXIA, and other types of LEARNING DISABILITY.

printing instruction   While computer keyboarding skills are becoming more and more a part of writing, printing remains an essential skill. Printing instruction begins in kindergarten where children are taught to write the letters of the alphabet, and continues through third grade until CURSIVE WRITING is introduced. Problems in forming letters accurately may be caused by poor visual and motor skills. Extreme printing difficulties are called dysgraphia.

problem solving   In relation to schoolwork, problem solving refers to finding the answer to mathematical word problems. It requires a type of thinking in which an individual must analyze and interpret information and then make decisions about how to find a solution. The complexity in problem solving can be particularly difficult for individuals with LANGUAGE DISORDERS, since it requires one to combine language and thinking before applying the appropriate mathematical computation in a variety of settings.

problem-solving skill   The ability to consider the probable factors that can influence the outcome of each of various solutions to a problem, and to select the best solution. Patients with deficits in this skill may become "immobilized" when faced with such a problem. By being unable to think of possible solutions, they respond by doing nothing.

program specialist   A specialist who works within an educational system and provides consultation and assessment in special needs areas.

proofreading   The process in which an individual reviews a completed piece of work for mistakes. For many individuals with a LEARNING DISABILITY, finding errors can be difficult. Unlike most students, who check over their work for accuracy, many students with learning disabilities and ADHD never bother with proofreading unless they receive specific practice in it. Such students do not understand the proofreading process and must be taught the specific skills involved in proofreading in detail.

New software programs and computer tools may make proofreading easier by identifying grammatical and/or spelling errors. People with learning disabilities may find it helpful to proofread for one skill at a time. For example, an individual may read over a homework essay to be sure sentence structure is cohesive, followed by a second reading for spelling errors. Another proofreading strategy is to let time lapse between writing and proofreading.

proprioceptive system   A person's sensory system that uses receptors in joints, muscles, and tendons to help perceive the body's position in space.

prosody   The inflections and intonations of speech.

pseudoword decoding   A type of phonological awareness test in which individuals are asked to decode nonsense words such as *pid, frap, theap,* and *phing*. Nonsense word decoding is often a subtest on achievement tests or reading tests.

The task is useful because it differentiates the skill of decoding (sound-symbol relationship) from SIGHT WORD recognition (in which an individual may simply have remembered the shape of a word).

When used effectively, a great deal can be learned diagnostically about what letter patterns an individual has not yet mastered, so that remediation can be designed accordingly.

Other than for the purpose of assessing decoding skills, pseudoword decoding—the ability to read nonsense words—is not a particularly useful skill.

psychiatrist A physician who specializes in the diagnosis, treatment, and prevention of disorders of thinking, feeling, or behavior. Typically, either a psychiatrist or a pediatrician will be involved when medication for ATTENTION DEFICIT HYPERACTIVITY DISORDER is prescribed. Psychiatrists must complete four years of medical or osteopathic school (earning an M.D. or O.D.). Then they spend at least three years of residency training in medicine, NEUROLOGY, and general psychiatry with adults, in an accredited residency in psychiatry. After completing medical school, graduates must pass a licensing test given by the board of medical examiners for the state where they want to work. To get board-certified, psychiatrists then must take and pass the certifying examination given by the Board of Psychiatry and Neurology.

Many psychiatrists undergo additional training so that they can further specialize in such areas as child and adolescent psychiatry, geriatric psychiatry, forensic psychiatry, psychopharmacology, and/or psychoanalysis. This extensive medical training enables the psychiatrist to understand the body's functions, and the complex relationship between emotional illness and other medical illnesses.

psychological evaluation A set of procedures that is sometimes used as part of a general ASSESSMENT of an individual's learning difficulties, especially when there are other significant behavioral, social, or emotional elements involved. A psychological evaluation is necessary to determine whether psychological or emotional factors may be involved in an individual's performance or behavior. It is also useful to rule out such conditions as DEPRESSION, OBSESSIVE-COMPULSIVE DISORDER, or a personality disorder, in cases where symptoms or behavior might indicate the presence of a significant psychological problem.

A psychological evaluation will involve the administration of multiple psychological tests, gathering anecdotal information, and any other information about psychological functioning. Psychological ethics as well as the Standards for Educational and Psychological Testing state that no single test or procedure constitutes a complete psychological evaluation.

psychologist A mental health expert who specializes in the diagnosis and treatment of mental or emotional problems. Clinical psychologists often use a range of ASSESSMENT tools, including INTELLIGENCE TESTING, to assess, diagnose, and treat patients. Psychologists can treat LEARNING DISABILITIES by helping the person explore upsetting thoughts and feelings so as to help find more positive ways to channel emotions.

A psychologist usually holds a doctoral degree (Ph.D., Psy.D., or Ed.D.) from a university or professional school. Generally, a psychologist in clinical practice will have a degree in clinical psychology (although it might be in counseling psychology). The American Psychological Association (APA), the largest organization representing psychologists in the world and that accredits doctoral training programs in psychology, has adopted the "scientist-practitioner" model of psychological training. That is, all psychologists trained under this model are expert in the theoretical issues and practical applications of psychology. With the exception of the Psy.D. (a purely clinical degree), all psychologists have had extensive training in research, having completed a doctoral dissertation as a major part of the training. In fact, the psychologist's training in research is what most distinguishes a psychologist from other providers of mental health treatment. In addition to research training, the psychologist must complete one or more clinical internships.

A psychologist studies and understands brain and behavior processes from a scientific viewpoint and applies this knowledge to help people understand, explain, and change behavior. Psychologists study the biological and social principles of learning, behavior, emotion, and human development and their interaction with environmental and biochemical/genetic factors to answer research questions about how people respond in various facets of their lives.

Psychologists develop standardized assessment tools to measure behavior and therapeutic interventions to help people improve their ability to function as individuals and in groups.

The APA believes that psychologists must be trained first in the core knowledge of psychology, including a comprehensive set of psychological ethics and practices. Only after they have been trained in the core knowledge of psychology do they specialize. Although there are many subspecialties within psychology, the APA advocates licensure in four major psychological specialties and provides training and practice guidelines in each: clinical psychology; counseling psychology; school psychology; and industrial psychology.

psychologist, educational A Ph.D.-level mental health expert who specializes in ASSESSMENT and consultation relating to educational issues, including the assessment of LEARNING DISABILITIES. Educational psychologists use a range of assessment tools, including intelligence and academic achievement testing.

Special educational needs, learning difficulties, DYSLEXIA, behavior problems, and gifted children all fall within the scope of the educational psychologist's expertise. The educational psychologist is qualified to give advice based upon expert assessment and observation of the child's strengths and weaknesses, drawing upon a knowledge of child psychology, child development, and education.

Psychologists use a range of techniques to put together a picture of the child's strengths and difficulties and identify important factors affecting the child's learning and behavior. Individual tests of intelligence will give a profile of the child's verbal and nonverbal thinking skills and may identify specific areas of strength and weakness that need to be taken into account. Tests of reading, spelling, and number are used to measure the child's achievement against expectations and potential. Information is also gathered through structured classroom observation, and interviews with teachers and parents. Getting an objective picture helps understanding and provides a framework for discussing solutions to problems.

psychologist, school A professionally trained PSYCHOLOGIST who specializes in working with preschool and school-aged children, adolescents, their teachers and families to help make education for students a positive and rewarding experience.

School psychologists address many issues, such as crisis intervention, social skills training, behavioral management techniques, SELF-ESTEEM, ATTENTION DEFICIT DISORDERS, post-traumatic stress disorders, and SPECIAL EDUCATION regulations. A school psychologist is also trained in counseling and crisis intervention and is often involved in one-on-one counseling and in group counseling with elementary and high school students.

In addition, school psychologists administer and interpret INTELLIGENCE TESTS and achievement tests, and complete social-emotional assessments such as tests of personality or DEPRESSION. They are primarily responsible in helping schools make an educational diagnosis of a LEARNING DISABILITY such as attention deficit disorder. One of the main roles of the school psychologist is to administer a variety of psychoeducational tests to students who are experiencing academic or behavioral problems in the classroom. Based on these test results and information collected from the student's teachers and parents, the school psychologist helps the schools determine if a student is eligible for special education services.

School psychologists work with students who have vastly different educational problems and needs, including learning disabilities, traumatic brain injuries, emotional and behavioral disorders, AUTISM, intellectual disabilities, and developmental delays.

There are several differences between a school psychologist and a school counselor. There is an ongoing controversy surrounding the nature and degree of training a person must have to be a school psychologist. At a bare minimum, school psychologists must have a specialist degree (that is, masters degree plus 30 graduate hours, advocated by NASP) or a doctoral degree (advocated by the American Psychological Association (APA)). Most school counselors, in contrast, have earned a bachelor's degree and a few have a master's. In addition, counselors are not trained or qualified to administer and interpret psychological and social-emotional assessments, nor are they able to make educational diagnoses of handicapping conditions as required by federal law. Many counselors spend their school day doing guidance in the classrooms.

School psychologists earn a bachelor's degree followed by an advanced degree—usually a master's degree plus 30 graduate credits. Many school psychology programs across the country offer a specialist degree as well, which is a master's degree plus 30 credits. The specialist degree is an intermediary degree between a master's and a Ph.D. In fact, most states require a specialist degree (or its equivalent) in order to become certified as a school psychologist. Certification allows the practitioner to work in a public school setting but is insufficient in most states to qualify the person for a license for private practice. Licensure for private practice in psychology, including school psychology, requires at minimum a doctorate in most states, although a few states allow a restricted form of licensure for associate-level school psychologists. Training focuses on mental health, child development, learning, and motivation.

School psychologists must be certified to work in the schools or licensed for private practice or to work as a supervising psychologist in most other settings in the state in which services are to be provided. The National Psychology Certification Board (NPCB) and the National Association of School Psychologists (NASP) are trying to establish a national certification in school psychology. However, the training requirements for this certification only requires associate-level training, not the doctoral training advocated by APA. Hence, doctoral-level school psychologists, many of whom were trained under and support the APA model, do not support the current national certification because the training requirements are lower than those advocated by the APA. Each state has different requirements for certification to work in the schools, although most follow the APA guidelines for licensure as professional school psychologists.

Public Law 94-142   See EDUCATION FOR ALL HANDICAPPED CHILDREN ACT OF 1975.

raw score   The number of correct responses on a NORM-REFERENCED TEST, a test that compares the performance of the test taker to the performance of a preselected group of children whose performance on the test becomes the standard against which test companies compare all other children's performances.

Generally, raw scores are converted into more precise quantitative measurements based on various factors. In themselves, raw scores provide only partial information and should not be used to determine a diagnosis or educational intervention.

readability   A measure of how easy it is to comprehend a text depending on a number of variables. These include vocabulary, sentence complexity, format, writing style, and topic, plus the READING COMPREHENSION level, interest, background information, and DECODING skills of the reader.

Some methods of predicting the readability of a text are used to gauge whether an individual can successfully read and comprehend a passage. One such method is to read a section of a passage and count the number of words that are unfamiliar to the reader. If, for example, the reader encounters more than three unfamiliar words, the readability may be too difficult.

In educational settings, a text's readability is often measured in grade level. For example, a history textbook with a readability of 9.3 means an average ninth grade, third month student should be able to read and comprehend it.

readiness   The degree to which an individual is prepared developmentally to learn a new skill. Readiness is a term often used in early education to describe a child's acquisition of prerequisite emo-tional, social, and cognitive skills for academic learning.

For example, reading readiness would include pre-reading skills such as letter identification, print awareness, and rhyming. When a child has demonstrated mastery of such skills, that child would be ready to learn to read.

However, the concept of readiness can be applied to any stage of learning. For example, readiness for algebra must mean an individual has mastered certain mathematical computations.

Normal three- to six-year-olds acquire academic and social readiness skills naturally when brought up in a literate environment, but developmentally delayed, learning disabled, or environmentally deprived children may need extra training or early intervention to prepare them for learning. Early school failure or unnecessary referrals can be prevented with some extra attention in early education to bolster children's readiness for school.

See also EARLY INTERVENTION PROGRAM; READINESS TESTS.

readiness tests   Tests that measure whether an individual has achieved a level of development or acquired the skills and information required to begin a new level of educational activity. For example, children are often given a reading readiness test that assesses whether they have reached a stage where it is appropriate for formal reading instruction to begin.

Readiness tests may be administered individually or in groups, usually at the end of kindergarten or the beginning of first grade, to determine which children are prepared for academic learning and who needs time to develop pre-academic skills. There are many types of readiness skills that vary from informal requests such as "draw a person" or "write the alphabet," to commercial inventories and examinations. The goals of these tests are to assess various skills deemed necessary for school success.

reading Students learn to read by knowing the sounds of letters and knowing the meanings of words (vocabulary), word parts, and groups of words (overall meaning, or semantics). To build this foundation, children need effective reading instruction.

The two main approaches to teaching reading today are WHOLE LANGUAGE and PHONICS. The "whole language" approach focuses on COMPREHENSION and is based on the understanding that reading is about finding the meaning in written language. Children learn meanings of words by multiple experiences with words, both written and spoken. A whole language approach to teaching reading can include teaching reading and writing throughout the day in the context of the lesson topics and also emphasizing storybooks rather than worksheets. Many writing opportunities are also important in the whole language approach.

In contrast, phonics focuses on the sounds of letters and words. A phonics approach focuses instruction on learning to associate printed letters and combinations of letters with their corresponding sounds. Phonics instruction gives students strategies to unlock or decode words.

A phonics approach to teaching reading can include "sounding out" words as a way of figuring out new words. For example, in a phonics lesson, the word "cat" would be sounded out as "cc-aa-tt." Practice worksheets or exercises focus on letter sounds, matching pictures with spoken words, short vowel/long vowel, or "letter of the week."

Many schools combine both approaches because of a decade of research suggesting that there is no one best way to build students' LITERACY skills. A balanced approach to teaching reading combines a strong foundation in phonics with whole language methods. Only through more than one kind of instruction can students gain the skills to recognize and manipulate the sounds of letters and words and the skills to understand what they read. Since all children learn differently, only a balanced approach to teaching reading can give all children the skills they need to read well.

Students learn to read in a certain order: first they must understand that words are made up of different sounds, then associate those sounds with written words, and finally decode words and read groups of words. Students who have trouble learning to read need to be specifically taught the relationships of letters, words, and sounds, since being aware of letter/sound relationships is the main tool good readers use to decode unfamiliar words.

Each child needs practice to be a fluent reader. Research at the National Institutes of Health has found that phonics instruction should be taught as part of a comprehensive, literature-based reading program. Many opportunities for children to read at their own reading level help them to learn to read for meaning and enjoy reading. Highly trained teachers can help children develop good, overall literacy skills, with good vocabularies, knowledge of correct syntax and spelling, reasoning and questioning skills.

Children with a language-based LEARNING DISABILITY have a harder time learning to read because they have a harder time with sounds of letters and words than other children. Research indicates that because phonics instruction focuses on recognizing and manipulating sounds of letters and words, more intense phonics instruction may be helpful for children with learning disabilities.

The ability to read is a fundamental skill for success in life. Reading research has found compelling evidence that children who have a poor start in reading have trouble catching up and develop negative attitudes toward reading, poor vocabulary growth, and missed opportunities for development of reading comprehension strategies.

Most children who are poor readers experience early and continuing difficulties in learning how to accurately identify printed words. These students have problems with "sounding out" unfamiliar words, and with developing "sight vocabulary" of words they are able to read fluently and automatically. The ability to develop these skills is necessary for fluent reading and good reading comprehension.

Diagnostic tests can predict with a high degree of accuracy which students in kindergarten and first grade will have difficulty learning to read. These tests can distinguish, with 92 percent accuracy, those children who will read below the 20th percentile at the end of second grade. These tests take as little as 10 to 15 minutes per child, and can be administered by classroom teachers. Prediction of reading disabilities from tests given at the beginning of first grade are more accurate than those administered during the first semester of kindergarten. The results from these objective tests can be supplemented by teacher ratings of behavior and attention.

Experts suggest a combination of types of tests to identify students who will experience reading problems—knowledge of letter names or sounds, and understanding of sounds (PHONEMIC AWARENESS).

Letter name and sound knowledge   Knowledge of letter name (a test better suited to kindergarten) is measured by asking for the name of each letter presented in uppercase type on a single card. Letter sound knowledge is measured by presenting all letters in lowercase type and asking for the "sound the letter makes in words." If a consonant letter can represent two different sounds (such as "c" or "g"), then the tester probes for the second sound and asks for the short and long pronunciation of each vowel. This test is better suited for children in first grade.

Understanding of sounds   A test to measure phonemic awareness (the ability to identify, think about, or manipulate the individual sounds in words) comes in a variety of measures divided into three broad categories:

Sound comparison   This test includes tasks that require a child to make comparisons between the sounds in different words (such as "which word begins with the same first sound as *can: bag, cat, or fish?*"). The test also includes tasks that require children to generate words that have the same first and last sound as a target word.

Phoneme segmentation   This test includes tasks that involve counting, pronouncing, deleting, adding, or reversing the individual sound in words (such as "say 'card' without the 'd' sound or say the sounds in 'hat' one at a time").

Phoneme blending   In this test, the tester pronounces a series of sounds in isolation and asks the child to blend them together to make a word ("What word do these sounds make /c/-/a/-/t/?").

A number of tests can be used for early screening purposes, including

- Phonological Awareness Test: five different measures of phonemic awareness plus a measure of sensitivity to rhyme; nationally normed on children ages five through nine
- Test of Phonological Awareness: a group-administered test for kindergarten and first grade children nationally normed on children ages five through seven
- Yopp-Singer Test of Phoneme Segmentation: a brief test of children's ability to isolate and pronounce the individual phonemes in words
- Letter identification subtest of the Woodcock Reading Mastery Test Revised
- Graphemes subtest of the Phonological Awareness Test: a comprehensive assessment of letter sound knowledge

Identifying reading difficulties early means children have more time to learn to be successful readers. Since reading is learned more easily and effectively during the early years, identifying language-based learning disabilities and providing appropriate interventions gives children more time to learn to read well.

A child identified as needing help will require careful and direct instruction in reading. An effective preventive program may involve several levels of instructional intensity ranging from small groups to one-on-one teaching, depending upon the severity of the difficulties for each child. In this way, a preventive program can be focused on the children who are most in need. Children with a reading disability/DYSLEXIA will have a positive beginning to their education and a much greater chance for success. Up to 90 percent of poor readers can increase their skills to "average" with prevention and intervention programs that combine instruction in phonemic awareness, phonics spelling, reading fluency, and reading comprehension strategies provided by well-trained teachers.

Kindergarten   In kindergarten, children begin to

- recognize some common words
- name uppercase and lowercase letters
- begin to associate letters and sounds
- recognize poetry

- distinguish reality from fantasy
- can match simple words to pictures
- aware of whether words begin or end with same sound
- beginning to be able to break words into syllables
- understand that reading goes from left to right and top to bottom on the page
- be aware of time sequence in a story

First Grade   In first grade, children begin to
- read long and short vowels
- read word families (hat, bat, cat)
- follow simple written directions
- develop larger sight vocabulary
- be aware of author, title, and table of contents
- recognize a play
- interpret maps and globes
- identify consonants in words
- break dictated words into individual sounds
- be aware of root words, endings, compound words, and contractions
- recognize main idea and cause/effect
- draw conclusions

Second Grade   In second grade, children begin to
- sound out unfamiliar words based on individual letter sounds
- identify words from contextual clues
- vary pitch and stress when reading aloud
- recognize character, setting, and motive of story
- use library for research
- interpret graphs
- use dictionary
- master harder phonetic skills
- understand root words and endings
- be aware of syllabication

Third Grade   In third grade, children begin to
- increase sight vocabulary and word-analysis ability
- understand homophones

- increase reading speed
- develop silent reading skills
- distinguish fiction and nonfiction, fact versus opinion
- understand synonyms and antonyms
- recognize author's purpose
- use index
- use encyclopedia
- interpret diagrams

Fourth Grade   In fourth grade, children begin to
- develop different reading styles for different types of reading
- expand vocabulary
- understand plot and main idea
- summarize a book or article
- organize study materials
- understand different genres (biography, folk tales, science fiction, and so on)
- understand author's point of view
- read a newspaper

reading comprehension   The ability to understand what is read. Reading involves two processes: DECODING (word recognition) and COMPREHENSION (understanding). In order to understand the text, an individual must be able to first recognize the words. Often, individuals with LEARNING DISABILITIES will be better at understanding than recognizing words. However, both skills are necessary for reading competence.

There is a relationship between vocabulary and comprehension—messages are composed of ideas, and ideas are expressed in words. Many studies have shown a close link between vocabulary knowledge and reading comprehension.

Good readers are active readers who have clear goals in mind for their reading, and they typically look over the text before they read, noting such things as the structure of the text and text sections that might be relevant to their goals. As they read, good readers frequently make predictions, reading selectively, continually making decisions about their reading—what to read carefully, what to read quickly, what not to read, what to reread, and so on. Good readers construct, revise, and question the meanings they make as they read. They draw upon, compare, and integrate their prior knowledge with material in the text. They think about the authors of the text, their style, beliefs, intentions, historical milieu, and so on. They monitor their understanding of the text, making adjustments in their reading as necessary. Good readers try to determine the meaning of unfamiliar words and concepts in the text, and deal with inconsistencies or gaps as needed. They evaluate the text's quality and value, and react to the text in a range of ways, both intellectual and emotional.

Moreover, good readers read different kinds of text differently. For example, when reading narrative, good readers attend closely to the setting and characters; when reading expository text these readers frequently construct and revise summaries of what they have read. Comprehension is a complex process, but one that for good readers is both satisfying and productive.

Research suggests that it is possible to help students learn the comprehension strategies used by good readers, and that this improves their overall comprehension of text, both the texts used to teach the strategies and texts they read on their own in the future.

Good comprehension instruction includes both explicit instruction in specific comprehension strategies and a great deal of time and opportunity for actual reading, writing, and discussion of text. It depends on many factors. Individuals with learning disabilities may have a weakness in one or more of the following six subskills of reading comprehension:

1. fluent decoding—the ability to accurately and quickly read each word in a passage

2. broad background knowledge—exposure to a wide variety of language experiences (stories, books, culture) often gained through reading and vocabulary development

3. oral vocabulary development—exposure to rich vocabulary

4. oral language comprehension—understanding oral syntax

5. knowledge of language conventions—can grasp main ideas, paraphrasing, topic sentences, dialogue, irony, and so on

6. reasoning skills—can make inferences, and predict, clarify, summarize information

Research has revealed information about good comprehension that contradicts many earlier beliefs held by proponents of whole language instruction. In the 1970s, experts believed that good readers made a lot of "guesses" while reading based on semantic and syntactic cues. In fact, experts now realize there is very little guessing involved in reading comprehension. Instead, individuals with strong reading comprehension skills actually process every letter in a word, but they do so very quickly and effortlessly. Efficient readers depend on the sounds of the letters to read accurately, and they spend little energy rereading words.

recall   A term used to denote the ability to retrieve information from LONG-TERM MEMORY. Recall is involved in a broad range of tasks, from remembering a phone number to recalling information for a school exam. While useful as a descriptive term, it does not refer to a specific area of cognitive function.

Difficulty recalling information may be caused by a number of different learning problems. This may include problems imprinting information during processing because of poor ATTENTION or short-term memory, as well as difficulty with rapid retrieval tasks that are typically found in EXPRESSIVE LANGUAGE DISORDERS.

receptive language   The forms of language that are received as input from listening and reading. Listening and reading are receptive skills that involve feeding information into the brain, as opposed to speaking and writing, which are the expressive forms of language. Most individuals maintain a fairly similar set of receptive and expressive, oral and written language function, but those with learning problems may have specific deficits in one or more of these areas.

Individuals with DYSLEXIA or specific reading disabilities have problems with receptive language, involving deficits in both ORAL LANGUAGE and processing sounds (PHONOLOGICAL PROCESSING), and significant problems in DECODING and understanding texts. Some individuals with these problems still have relatively strong oral expression, although most will have problems with written expression due to problems with reading written language.

reciprocal reading/teaching A situation in which teachers and students take turns in reading or discussing a written passage. Reciprocal reading is useful because teachers model good reading such as pausing at punctuation, using intonation, and tracking with a finger. Reciprocal teaching also can involve shared discussion where the teacher can model good COMPREHENSION and questioning strategies to promote critical thinking.

In reciprocal teaching and learning, teachers and students share in the process of a learning activity and teachers can also monitor and assess students while they try out new reading/thinking strategies.

referral process When a teacher becomes concerned about a child struggling with daily schoolwork, he or she refers that student to the school's CHILD STUDY COMMITTEE for consideration of appropriate interventions. Frequently, the child study team's interventions will result in significant alleviation of the problems that brought the student to their attention. If, however, the interventions do not help, and the child still has significant difficulties, the committee may refer the student for a multidisciplinary evaluation. A referral to the child study team can be made by the student or a parent, teacher, or other professional. Schools frequently receive "prescriptions" from outside psychologists, reading tutors, and physicians demanding an immediate multidisciplinary evaluation. And many parents seek to bypass the child study team referral and demand that their child receive a referral without first trying to solve the problems by appropriate interventions. However, such demands cannot bypass the requirement that the child first be referred to the child study team for consideration of appropriate interventions before resorting to a multidisciplinary evaluation.

Once a referral has been made, school personnel must begin a process that begins with notifying the parents of the referral. Parents must give written permission for an evaluation to be carried out by the MULTIDISCIPLINARY TEAM.

Strict federal and state laws outline what happens once a referral has been made. Once written permission has been received by the child's parents, the student is evaluated by a multidisciplinary team. The evaluation is then reviewed by the team, which must decide if the student is eligible for special services. Once the team has decided if services are needed, parents (and the student, when appropriate) are called to discuss the situation at a case conference. At this conference, the committee formulates the student's INDIVIDUALIZED EDUCATION PROGRAM, a document that summarizes a child's educational performance, plans the short-term educational goals, and outlines annual goals. It also gives methods for measuring progress.

If the child does not qualify for SPECIAL EDUCATION, it is still important for the parents to work with the teacher to create an informal program that meets the child's needs.

reflex test The testing of reflexes is necessary to ensure that a child's motor system is working properly. Tested reflexes are correlated with specific nerves in the spinal cord.

regular education Non–special education classes.
See also GENERAL EDUCATION.

Rehabilitation Act of 1973 (Public Law 93-112, Section 504) A major piece of legislation requiring that schools not discriminate against children with disabilities (including a LEARNING DISABILITY) and that they provide children with reasonable ACCOMMODATIONS. Under some circumstances, these "reasonable accommodations" may include the provision of services.

While the INDIVIDUALS WITH DISABILITIES EDUCATION IMPROVEMENT ACT (IDEIA) focuses on "free appropriate public education" for children with disabilities, Section 504 of the Rehabilitation Act (ERA) is intended to prohibit discrimination against individuals with handicaps in programs receiving federal financial assistance. The RA is more general in scope, and its definition of "disabled" is somewhat broader than that of "handicapped" in the IDEIA.

Unlike the IDEIA, which applies primarily to public elementary and secondary education for children with disabilities, the Rehabilitation Act also applies to postsecondary institutions that receive federal funds in any form. To fall under the protection of the RA, an individual must meet the definition of "disabled" in the act and be "otherwise qualified," and establish that he or she was denied employment or education "solely by reason" of the disability. In addition, the act requires that an employer or educational institution must make "reasonable accommodations" for the disability.

Eligibility   Eligibility for Section 504 is based on the existence of an identified physical or mental condition that substantially limits a major life activity. As learning is considered a major life activity, children diagnosed with ATTENTION DEFICIT HYPERACTIVITY DISORDER (ADHD) are entitled to the protections of Section 504 if the disability is substantially limiting their ability to learn. Children who are not eligible for special education may still be guaranteed access to related services if they meet the Section 504 eligibility criteria.

Evaluation   Although Section 504 requires nondiscriminatory testing, there are far fewer regulations placed on the testing procedure than are required for IDEIA. In addition, unlike IDEIA, Section 504 does not discuss the frequency of testing; the role outside evaluations may play; nor require parental consent for testing. It does require that an evaluation be conducted before a child receives a remediation plan and before any changes are made to the plan.

Section 504 plan   If the child is eligible for services under Section 504, the school district must develop a "Section 504 plan." However, the regulations do not dictate the frequency of review of the 504 plan, and do not specify the right of parents to participate in its development.

In general, Section 504 provides a faster, more flexible and less stigmatizing procedure for obtaining some accommodations and services for children with disabilities. By virtue of the looser eligibility criteria, some children may receive protection who are not eligible for services or protection under IDEIA, and less information is needed to obtain eligibility. For example, a student with a broken leg who must ride an elevator to the third floor science class qualifies for a Section 504 plan until the leg has healed. Or, a student with a serious hearing loss who can participate in group stan-dardized testing if there is an aide to sign the test proctor's spoken instructions will qualify for a Section 504 plan providing an interpreter. Thus, Section 504 can provide an efficient way to obtain limited assistance without the stigma and bureaucratic procedures attached to IDEIA.

There are some benefits under IDEIA, however

- a wider range of service options
- procedures for parent participation and procedural safeguards that are far more extensive
- a degree of regulation far more specific than that found in Section 504
- a more stringent enforcement mechanism to ensure that the requirements of the law are met

If a child has behavioral problems that could lead to the possibility of excessive discipline, suspension, and expulsion, parents should be particularly aware of the less rigorous safeguards provided by Section 504.

reliability   A statistical term that refers to the consistency of test scores in different contexts or with different populations. A judgment of a high degree of reliability indicates that a test is dependable and relatively free from random errors of measurement.

remedial programs   Programs designed to address specific weaknesses for individuals who are not achieving up to grade-level expectations. Remedial programs take place outside the regular or general classroom and are typically tailored to meet individual needs. Remedial programs can also take place in clinics or in private tutoring centers.

Remedial programs in public schools (such as resource room instruction) that are indicated on an INDIVIDUALIZED EDUCATION PROGRAM are free. Remediation of skills through intensive instruction and practice occurs in remedial programs.

resource room   An educational setting within a school that offers remedial instruction to students with a LEARNING DISABILITY (LD) or other handicaps. Students generally spend most of their day in general or regular education classes, but visit the resource room for a portion of their day (often 45–60 minutes) for individual or small-group instruction on specific areas outlined on the student's INDIVIDUALIZED EDUCATION PROGRAM.

The resource room teacher often supports the regular education curriculum while also providing remediation. Certain considerations must be taken into account when scheduling students in the resource room. For example, if a student excels in or enjoys physical education class, care should be taken to avoid pulling the student out of that class for resource room time.

The resource room does not necessarily serve only students within a single class of handicap, such as an all-LD or an all–seriously emotionally disturbed class. Rather, many serve students with a mixture of handicaps such a few LD, a few with hearing problems, several with emotional disturbance, and so on.

One way most states distinguish a resource room from a self-contained placement is that students are considered to be in a resource room placement if they attend that SPECIAL EDUCATION class for at least one instructional period per day but attend special education classes for less than half of the day.

The different types of remedial instruction settings include

Consultative: The child never physically enters the special education class, but a special education teacher consults with the regular classroom teacher who actually provides the instruction.
Itinerant: The student attends less than one period of special education per day, such as one period once a week, half a period two days per week, and so on.
Resource: The student attends special education classes for at least one instructional period per day but less than half of the school day.
Self-Contained: The student attends special education classes for more than half of the school day, but the student remains in the same school he or she would attend if not handicapped.
Self-Contained with School Transfer: The student attends a self-contained class but must transfer to another school than he or she would attend if not handicapped. School districts frequently resort to this if there are not enough students in

each school for that school to have its own self-contained class, but, pooled together, there are enough students to make a class if two or more schools combine their students who need that class.
Homebound: The child is sent home and receives one to five instructional periods per week from a special education teacher who visits the home. This arrangement occurs if there is some factor (such as severe medical fragility) that endangers the student if he or she attends school, or that endangers others (such as a student classified as handicapped but whose behavior consistently prevents others from learning or endangers others).
Segregated, Other Facility: The student is removed from the local school and placed in a facility educating only students with handicaps, but the student goes home each night. This is the type of program that many school districts provided prior to Public Law 94-142, which required that schools educate students with handicaps in the LEAST RESTRICTIVE ENVIRONMENT.
Institutional Placement: Placement in an institution such as a state mental hospital, used only in severe circumstances, such as severe medical disorders, psychoses that cause the student to be a danger to self or others, or when a student has been committed to a juvenile facility following criminal charges.

resource teacher   A SPECIAL EDUCATION teacher who works with students with disabilities. Usually, these children spend part of their school day in a RESOURCE ROOM staffed with trained teachers in order to receive individualized attention.

reticular activating system (RASY)   The part of the brain that filters out extraneous stimuli and helps a person stay focused. A network of nerve fibers (also known as the reticular formation) located in the brain stem moderates the level of central nervous system activity, controlling arousal, consciousness, and attention. It is also involved in breathing and cardiac functions, movement, awareness, and sleep. Many neurologists and neuropsychologists believe that a dysfunction in the RASY plays an important role in ATTENTION DEFICIT HYPERACTIVITY DISORDER (ADHD). Theoretically, the way that stimulant drugs such as Ritalin (see METHYL-PHENIDATE) work to control the symptoms of ADHD is to stimulate the RASY to exert proper control over the individual's arousal, consciousness, and attention.

retrieval   The searching and finding process that leads to recognition and recall, bringing information out of LONG-TERM MEMORY.

Rett syndrome   A progressive neurological disorder in which individuals exhibit a LEARNING DISABILITY, poor muscle tone, autistic-like behavior, useless hand movements, lessened ability to express feelings, avoidance of eye contact, a lag in brain and head growth, walking abnormalities, and seizures. Loss of muscle tone is usually the first symptom. Rett syndrome is one of five disorders typically included the AUTISM SPECTRUM DISORDERS umbrella (the other conditions include AUTISM, ASPERGER'S SYNDROME, CHILDHOOD DISINTEGRATIVE DISORDER, and PERVASIVE DEVELOPMENT DISORDER—NOT OTHERWISE SPECIFIED. Each of these disorders has specific diagnostic criteria as outlined by the *DIAGNOSTIC AND STATISTICAL MANUAL OF MENTAL DISORDERS—FOURTH EDITION, TEXT REVISION.*

The syndrome occurs in about one of every 10,000 to 15,000 live female births, with symptoms usually appearing in early childhood, between the ages of six and 18 months. Experts believe that while boys can get Rett syndrome, in boys the condition is fatal and they do not survive much past birth. This is because of the difference in sex chromosomes. Girls have two X chromosomes, but only one is active in any particular cell. That means that only about half the cells in a girl's nervous system will actually be using the defective gene. Because boys have a single X chromosome, all of their cells are obliged to use the faulty version of the gene, which presumably results in fatal defects.

Rett syndrome follows a tragic and irreversible course. Although the child develops normally for the first six months to 18 months of life, she begins to gradually deteriorate mentally and physically. As the damage to the nervous system worsens, she loses the ability to speak, begins to have trouble walking or crawling, and is shaken by seizures. One of the most striking symptoms is loss of conscious control of the hands, leading to continual, compulsive hand-wringing. Although rarely fatal, Rett syndrome nevertheless leaves girls permanently impaired.

Most researchers now agree that Rett syndrome is a developmental disorder rather than a progressive, degenerative disorder as once thought. In October 1999, scientists discovered a genetic mutation on the X chromosome that has been linked to Rett syndrome. This mutation has been found in up to 75 percent of typical and atypical cases of Rett. Continued research will focus on other still unidentified genetic factors that contribute to the condition. Researchers agree that its severity is probably not linked to the exact location of individual mutations on the gene, but to the X inactivation patterns in each affected girl.

The gene produces part of a switch that shuts off production of as yet unidentified proteins. Experts suspect that overproduction of some proteins might cause the nervous system deterioration characteristic of the disease. Discovery of the gene will enable the unraveling of the steps of the disease process and could eventually lead to drugs that will lessen the damage.

First described by Dr. Andreas Rett, the condition received worldwide recognition after research by Bengt Hagberg and colleagues was published in 1983.

Symptoms and Diagnostic Path
The child with Rett syndrome usually shows an early period of apparently normal or near-normal development until six months to 18 months of life. A period of temporary stagnation or regression follows during which the child loses communication skills and purposeful use of the hands. Soon, stereotyped hand movements, gait disturbances, and slowing of the rate of head growth become apparent.

Most girls do not crawl typically, but may "bottom scoot" without using their hands. Many girls begin independent walking within the normal age range, while others show significant delay or inability to walk independently. Some begin walking and lose this skill, while others continue to walk throughout life. Still others do not walk until late childhood or adolescence.

A girl's problems may include seizures, which can range from nonexistent to severe, but do tend to lessen in their intensity in later adolescence. Disorganized breathing patterns also may occur and tend to decrease with age. While scoliosis is a prominent feature of RS, it can range from mild to severe.

APRAXIA (dyspraxia), the inability to program the body to perform motor movements, is the most fundamental and severely handicapping aspect of the condition. It can interfere with every body movement, including eye gaze and speech, making it difficult for the child to do what she wants to do. Due to apraxia and lack of verbal communication skills, an accurate assessment of intelligence is difficult. Most traditional testing methods require use of the hands or speech, which may be impossible for the girl with Rett. Some children start to use single words and word combinations before they lose this ability.

Diagnosing the disorder before the child is four or five years old is often difficult. However, the discovery of the genetic mutation will lead to a genetic test to improve the accuracy of early diagnosis. If combined with an effective therapy, the test might allow doctors to forestall the drastic consequences of the disease.

The condition is most often misdiagnosed as AUTISM, CEREBRAL PALSY, or nonspecific developmental delay. While many health professionals may not be familiar with Rett syndrome, it is a relatively frequent cause of neurological dysfunction in females.

Treatment Options and Outlook

There is no cure for Rett syndrome; however, there are several treatment options, including treatments for the learning disabilities and seizures that may occur, and treatments aimed at slowing the motor problems. Some children may require special nutritional programs to maintain adequate weight.

Predicting the severity of Rett syndrome in any individual is difficult, but in spite of the severe impairments that characterize this disorder, most children with Rett syndrome survive into their 40s. Girls and women with Rett can continue to learn and enjoy family and friends well into middle age and beyond. They experience a full range of emotions and show engaging personalities as they take part in social, educational, and recreational activities at home and in the community. However, the risk of death increases with age, and sudden, unexplained death often occurs, possibly from brainstem problems that interfere with breathing.

reverbalization   A strategy in which an individual restates a message out loud to enhance memorization and ensure understanding. Similar to paraphrasing, where individuals restate a message using their own words (usually in writing); in reverbalizing, the individual repeats information out loud to promote LONG-TERM MEMORY.

For individuals with short-term memory or AUDITORY PROCESSING difficulties, reverbalizing information can enhance learning through rehearsal.

Diagnostically, reverbalizing can be an effective way for instructors to monitor whether students have accurately received information.

reversals   A reading or writing error in which similar-shaped letters or words are reversed. For example, a student would reverse "b" for "d" or "was" for "saw."

Reversal errors in emergent readers and writers are common and disappear with more experience; however, reversals that continue to interfere with a student's progress indicate a language processing difficulty that may require treatment.

Remediation for reversals could include using multimodal strategies such as tracing, color-coding, speaking, or using mnemonic devices.

rhetorical patterns   The way in which prose is organized, using six common structures:

- definition
- chronology
- compare-contrast
- cause-effect
- problem-solution
- enumeration

By recognizing a rhetorical pattern when reading, an individual may find it easier to comprehend the passage and predict what might happen next.

Recognizing rhetorical patterns is also important in writing because the patterns provide clear structures around which the writer can organize main ideas and details. Rhetorical patterns may be used alone or in combinations.

Ritalin   See METHYLPHENIDATE.

rule-governed behavior The ways in which humans are able to use LANGUAGE or other symbolic stimuli to govern or control behavior. Language use is rule-governed behavior, rather than simply a skill.

Assessment of language problems must take into account the ways in which an individual may have failed to learn specific language rules, or may have substituted self-generated rules for the standard rules governing usage.

saliency   The relevance of an item or phenomenon to a task or activity. For example, the homework assignment that a teacher writes on the blackboard is highly salient to a student in the class, while the sounds of an activity out in the hallway are nonsalient. Problems with determining saliency (what is relevant or important to a particular task) are a significant issue in individuals with attention disorders.

scale scores   Scale scores provide a statistical method of giving relative meaning to a student's STANDARDIZED TEST scores. Scale score reporting systems have been used more and more often in recent years.

A scale used for a test score usually refers to numbers assigned to students based on how well they did on the test. The higher the number, the better their test performance. Therefore, a scale might be made up of a set of raw scores, in which each test item that is correctly answered adds one more point on the raw score scale. However, raw scores alone are very hard to interpret—a student's score on a raw score scale provides no hint of the child's relative performance. A raw score of "53" means nothing in itself. As a result, testing experts developed scales—like the scale score—to help interpret test results.

Scale scores are converted raw scores using an arbitrarily chosen scale that represents achievement (or ability). A scale-score system is created when a test manufacturer invents a new numerical scale; students' raw scores are then converted to this new scale. For example, in a test of 50 items, a student could achieve a raw score ranging from 0 to 50; a new converted scale of 500 to 1,000 is assigned to correspond to the raw scores. If a student achieves a perfect raw score of 50, the scale score will be 1,000.

One of the reasons that scale scores are used is because it may be necessary to test a student several times using different tests. For example, if one school requires a student to pass a basic skills test before graduating, a student who failed this test would be given another chance to pass it. A retake of this test is not the same exam, but it is almost impossible to create two identical but different tests. To be fair, scale scores can help solve the problem. Scores on two tests can be statistically adjusted so that the new scale scores represent a student's performance as if the two tests had been perfectly equal.

scatter   A term that describes marked variance in a child's subtest scores on any one assessment. Significant scatter within the subtest measurements may indicate a pattern of strengths and weaknesses that should be explored to determine the most effective educational accommodations.

For example, clinicians study profiles of subtest scores from major intelligence tests such as the WECHSLER INTELLIGENCE SCALE FOR CHILDREN—III to determine what test score patterns reveal about students' strengths and weaknesses. A pattern in which the student scores lowest on the digit-span and coding subtests, for example, may indicate a significant weakness in short-term memory.

Scholastic Aptitude Test (SAT)   A comprehensive test used to determine college admissions, taken by high school juniors and seniors across the United States. The SAT measures the kind of reasoning skills needed for college by assessing how students apply what they have learned in school. Colleges use the SAT as a common yardstick that complements a student's high school record in a consistent way. The SAT changed in March 2005; the class of 2006 was the first class to take the new

SAT for college admissions. Changes to the test include the addition of third-year college preparatory math, more critical reading, and a new writing section. The College Board made these changes to better reflect what students study in high school.

In the writing section, students must write an essay that requires them to take a position on an issue and use reasoning and examples to support their position. The essay is similar to the type of writing required on in-class college essay exams. Multiple-choice questions measure a student's ability to identify sentence errors, improve sentences, and improve paragraphs. The new math section includes topics from third-year college-preparatory math, such as exponential growth, absolute value, functional notation, and negative and fractional exponents. Quantitative comparisons have been eliminated. The critical reading section, previously known as the verbal section, includes short and long reading passages. ANALOGIES have been eliminated, but sentence-completion questions remain.

The SAT is developed by the College Board, a not-for-profit association composed of more than 4,700 schools, colleges, universities, and other educational organizations. Among its best-known programs are the SAT, the PSAT/NMSQT, and the Advanced Placement (AP) Program.

SAT with Accommodations   Students with a variety of disabilities may be eligible to take College Board tests (SAT, SAT Subject Tests, AP, PSAT) with ACCOMMODATIONS. To be eligible, a student must

- have a disability that necessitates testing accommodations
- have documentation on file at school that supports the need for requested accommodations and meets the *Guidelines for Documentation*
- receive and use the requested accommodations, due to the disability, for school-based tests

There are many disabilities that affect a student's academic functioning, including LEARNING DISABILITIES, blindness or vision impairment, ATTENTION DEFICIT HYPERACTIVITY DISORDER (ADHD), deafness/hearing problems, certain medical conditions, physical disabilities, and psychiatric conditions.

screening   Informal assessments and data collection used to identify individuals who may require further assessment to determine if they have LEARNING DISABILITY or developmental delays. Screening is usually done in a group setting with the goal of identifying individuals at risk of having a learning disability. Screening is used also in early education to identify children who may be developmentally delayed in vision, hearing, motor skills, cognitive ability, or social-emotional maturity.

Many school districts use these types of screening for all incoming kindergarten students as a low-cost way of identifying and implementing early intervention strategies. Students with learning problems will typically be screened to determine whether more extensive evaluations to establish learning disabilities are needed.

screen reading program   See KURZWEIL READING MACHINE; SPEECH SYNTHESIZER/SCREEN READERS.

script   See CURSIVE WRITING.

segregated other facility   A SPECIAL EDUCATION placement in which students are removed to a separate school or clinic where they are no longer exposed to nonhandicapped students. The students go home every day rather than live at the facility. A segregated other facility is considered to be less restrictive than an institutional placement, but more restrictive than a SELF-CONTAINED CLASSROOM.

selective attention   Picking out the most relevant cue among stimuli in the environment, and excluding the rest. It is well established that people do not pay attention to everything; for example, at a party an individual can focus on the voice of one person with whom he or she is conversing.

Yet while it is clear that people do filter out a great number of stimuli, it is not at all clear how this is done, nor what information is noted unconsciously. In an attempt to find out, PSYCHOLOGISTS have often used dichotic listening experiments (that is, two different messages are presented separately to each ear), roughly along the lines of the situation at a party.

If a child's "attention" problems are selective—that is, appearing only in certain subjects—it suggests that he or she is capable of paying attention when the subjects are comprehensible and meaningful.

self-advocacy An individual's ability to discuss a personal LEARNING DISABILITY and request appropriate ACCOMMODATIONS and services. Self-advocacy skills are important to develop in people with learning disabilities so they can take responsibility for their own learning and become empowered in school, work, and life. Individuals with disabilities should be familiar with their learning profile as well as relevant legislation.

Self-advocacy skills should be developed as soon as an individual is old enough to understand the learning process. Parents have a right to include their children who are being considered for special education classification in the multidisciplinary team meeting and in development of the INDIVIDUALIZED EDUCATION PROGRAM. Many high schools encourage students to become self-advocates by discussing their learning style and needs with teachers, and by actively making transition plans from high school to the next environment.

Self-advocacy skills become even more important once an individual leaves school and begins a job or college, where there are no special educators or parents to advocate for them.

self-concept The way a person sees himself or herself including all the beliefs, feelings, and attitudes. Self-concept also can affect how one feels about others.

Self-concept is a subject that has fascinated philosophers from earliest times. In the field of psychology, self-concept has always been an important and sometimes controversial subject. Both psychologists William James and Mary Calkins used methods of introspection to study the self, while Sigmund Freud, Carl Jung, and Alfred Adler all discussed the development of the self in their writing.

During the 1950s and 1960s, the "self-concept" was a central idea in the work of both Abraham Maslow and Carl Rogers. Maslow believed that building SELF-ESTEEM, an individual's evaluation of self-worth, was a key step in the self-actualization process. Rogers believed that if one had a positive view of the self then one would view the world in a positive way. If the self-view were negative, one would fall short of the goals related to the ideal self. As a part of this perspective, Donald Super

developed a related theory of vocational choice. He believed that career satisfaction was related to the degree to which someone could implement his self-concept in the workplace.

Social psychologists argue that an individual's self-concept develops through associations with others. Cognitive psychologists study how people think about themselves and how they think about their own thinking. Although many criticize the term and its usefulness because it is difficult to quantify or measure consistently, it remains an important concept among educators and developmental psychologists. Both groups are concerned with the effects of the educational setting, peers, and family on a child's developing self-concept.

Individuals with LEARNING DISABILITY, not surprisingly, often rate themselves lower than typically achieving students on COGNITIVE ABILITY. Because academic performance is a culturally valued domain, it makes sense that individuals with learning disabilities would also place importance on academic performance.

Some research suggests that for college students with learning disabilities, the availability of a social support network, including clubs, disability services, and interactions with professors, is a correlate of self-esteem. Other research of successful adults with learning disabilities gives insight into how to nurture emotional health while managing the challenges that a disability entails. Researchers studied moderately successful and highly successful adults with learning disabilities to identify factors related to their success. Success was defined as high ratings in the following categories: income level, job classification, education level, career prominence and job satisfaction.

Other research focuses on resilience—the healthy adaptation in the context of severe stress. Despite the challenges and hardships that can accompany having a learning disability, some individuals maintain a positive outlook, achieve success, and avoid emotional problems. Important characteristics of resilient individuals include accuracy of self-appraisal, self-determination, and help from a significant supportive person.

self-contained classroom A separate classroom within a school designed especially for students with disabilities, to provide a more structured environment and intensive instruction. Most self-contained classes have 12 or fewer students.

Students are placed in a self-contained classroom as the LEAST RESTRICTIVE ENVIRONMENT, if their needs cannot be met in a regular classroom with resource room remedial work and they do not need to be placed in a special school. Students placed in a self-contained classroom spend more than 60 percent of their day in this classroom.

There are two types of self-contained classrooms (sometimes referred to as special classrooms). A classroom designed for only one type of disability is called a categorical classroom; classrooms that contain a variety of children with disabilities (such as emotional, learning, or physical) are called cross-categorical classrooms.

Self-contained classrooms offer some advantages to students with a more severe LEARNING DISABILITY, such as highly specialized learning environments and individual or small-group instruction. This type of classroom allows some students to be mainstreamed with non–SPECIAL EDUCATION peers for certain classes, such as art or music.

self-correction A student's ability to detect and correct errors. The term is often used while students read aloud and hear themselves make errors but correct it. Some reading tests consider a self-correction to be an error, which can result in a misleading oral reading score.

self-efficacy The belief that an individual can produce effects through personal effort. Like SELF-ESTEEM, self-efficacy is important in setting and meeting goals for students of all ages.

self-esteem A particularly positive way of experiencing the self that involves emotional, evaluation, and thinking components.

Self-esteem is the ability to experience oneself as being competent to cope with the basic challenges of life, and of being worthy of happiness. By extension, it is confidence in the ability to learn, to make appropriate choices and decisions, and respond effectively to change. It also involves the experience that success, achievement, fulfillment, and happiness are right and natural.

While many things can make a person feel good temporarily, if self-esteem is not grounded in reality, it is not self-esteem.

If a teacher treats students with respect, avoids ridicule, deals fairly, and projects a benevolent conviction about every student's potential, then that teacher is supporting both self-esteem and the process of learning and mastering challenges. On the other hand, if a teacher tries to nurture self-esteem by empty praise that bears no relationship to the students' actual accomplishments, then self-esteem is undermined and so is academic achievement.

Research indicates that there is a significant relationship between self-esteem and academic achievement, and that if a student's self-esteem can be improved, academic improvement tends to follow. Many factors influence self-esteem, including parents, teachers, and other adults, and biology and life experiences.

Many students with a LEARNING DISABILITY experience poor self-esteem due to years of academic failure. This is why it is especially important to build positive self-esteem by creating opportunities for success, giving sincere praise, and cultivating talents and strengths in individuals with learning disabilities.

See also SELF-CONCEPT.

self-monitoring A strategy in which a student reviews his work to check for errors.

self-regulation The ability to regulate and monitor a person's own actions and behavior. Problems with effective self-regulation are a primary struggle for students with attention and EXECUTIVE FUNCTION problems.

Effective self-regulation depends on a complex interaction of thinking, feeling, and perception.

Problems with self-regulation may stem from many different sources. Individuals with ATTENTION DEFICIT HYPERACTIVITY DISORDER typically have problems with self-regulation due to underlying brain processing difficulties with MEMORY, ATTENTION, and executive function, particularly as these affect the ability to control impulses and restrain and monitor internal thoughts. Problems with self-regulation also may be caused by other psychological conditions, such as BIPOLAR DISORDER, CONDUCT DISORDERS, or OBSESSIVE-COMPULSIVE DISORDER.

Development of more effective ways to self-regulate is part of an effective coaching and strategy development program for individuals with ADHD. In general, while self-regulation may be seen as an underlying brain function, it also is learned behavior. Therefore, it is possible to teach individuals how to change patterns of impulsive and reckless behavior.

semantic cueing A strategy used to help an individual retrieve or read a word by giving hints with words of similar meaning. For example, if an individual is trying to remember the word *compliment,* giving the semantic cue *praise* may help make a meaningful connection to the word in question.

Similarly, semantic cueing can be used to help an individual read an unfamiliar word. For example, if a reader stumbles on the word *psychologist,* an instructor may give the semantic cue *a therapist* or *a doctor for your mind* rather than providing a phonetic or DECODING cue, such as "*psych* is pronounced 'sike'."

semantic knowledge Data stored in LONG-TERM MEMORY regarding general information and concepts.

semantic memory Memory for facts, such as the information that would be contained in a dictionary or encyclopedia with no connection to time or place. People do not remember when or where they learn this type of information.

Semantic memory registers and stores knowledge about the world in the broadest sense; it allows people to represent and mentally operate in situations, objects, and relations in the world that are not present to the senses. A person with an intact semantic memory system can think about things that are not here now.

Because semantic memory develops first in childhood, before episodic memory, children are able to learn facts before they can remember their own experiences.

The seat of semantic memory is believed to be located in the medial temporal lobe and diencephalic structures of the brain.

See also MEMORY.

semantic network Chunks of information connected into networks by associated meanings. Activation of any one chunk automatically "readies" others that are closely associated with it, with lessening degrees of activation spreading from one network to another. Some scientists believe the semantic network may be the main structural component of long-term memory.

semantics The study of words and sentences and their meanings. An individual with a weak vocabulary may be considered to have a *semantic disorder.* An individual with a semantic disorder may understand concepts, but have difficulty finding the word to express it. Informal activities such as quizzing verbal opposites, word categorization, and classification tasks can be useful ways in which to assess semantic skills.

sensorimotor stage A developmental stage in which a child has little ability with LANGUAGE or the use of symbols, but experiences the world through sensation and movement. It is the first of four stages in the theory of cognitive development as described by child psychiatrist JEAN PIAGET. The sensorimotor stage lasts from birth to about age two.

Infants are normally born with a range of reflexes that ensures their survival, such as sucking and grasping. As the infant adapts these reflexes over time, the child can begin to interact with the environment with greater efficiency. By the end of this stage, the child is able to solve simple problems, such as looking for a lost toy or communicating simple needs to a parent or another child. It is also during this stage that the infant develops a sense of object permanence—the awareness that things and people continue to exist even when they cannot be perceived. For example, before the age of two if a parent hides a toy under a pillow in front of the child, the child will not understand that the toy still exists under the pillow. Once a sense of object permanence is developed, the child will understand that the toy hidden under the pillow still exists, and will lift up the pillow to retrieve the toy.

Modern technology was not available in Piaget's time, so he often used motor tasks to test the cognitive understanding of an infant. With the availability of more advanced techniques that can track an infant's eye movements or rate of sucking in response to stimuli, researchers now know that infants reach cognitive milestones such as object permanence at a younger age than Piaget had suspected. However, Piaget's view of the infant as a "little scientist" who comes to understand the world through trial and error experiments remains consistent with recent findings.

sensory diet   A management plan developed by a child and an OCCUPATIONAL THERAPIST to help the child learn skills and activities that ease the effects of SENSORY INTEGRATION DYSFUNCTION.

See also SENSORY INTEGRATION.

sensory impairment   Any impairment of the sensory system; the most prominent and predominant forms of sensory impairment are hearing and visual problems. All standard and legal definitions of LEARNING DISABILITY rule out sensory impairment as a contributing cause because those sensory impairments are classified separately in their own handicap categories. However, it is possible for a child with a sensory impairment to also have a learning disability. It is also difficult to tell the difference between the effects of a sensory impairment on learning and those effects that may be associated with a learning disability. It is likely that children with significant sensory problems who also have learning disabilities may generally be underdiagnosed and largely overlooked.

sensory integration   The process of taking in sensory information, organizing this information in the central nervous system, and using the information to function smoothly in daily life. Sensory integration is a continual process: as children gain competence, their sensory integration improves, so that the more children do, the more they can do.

Sensory experiences include touch, movement, body awareness, sight, sound, and the pull of gravity; as the brain organizes and interprets this information, it provides a crucial foundation for later, more complex learning and behavior. This critical function of the brain is responsible for producing a composite picture of a person's existence, so that the person can understand who he or she is physically, where he or she is, and what is going on in the environment around him or her.

For most people, effective sensory integration occurs automatically and unconsciously, without effort. For others, however, the process is inefficient, demanding effort and attention with no guarantee of accuracy.

For most children, sensory integration develops in the course of ordinary childhood activities. But for some children, sensory integration does not develop as efficiently as it should. When the process breaks down, a number of problems in learning, development, or behavior may develop.

The concept of sensory integration comes from a body of work developed by OCCUPATIONAL THERAPIST A. Jean Ayres, Ph.D., who was interested in the way in which sensory processing and motor planning disorders interfere with daily life function and learning. This theory has been developed and refined by the research of Dr. Ayres, as well as other occupational and physical therapists. In addition, literature from the fields of NEUROPSYCHOLOGY, NEUROLOGY, physiology, child development, and psychology has contributed to theory development and treatment strategies, although the theory is not yet fully accepted by all experts.

The theory states that children with sensory integration problems may be bright, but they may have trouble using a pencil, playing with toys, or taking care of personal tasks, such as getting dressed. Some children with this problem are so afraid of movement that ordinary swings, slides, or jungle gyms trigger fear and insecurity. On the other hand, some children whose problems lie at the opposite extreme are uninhibited and overly active, often falling and running headlong into dangerous situations. In each of these cases, some experts believe a sensory integrative problem may be an underlying factor. Its far-reaching effects can interfere with academic learning, social skills, even SELF-ESTEEM.

Research clearly identifies sensory integrative problems in children with developmental or learning difficulties, and independent research shows that a sensory integrative problem can be found in some children who are considered learning disabled by schools. However, sensory integrative problems are not limited to children with LEARNING DISABILITIES; they can affect all ages, intellectual levels, and socioeconomic groups.

A number of situations can trigger sensory integration problems, including prematurity, developmental disorders, learning disabilities and brain injury.

Prematurity As more premature infants survive today, they enter the world with easily over-stimulated nervous systems and multiple medical problems. Parents need to learn how to give their premature infant the sensory nourishment their child requires for optimal development, and how to avoid harmful over-stimulation.

Developmental disorders Severe problems with sensory processing is a hallmark of AUTISM. Autistic children seek out unusual amounts of certain types of sensations, but are extremely hypersensitive to others. Similar traits are often seen in other children with developmental disorders. Improving sensory processing will help these children develop more productive contacts with people and environments.

Learning disabilities As many as 30 percent of school-age children may have learning disabilities. While most of these children have normal INTELLIGENCE, many are likely to have sensory integrative problems. These children are also more likely than their peers to have been born prematurely, to have had early developmental problems, and to have poor motor coordination. Early intervention can improve sensory integration in these children, minimizing the possibility of school failure before it occurs.

Many studies indicate that children with learning disabilities are at risk for later delinquency, criminal behavior, alcoholism, and drug abuse because of repeated failure in school. By interrupting the vicious cycle of failure, intervention to help children with sensory integration and learning problems may also prevent serious social problems later in life.

Brain injury Trauma to the brain as a result of accidents and strokes can have profound effects on sensory functioning. People who suffer from these effects deserve treatment that will lead to the best possible recovery. In order for this to occur, their sensory deficits must be addressed.

See also SENSORY INTEGRATION DYSFUNCTION.

sensory integration dysfunction (SID) The inefficient brain processing of information received through the senses. A child with SID has trouble detecting, discriminating, or integrating sensations. This complex neurological problem leads to either sensory seeking or sensory avoiding patterns, or a motor planning problem called DYSPRAXIA.

Symptoms and Diagnostic Path

Sensory seekers These children have nervous systems that do not always process sensory input that is sent to the brain. As a result, they respond too strongly to sensations. Children who are underresponsive to sensation seek out sensory experiences that are more intense or of longer duration. They may

- be hyperactive as they seek more and more movement input
- be unaware of touch or pain, or touch others too often or too hard (may seem aggressive)
- engage in unsafe behaviors, such as climbing too high
- enjoy sounds that are too loud, such as TV or radio volume

Sensory avoiders At the other end of the spectrum of this disorder are those children who have nervous systems that feel sensation too easily or so much so that they are overly responsive to sensation. As a result, they may have "fight or flight" responses to sensation, a condition called "sensory defensiveness." They may

- respond to being touched with aggression or withdrawal
- be afraid of, or become sick with, movement and heights
- be very cautious and unwilling to take risks or try new things
- be uncomfortable in loud or busy environments such as sports events or malls
- be very picky eaters or overly sensitive to food smells, texture, or temperature

Dyspraxia These children are clumsy and awkward. They have particular problems with new motor skills and activities. They may have

- very poor FINE MOTOR SKILLS, such as handwriting

- very poor GROSS MOTOR SKILLS, such as kicking, catching, or throwing balls
- trouble imitating movements, such as in the game "Simon Says"
- trouble with balance, sequences of movements, and bilateral coordination

Treatment Options and Outlook

To proponents, sensory integration dysfunction appears to be a neurological problem that affects behavior and learning. Medicine cannot cure the problem, but occupational therapy can address the child's underlying problems in processing sensations. Not stimulant drugs, but a good sensory treatment plan may be a major component in treating the child with SID. Taking a conservative approach often helps the inattentive child whose problem is not ADD, but developmentally delayed sensory processing.

If a child is suspected of having a sensory integrative disorder, a qualified occupational or physical therapist can conduct an evaluation. Evaluation usually consists of both standardized testing and structured observation of responses to sensory stimulation, posture, balance, coordination, and eye movements. After carefully analyzing test results and other ASSESSMENT data along with information from other professionals and parents, the therapist will recommend appropriate treatment.

If therapy is recommended, the child will be guided through activities that challenge the child's ability to respond appropriately to sensory input by making a successful, organized response. Training of specific skills is not usually the focus of this kind of therapy. Instead, adaptive physical education, movement education, and gymnastics are examples of services that typically focus on specific motor skills training. Such services are important, but they are not the same as therapy using a sensory integrative approach.

Occupational therapy usually takes place in a large, sensory-enriched gym with lots of swinging, spinning, tactile, visual, auditory, and taste opportunities.

The motivation of the child plays a crucial role in the selection of the activities in a sensory integrative approach. Most children tend to seek out activities that provide the best sensory experiences at that particular point in their development. It is this active involvement and exploration that enables the child to become a more mature and efficient organizer of sensory information.

The most important step in promoting sensory integration in children is to recognize that it exists and that it plays an important role in the development of a child. By learning more about sensory integration, proponents say, parents, educators, and caregivers can provide an enriched environment that will foster healthy growth and maturation.

The goal of occupational therapy is to enable children to take part in the normal "job" of childhood, such as playing, enjoying school, eating, dressing, and sleeping—activities that are often a problem for children with SID. Each child is provided with an INDIVIDUALIZED TREATMENT PLAN that directly involves parents.

See also SENSORY DIET.

sequencing skills The ability to order elements correctly. Sequencing skills may be motor (sequencing body movements smoothly) or linguistic (sequencing words appropriately into sentences), as well as keeping track of the correct order of stimuli.

shaken baby syndrome Forceful shaking of an infant or young child by the arms, legs, chest, or shoulders. This shaking can cause brain damage leading to MENTAL RETARDATION, speech and LEARNING DISABILITIES, paralysis, seizures, hearing loss, or death. It may cause bleeding around the brain and eyes, resulting in blindness.

A baby's head and neck are especially vulnerable to injury because the head is so large and the neck muscles are still weak. In addition, the baby's brain and blood vessels are very fragile and are easily damaged by whiplash motions such as shaking, jerking, and jolting.

About 50,000 cases of shaken baby syndrome occur each year in the United States; one shaken baby in four dies as a result of this abuse. Head trauma is the most frequent cause of permanent damage or death among abused infants and children, and shaking accounts for a significant number of those cases. Some studies estimate that 15 percent of children's deaths are due to battering or shaking and an additional 15 percent are possible cases of shaking. The victims of shaken baby syndrome range in age from a few days to five years, with an average age of six to eight months.

While abusers are not limited to any special group of people, 65 percent to 90 percent of shakers are men. In the United States, men in their early 20s who are the baby's father or the mother's boyfriend are typically the shaker. Women who injure babies by shaking them are more likely to be baby sitters or childcare providers than mothers.

Severe shaking often begins in response to frustration over a baby's crying or toilet problems. The adult shaker also may be jealous of the attention that the child receives from a partner.

Shaken baby syndrome is also known as abusive head trauma, shaken brain trauma, pediatric traumatic brain injury, whiplash shaken infant syndrome, and shaken impact syndrome.

Symptoms and Diagnostic Path

Shaken baby syndrome is difficult to diagnose unless someone accurately describes what happens. Physicians often report that a child with possible shaken baby syndrome is brought for medical attention due to falls, difficulty breathing, seizures, vomiting, altered consciousness, or choking. The caregiver may report that the child was shaken to try to restart breathing. Babies with severe or lethal shaken baby syndrome are typically brought to the hospital unconscious, with a closed head injury.

To diagnose shaken baby syndrome, physicians look for bleeding in the retina of the eyes, blood in the brain, or increased head size indicating buildup of fluid in the tissues of the brain. Damage to the spinal cord and broken ribs from grasping the baby too hard are other signs of shaken baby syndrome. Computed tomography (CT) and magnetic resonance imaging (MRI) scans can reveal injuries in the brain, but are not regularly used because of their expense.

A milder form of this syndrome may be missed or misdiagnosed. Subtle symptoms, which may be the result of shaken baby syndrome, are often attributed to mild viral illnesses, feeding dysfunction, or infant colic. These include a history of poor feeding; vomiting or flu-like symptoms with no accompanying fever or diarrhea; lethargy and irritability over a period of time. Without early medical intervention, the child may be at risk for further damage or even death, depending on the continued occurrences of shaking.

Treatment Options and Outlook

The treatment of survivors falls into three major categories—medical, behavioral, and educational. In addition to medical care, children may need speech and language therapy, vision therapy, physical therapy, occupational therapy, and SPECIAL EDUCATION services. Some may need the assistance of feeding experts and behavioral consultants.

Immediate medical attention can help reduce the impact of shaking, but many children are left with permanent damage. Fewer than 10 to 15 percent of shaken babies recover completely; the rest have a variety of disabilities, including partial or complete loss of vision, hearing problems, seizure disorders, CEREBRAL PALSY, sucking and swallowing disorders, DEVELOPMENTAL DISABILITIES, AUTISM, cognitive or behavior problems, or a permanent vegetative state.

sight-word approach A method of teaching reading and spelling in which small numbers of instantly recognizable SIGHT WORDS are presented until the child masters them.

While many early readers naturally learn to read words through frequent exposure to them in stories, sight words often should be explicitly taught to individuals with a LEARNING DISABILITY. Sight words can be hard to learn for these children because they frequently have trouble following common spelling and pronunciation patterns, such as *are, were, been,* and *some,* and require a strong VISUAL MEMORY for words.

To avoid such confusions when using the sight-word approach to teach reading and spelling, words should be carefully selected initially to follow consistent spelling patterns.

sight words Words that are recognized instantly, without using word attack skills. The larger the sight-word vocabulary, the more fluent the reading process. Sight words are frequently used words that make up the majority of written text, such as

- the
- just
- had
- from
- about

The Dolch List is a well-known compilation of the 220 most often used sight words that average learners should know by the end of third grade. When an individual has difficulty recognizing common words by sight, reading is slow and laborious.

See also SIGHT-WORD APPROACH.

simultaneous retrieval memory Recalling multiple items or procedures at the same time. This form of recall is particularly involved in writing tasks. For example, in writing a sentence one must simultaneously recall information about correct spelling, word order and syntactic patterns, and appropriate punctuation. For many individuals with LEARNING DISABILITIES, difficulties in this area may result in performance that does not reflect their actual knowledge of such elements as spelling or punctuation rules. The presence of errors can reflect difficulty in accessing knowledge in LONG-TERM MEMORY on demand and simultaneously, rather than in isolation and with time for thought and reflection.

Sixteen Primary Factor Inventory (16PF) Also known as the Cattell 16PF, this personality test evaluates personality traits and identifies the test taker's strengths. Developed by Raymond Cattell, it is used primarily for job seekers and to assess relationship strengths and weaknesses. A children's and teen version of the 16PF are also available.

social cognition A term used by social and developmental psychologists to refer to how people come to be concerned about the actions, thoughts, and feelings of others. This area of study examines how social perceptions develop, how individuals make social judgments, and how others affect an individual's SELF-CONCEPT. Many children with LEARNING DISABILITIES have significant deficits in social cognition as well as academic difficulties.

social maladjustment A vague term for a child's chronic misconduct in the absence of emotional disturbance. The INDIVIDUALS WITH DISABILITIES EDU-

CATION IMPROVEMENT ACT specifically prohibits the classification of children as handicapped because of social maladjustment, although social maladjustment may occur together with legally defined handicaps.

In the past, it was a common practice for schools to place children into SPECIAL EDUCATION classes based on their misconduct rather than in the presence of a handicap. Many alleged that public school special education classes became "dumping grounds" for the children whom no one wanted to teach, such as juvenile delinquents and those who defied authority.

social skills problems Children with a LEARNING DISABILITY (especially nonverbal disabilities) may have trouble with social skills as a result of problems with perception. Children in this situation tend to be isolated, with few close friends, and only rarely participate in school activities. They are often rejected by children their own age because of odd behavior or poor school performance.

Teachers tend to rate these children as being easily led and with poor social adjustment. These problems may be caused by poor social comprehension, the inability to understand another's point of view, poor language skills, or misinterpretation of body language.

social skills training A type of behavioral therapy in which a therapist describes and models appropriate behaviors (such as waiting for a turn, sharing toys, asking for help, or responding to teasing). Through role-playing, a child has an opportunity to practice these skills in a therapeutic setting.

social worker A mental health professional who provides intervention and treatment to clients who are referred to an agency or through typical school channels. These professionals typically work as part of a team, providing consultation regarding further assessment or actions for individuals with medical and/or psychological issues. Social workers must have a degree in social work from a college or university program accredited by the Council on Social Work Education.

Degrees in social work include the bachelor of social work (B.S.W.), the master of social work

(M.S.W.), and the doctorate in social work (D.S.W. or Ph.D.). A minimum of an M.S.W. is required to provide therapy. Degree programs involve classroom study as well as practical field experience. The bachelor's degree prepares graduates for generalist entry-level work, whereas the master's degree enables the social worker to engage in advanced clinical practice. A D.S.W. or Ph.D. is useful for doing research or teaching at the university level.

Most states require practicing social workers to be licensed, certified, or registered, although standards vary.

sociocultural perspective A psychological approach that explores the social and cultural influences on behavior and learning.

socioeconomic status Class distinctions based on the social and economic status of an individual. Considerations that factor into an individual's socioeconomic status may include level of education, race, social class, or level of income.

Statistics show that families living in poverty have inadequate housing and healthcare, which puts their children at higher risk for learning disabilities.

sociolinguistics The study of the way people use language in different social situations and the connection between language and society.

Sociolinguistics studies how language influences the social roles in a community. It ranges from the study of the wide variety of dialects across a given region to the analysis of the way men and women speak to one another. Sociolinguistics often reveals the humorous realities of human speech and how a dialect of a given language can often describe the age, sex, and social class of the speaker; it codes the social function of a language.

soft neurological signs Any of a number of minor abnormalities that emerge in childhood and are used as diagnostic indicators of minimal brain damage.

Soft signs are subtle and difficult to detect reliably; they tend to run their developmental course with no clear cause and are not regarded as indicators of any specific neurological disease. The *soft* in

the term comes from the difficulties of interpretation and the uncertain association with structural brain damage.

Certain soft signs, like those related to fine and GROSS MOTOR SKILLS, may be used to help diagnose LEARNING DISABILITIES. Neuropsychological evaluations and psychological evaluations for learning disabilities typically include soft signs assessments such as the ability to walk a straight line, the ability to tell left from right, and the ability to track objects horizontally and vertically.

sound blending The ability to hear sounds in isolation and then blend them into a continuous word. Sound blending requires auditory perception skills to take in information and reproduce the sounds fluently. For example, an instructor may say "put /m/ /a/ /t/ together" to assess if the student can say *mat*. Sound blending is an important skill to develop the awareness of word sounds.

sound/letter/word retrieval The process of reading requires a student to quickly retrieve sounds, letters, and words. Research has shown that a delay in naming pictures, symbols, letters, and words is an accurate predictor of reading problems. Problems in retrieving are probably due to MEMORY retrieval problems that make it difficult to access phonological and verbal information.

Sound, letter, and word retrieval interventions are available, such as computer software programs that slow the pace of language to allow individuals to retrain the pace of language processing.

sound/symbol association The idea that certain sounds are paired with specific symbols.

source memory The memory of where a person obtained information. For example, a child might know that Harrisburg is the capital of Pennsylvania, but not recall where he or she obtained that information. Many students with LEARNING DIS-ABILITIES have deficient source memory.

space perception The ability to understand on a perceptual level the way in which objects are facing or placed, the direction in which they are moving, and the relation of objects to each other, both in distance and orientation.

spasmodic dysphonia   A voice disorder (also called laryngeal dystonia) that causes the voice to break or to have a tight, strained or strangled quality, caused by involuntary movements of one or more muscles of the voice box (larynx). Individuals with this problem may have occasional trouble saying a word or two, or they may have such problems that it interferes with communication. There are three different types of spasmodic dysphonia: adductor spasmodic dysphonia, abductor spasmodic dysphonia, and mixed spasmodic dysphonia.

Spasmodic dysphonia can affect anyone, but it typically occurs most often in individuals between 30 and 50 years of age. More women appear to be affected by spasmodic dysphonia than men.

The cause is unknown. Because the voice can sound normal or near normal at times, spasmodic dysphonia was once thought to be all in a person's mind (psychogenic) rather than from a physical cause. However, while there are psychogenic forms of spasmodic dysphonia, research has found evidence that most cases of spasmodic dysphonia have to do with the nervous system.

In some individuals, the voice symptoms appear after an upper respiratory infection, injury to the larynx, a long period of voice use, or stress.

Spasmodic dysphonia may occur at the same time as other movement disorders, such as blepharospasm (excessive eye blinking and involuntary forced eye closure), TARDIVE DYSKINESIA (involuntary and repetitious movement of muscles of the face, body, arms, and legs), oromandibular dystonia (involuntary movements of the jaw muscles, lips, and tongue), torticollis (involuntary movements of the neck muscles), or tremor (rhythmic, quivering muscle movements).

In some cases, spasmodic dysphonia may be inherited; a possible gene on chromosome 9 may contribute to hereditary spasmodic dysphonia.

Symptoms and Diagnostic Path
In adductor spasmodic dysphonia, sudden involuntary muscle movements or spasms cause the vocal cords to stiffen and slam together, making it difficult for the cords to vibrate and produce the voice. Words are often cut off or hard to start because of the muscle spasms. Therefore, speech may be choppy and sound like STUTTERING. The voice of an individual with adductor spasmodic dysphonia is commonly described as strained or strangled and full of effort. Surprisingly, the spasms are usually absent while whispering, laughing, singing, or while speaking in a high pitch or while inhaling. Stress often makes the muscle spasms more severe.

In abductor spasmodic dysphonia, sudden spasms cause the vocal cords to open, which means they cannot vibrate. This also allows air to escape from the lungs during speech. As a result, the voice of a person with this problem often sounds weak, quiet, breathy, or whispery. As with adductor spasmodic dysphonia, the spasms are often absent during activities such as laughing or singing.

Mixed spasmodic dysphonia involves muscles that open and close the vocal cords, which is why the condition has features of both adductor and abductor spasmodic dysphonia.

A doctor can diagnose spasmodic dysphonia after identifying the way the symptoms developed, as well as by careful physical examination. Most people are evaluated by a team that usually includes an otolaryngologist (an ear, nose, and throat specialist), a SPEECH-LANGUAGE PATHOLOGIST, and a NEUROLOGIST. The otolaryngologist examines the vocal cords during speech using fiberoptic nasolaryngoscopy (a small, lighted tube through the nose and into the throat). The speech-language pathologist evaluates the patient's voice and voice quality, and the neurologist evaluates the patient for signs of other muscle movement disorders.

Treatment Options and Outlook
There is no cure for spasmodic dysphonia, but therapy can help reduce the symptoms. Voice therapy may reduce some mild symptoms. An operation that cuts one of the nerves of the vocal cords has improved the voice of many for several months to several years, but the improvement is often temporary. Others may benefit from psychological counseling to accept and live with a voice problem. Still others may benefit from job counseling to select a job more compatible with speaking limitations.

Currently the most promising treatment for reducing the symptoms of spasmodic dysphonia is injections of very small amounts of botulinum toxin (botox) directly into the affected muscles of the larynx. Botox weakens muscles by blocking the nerve impulse to the muscle and generally improves the voice for a period of three to four months. After this, the symptoms gradually return. Reinjections are necessary to maintain a good speaking voice. Initial side effects that usually subside after a few days to a few weeks may include a temporary weak, breathy voice or occasional swallowing difficulties. Botox may relieve the symptoms of both adductor and abductor spasmodic dysphonia.

spatial ability   The ability to imagine objects or symbols in space.

spatial judgment   The ability to judge spatial relationships, as between fixed objects or between a moving object and a fixed point. Spatial judgment is involved in activities such as driving a car or playing a sport. Individuals with LEARNING DISABILITIES may have problems with spatial judgment as part of an overall pattern of difficulty with visual-spatial abilities.

spatial-material organizational disorder   A problem with organizing materials so that the child constantly struggles for survival within an ordered environment.

A child with this problem has a hard time organizing information on paper. Margins are missing, spacing between words and letters is incorrect, centering is difficult, and the overall appearance of the work is messy. Teachers often have trouble reading the child's work. Often, a child with this problem forgets assignments or books needed to complete assignments. Assignments themselves may be incomplete, or the child cannot find completed assignments.

In addition, a child with this problem is often disorganized and has problems following routines or completing tasks. Desk and home environment are usually quite messy and disorganized, although the child may appear to have his own system of organization in his own space.

spatial orientation   The ability to maintain a sense of orientation in a physical space. Difficulties in spatial orientation may be part of a larger pattern of visual-spatial skills deficits that are linked with a LEARNING DISABILITY in some cases. These problems may have a profound effect on an individual's ability to follow physical directions or to locate information or objects within a space.

spatial relationships   The relative positions of objects in a space. Children learn about spatial relationships at an early age as they manipulate toys and other objects. Academically, spatial relationships are involved in the acquisition of reading skills and mathematics: a child must perceive the space between words in a sentence in order to understand the concept of a sentence. In math, understanding spatial relationships is essential for developing many types of math skills such as computation, graphing, and understanding a number line. For example, the child can recognize that the toy is on top of or above the bed; in looking at a picture, a child can recognize that the moon is above the ground. This understanding is often obvious in children's drawings.

spatial sequencing   Refers to the ability to recognize and organize objects in a pattern. For example, spatial sequencing is demanded in the copying of block patterns. Later, spatial sequencing is demanded in reading, in recognizing and interpreting the sequence of letters in words and the spaces between words. At this last level, the skill may be considered cognitive.

special education   Educational services and programs for students with abilities ranging from giftedness to MENTAL RETARDATION, and including various physical, emotional, or learning differences.

The history of special education can be traced at least as far back as Plato's recommendation that children with extraordinary intellectual ability should be provided special leadership training. In more modern times special education was practiced in the 16th century when Pedro Ponce de León taught deaf Spanish children to speak, read, and write. In the 18th century, Jean-Marc-Gaspard Itard (1775–1838) developed special education techniques with Victor, the so-called Wild Boy of Aveyron. During the late 18th and early 19th centuries, special education procedures for teaching some school skills to pupils with sensory handicaps were supported by Thomas Hopkins Gallaudet. For example, individuals with profound hearing loss were taught meanings for printed words by repeated simultaneous presentations of a printed word and a picture of what the word represented.

About the same time, attempts to educate individuals with mental retardation or with emotional or behavioral disorders increased in number and success, as exemplified in the work of the American educator Samuel Gridley Howe (1801–76). Successful attempts to educate the deaf and blind led to scientific methods to teach the mentally retarded in Europe. For example, Maria Montessori, a pediatrician and innovative educator, used multisensory methods to teach mentally retarded and culturally deprived children in Rome in the late 19th century.

In the 20th century, the enactment and implementation of compulsory education laws led to an increasing need for special education services. In the latter half of the 20th century, great gains have been made in special education. In most developed countries, addressing the educational needs of the disabled has become universal. However, it was not until the mid-1970s, with the passage of the EDUCATION FOR ALL HANDICAPPED CHILDREN ACT OF 1975 (PL 94-142), that the education of disabled children carried the force of law in the United States. This revolutionary legislation, guaranteeing a free and appropriate education for all children, paved the way for a rapid expansion of the field of special education that continues to this day.

Public Law 94-142, renamed INDIVIDUALS WITH DISABILITIES EDUCATION IMPROVEMENT ACT (IDEIA) in 1990, requires students with disabilities to be placed in the LEAST RESTRICTIVE ENVIRONMENT available in order to avoid segregating students with disabilities.

Schools that comply with the laws receive more money from the federal government to offset part of the costs of providing special education services. The federal government also requires that schools report the number of special education students they serve.

A child who seems to be struggling in school will be evaluated to see if special education services are needed. First, the child's teacher meets with the school's CHILD STUDY COMMITTEE (also called a student intervention team, or pupil assistance committee). Every public school is required by law to have such a team in place.

The school-based child study team usually meets on a regular basis to address the concerns of teachers or parents about students who are struggling in school in the regular education program. Meeting with this team is the first step to take when a child is having trouble in school, before a formal evaluation to see if a child needs special education.

The child study team can help identify children who need extra support, recommend what help the school might offer, and advise if testing or outside evaluation might be needed. The team, which typically includes teachers, an administrator, and the child's parents, reviews information about the child from parents, school records, administrators, counselors, and teachers.

If a school-related problem is suspected, team members might suggest testing of the child's IQ, academic skills, and information processing skills. Once all the observations and testing are completed, the team suggests ways to help the child improve, including ideas for the classroom teacher and the parents at home.

After a few weeks spent on these new strategies, the team will review the results. If no progress has been made, the team should discuss other ideas that might improve the situation. If these ideas still do not help, the team may ask for a special education evaluation (sometimes called a MULTIDISCIPLINARY TEAM EVALUATION or an INDIVIDUALIZED EDUCATION PROGRAM (IEP) evaluation, depending on the state).

This formal special education evaluation will determine if a child's problems are significant enough to legally qualify for special education services. The evaluation will include a detailed description of the problems the child encounters every day, samples of daily work, and examples of what ACCOMMODATIONS did and did not work.

The team also can consider other information, such as health screenings to rule out physical problems, or independent evaluations by private specialists. Depending on the child's problems, the special education evaluation may involve SCHOOL PSYCHOLOGISTS, special education teachers, speech-language therapists or other therapists, AUDIOLOGISTS, and vision or hearing education teachers.

At this point, legal guidelines and requirements ensure each child gets a good education, no matter what the problems. The three main federal laws that govern special education include the Education for All Handicapped Children Act of 1975, the Education and Handicapped Act Amendments of 1986, and IDEIA, which was updated in 2004. These laws require educators to identify children with LEARNING DISABILITIES (and certain other disabilities) so they can receive the best possible education.

As a result, more than 6 million children are receiving services who otherwise might not receive the support programs and services they need to be successful. To be legally placed in "special education," your child must fit the criteria for one of the 13 handicaps as outlined in IDEIA:

- autism
- deaf-blindness
- deafness
- hearing impairment
- mental retardation (sometimes called cognitive disability)
- multiple disabilities
- orthopedic impairment
- other health impairment limiting strength, vitality, or alertness
- serious emotional disturbance (sometimes called emotional-behavioral disability)
- specific learning disability
- speech or language impairment
- traumatic brain injury
- visual impairment, including blindness

The laws give parents the right to submit to the evaluation team independent evaluations by experts outside school, but a child is not automatically eligible for special education just because an independent evaluation report says the child should be eligible or that he or she needs special education. It is up to the child's school evaluation team to consider these independent evaluations along with current academic assessment, report cards, teacher input, student work samples, previous education or behavior interventions, and parent input. Then the team must make its own decision.

If the team finds that a child is eligible for special education, the school district must then provide an IEP that outlines all areas of the child's educational program. The IEP is required by law, and includes the child's current level of performance and annual goals. The IEP may spell out a variety of extra (called "related") services (such as occupational therapy) that the child will receive, including how often and from whom. The IEP also outlines the child's areas of impairment from the list of 13 federal categories.

However, sometimes a particular child's needs do not meet the specific legal criteria that the school district must follow. If a school's team decides a child is not eligible for special education services, the team may refer him or her back to the regular education child study team to help the classroom teacher with appropriate classroom interventions.

Federal handicapped law is not intended to provide all help children need in all areas of schooling. Rather, it is designed to ensure that children with one or more of the 13 specifically defined handicaps receive a free, appropriate public education in the least restrictive environment.

Special equipment is used extensively with students who have problems with vision or hearing. Equipment such as computers to convert printed materials into synthetic speech, and special desks, chairs, writing devices, and school buses may help students with physical handicaps. Special ramps and wide doors, swimming pools and schoolrooms specially equipped with hearing aid transmission equipment are all part of special education.

Special services for exceptional individuals include speech training, physical and occupational therapies, counseling, and vocational training for students with mental retardation.

The most common element of special education are the specialized instructional techniques, such as

- sign language
- programmed instruction procedures designed to present information in small steps
- behavior modification techniques such as token economies

While most special education takes place in regular public schools, some classes are provided in special public or private day or residential schools, public or private hospitals, and, in some cases, the homes of individuals whose disabilities prevent them from attending school. Most individuals with disabilities do not require an entire program of services apart from conventional instruction, but rather only a modification of features.

When children are considered able to benefit from participation with other children, they are usually taught in the normal school program. This process, known as MAINSTREAMING, was believed to be consistent with the legal mandate for education in the least restrictive environment. More than two-thirds of students with disabilities receive most of their education in regular education classes.

If a child's handicap is not severe, a special education teacher works with the regular classroom teacher to develop skills. In other cases, an assistant teacher may be able to care for a student's specific needs. For individuals with more serious problems, special education may be provided in a separate classroom for part of the school day; students with severe learning and behavioral problems may remain in a separate special education room all day. The ratio of students to teachers is usually much lower in a special education classroom than in an ordinary classroom.

Special education also includes enhancement for gifted and talented students, and includes special activities beyond the regular curriculum, conventional courses at a faster-than-normal pace, and the opportunity to take college-level courses earlier in the school career.

With the development of ASSISTIVE TECHNOLOGIES, the field of special education continues to evolve, although its goal remains the same as it was from the beginning—to educate and integrate individuals with disabilities into society.

specific language disability (SLD)   A severe problem with some aspect of listening, speaking, reading, writing, or spelling, while skills in the other areas are age-appropriate. It is also called specific language learning disability.

These problems vary in focus and intensity, ranging from mild to severe. Some have severe problems with listening and reading (or *receptive language*) while others struggle with speaking and writing (*expressive language*). Other problems that often appear together with an specific learning disability include mild to severe organization problems and difficulty with directions.

Specific language disability may be a disorder of the left hemisphere of the brain, or a dominant right hemisphere.

Treatment Options and Outlook
While there is no cure, the disability can be managed using educational methods and unconventional learning techniques. A multisensory approach is extremely important in teaching these students, making sure the person must hear, say, see, write, and use movement and feeling. For the reader with a specific language disability, this varied approach ensures that information will move from short- to LONG-TERM MEMORY. The approach is also called the VAKT (Visual, Auditory, Kinesthetic, and Tactile) method.

specific learning disabilities   A legal term that plays a central role in legislation governing LEARNING DISABILITIES. As described in Public Law 94-142 (amended by PL 101-76), "specific learning disability" means a disorder in one or more of the basic psychological processes involved in understanding or in using spoken or written language. This may manifest itself in an imperfect ability to listen, think, speak, read, write, spell, or to do mathematical calculations.

The term includes such conditions as perceptual handicaps, brain injury, MINIMAL BRAIN DYSFUNCTION, DYSLEXIA, and developmental APHASIA. The term does not include children whose conditions are primarily caused by visual, hearing, or motor problems; MENTAL RETARDATION; emotional disturbance; or due to environmental, cultural, or economic disadvantage.

speech disorders   Individuals express thoughts, feelings, and ideas out loud to one another through a series of complex movements that mold the basic tone created by the voice into specific sounds. Speech is produced by precisely coordinated muscle actions in the head, neck, chest, and abdomen;

this gradual process requires years of practice to master in order to produce understandable speech.

By first grade, about 5 percent of children will develop a noticeable speech disorder, most of which have no known cause. Most speech disorders in the preschool years occur in children who are developing normally in all other areas, although speech disorders also may occur in children who have developmental disabilities.

One of the most common categories of speech disorders is STUTTERING, a condition in which there is a disruption in the flow of speech. Stuttering is a condition that involves repetitions of speech sounds, hesitations before and during speaking, and the prolonged emphasis of speech sounds. More than 15 million individuals around the world have this problem, most of whom began stuttering at a very early age.

Children with specific speech sound disorders (also called articulation disorder or phonological disorder) have trouble producing the speech sounds of their language that would be expected for their age. The extent of these errors will affect how easy it is to understand their speech, in some cases making it impossible for others to understand what the child is saying.

speech-language pathologist   An expert who specializes in the assessment and treatment of speech, language, and voice disorders. Also known as a speech pathologist or speech therapist, the speech-language pathologist evaluates and treats individuals with communication problems resulting from a LEARNING DISABILITY, hearing loss, brain injury, cleft palate, emotional problems, development delays, or stroke. He also provides clinical therapy to help those with speech and language disorders, and helps them and their families understand the disorder and develop better communication skills.

Speech-language pathologists perform screening tests and make recommendations for the type of speech language treatment required. Treatment could include a specific program of exercises to improve language ability or speech, together with support from the client's family and friends.

They conduct research to develop new and better ways to diagnose and treat speech/language problems, work with children who have language delays and speech problems, and provide treatment to people who stutter and to those with voice and articulation problems.

Educational requirements include a master's degree in speech-language pathology, more than 300 hours of supervised clinical experience, and successful completion of a certifying exam. Those who meet the strict requirements of the American Speech-Language and Hearing Association are awarded the certificate of clinical competence.

speech-language specialist   An expert who works in the area of speech and LANGUAGE, typically providing individualized work on language areas for children who have been identified as needing services. A speech-language specialist identifies and treats students with speech, language, and related problems, and collaborates with parents, caregivers, teachers, and other professionals in monitoring a student's progress.

speech synthesizer/screen readers   Computers designed to convert text into computer-generated speech. Originally designed for individuals with vision problems, as the programs became more sophisticated and affordable, they have been marketed to students with and without a LEARNING DISABILITY.

Many students find screen readers helpful in wading through large reading assignments. For now, getting the reading assignments *into* the computer adds a cumbersome step to the reading process; however, the time saved using the reading software far exceeds the time students take to convert print text into digital text. As college and university publishers move toward Web-based textbooks, this accessibility to digital texts may become the standard, making screen readers an essential tool for many students.

Although the quality of computerized voices is continuously improving, at present they can take some adjustment for the user.

Screen readers can be built into a word processing program, or designed as a feature of a voice recognition program. Typically, text can be scanned in, accessed online, or imported from a file. To be used primarily as a reading tool, a scanner is essential in order to enter text that is not already in digital form (such as in a textbook). Many screen readers are used for both reading and writing, though, since they were originally designed to be readers, they tend to be limited as word processors. Screen readers can be invaluable for students with learning disabilities when used in conjunction with other technologies such as word prediction, word processing, and spell checking since they allow students to hear words on the screen.

As reading tools, research has indicated that they enhance both fluency and COMPREHENSION. Unlike a print text environment, screen readers empower low decoders by providing flexibility and manipulation of the text. Because users can control how fast the reader reads, and combine both visual and auditory channels for "reading," slow readers can set the speed to much faster than they can read, but not faster than they can comprehend. Since slow readers are exposed to much more text than they would be relying on with traditional reading, studies show that fluency improves.

Not only are screen readers powerful reading tools, they are also useful for students with learning disabilities in the writing process, to hear their papers for proofing and revising.

As with all assistive technology, there are limitations. Although research has shown that college students with learning disabilities were able to find and correct about one-third of their errors with the use of a screen reader, it will not help catch homophone errors such as their/there that are common for students with learning disabilities.

See also KURZWEIL READING MACHINE.

spell checkers An electronic computer tool that checks a document for correct spelling. Nearly all word processing programs come with a built-in spell checking tool that can be invaluable for students with a LEARNING DISABILITY, since many written language disabilities include a problem with spelling.

Spell checkers perform two important functions: first, they identify misspelled words and second, they suggest correct spellings.

The process for spell checking is fairly universal. It begins by scanning a document against the program's dictionary and then flagging misspelled words. (Automatic spell checks that identify misspellings as a person types can be visually disruptive for some students. With this system, as it scans the document and flags misspelled words, the spell check will display a list of spelling suggestions. The user then selects the intended word, and it automatically replaces the misspelled word in the document.)

While spell checkers are valuable, they are not without several limitations to students with learning disabilities. First, spell checkers cannot identify spelling errors that are real words. Since studies show that up to 40 percent of spelling errors are real words, this can be a problem. For example, in the following sentence the spell checker would miss the underlined words because they are correctly spelled, although incorrect in this context: "After the cloths our finished drying, if you do not fold them they will wriggle." One way to overcome this problem with spell check is to use it together with a synthesized speech program, so the student can hear the words.

Another significant problem with spell checkers for students with learning disabilities is they do not always offer spelling suggestions for badly misspelled words. If the student cannot estimate the spelling of the intended word closely enough, then the spell checker is of little use.

Spell checkers may cause problems for students with learning disabilities when a suggested list of words appears in which many words are visually similar. In this case, it is difficult for the user to identify the intended word. A student can avoid selecting the wrong word by cross-checking with a thesaurus or using synthesized speech.

Finally, spell checking tools often flag proper nouns as incorrect, which can be confusing for students with learning disabilities.

Since spelling is often one of the major barriers to writing for students with learning disabilities, most students gladly accept the limitations of spell checking. Spell checkers are most effective with students who have learning disabilities but ample awareness of word sounds, which allows them to approximate the sounds of the intended word. The system is also better suited for those who can distinguish between similar-looking words.

As with all ASSISTIVE TECHNOLOGY, it is extremely important that students with learning disabilities are trained to use the technology in a way that will most empower their writing potential.

spelling   Words in the English language can be difficult to learn to spell because of many irregular spelling patterns. For example, *do, due,* and *dew* are all pronounced exactly the same but differ in meaning. While English has 44 sounds, it has only 26 letters.

The letter-sound correspondence is essential for reading, as is the sound-letter correspondence for correct spelling. A difficulty in these relationships results in LANGUAGE DISABILITIES.

Spelling a word is more difficult than reading a word for several reasons. First, passive (receptive) skills such as reading tend to be easier than active, expressive skills such as spelling. In addition, there are no contextual or structural cues to help with spelling as there are for reading. While spelling can be difficult for average learners, it is particularly difficult for individuals with a weakness in DECODING.

SQ3R   An acronym for an active reading method that stands for Survey, Question, Read, Recite, and Review; developed by psychologist Francis Robinson in 1941. To develop this method, Robinson applied the principles of learning theory to the development of reading and study skills. Through extensive research and testing, SQ3R has proven to be an effective reading and study strategy that enhances understanding and recall.

Surveying a passage before reading prepares one mentally to read. Creating questions based on chapter titles, subheading, and vocabulary creates a purpose for reading. Reading, reciting (paraphrasing and margin noting), and reviewing provide repetition of information. Thus, SQ3R combines reading and studying to create an active learning activity.

standard deviation   The measure of how the distribution of test scores varies from the mean. When the scores are tightly bunched together around the mean, the standard deviation is small. When the examples are spread apart, the standard deviation is larger. Computation of the standard deviation is based upon the square of the deviation of each score from the mean.

standardized test   A test that is designed to be administered and scored in a consistent manner in order to provide objective information about performance, ability, or achievement in a specific academic area.

The development process for a standardized test is extensive. Standardized tests typically include comprehensive guidelines for administration and scoring in order to reduce elements that might influence test results. Scores are often NORM-REFERENCED. The STANFORD ACHIEVEMENT TEST (SAT) and ACT are examples of standardized tests.

Unfortunately, as pressure increases on elementary and high schools to provide evidence of success, standardized tests are being used in ways for which they were never designed. A standardized test should never be used as the only criterion in placing a child in a special class, nor as the sole criterion for passing, failing, or graduating.

The two major types of group standardized tests are CRITERION-REFERENCED TESTS and norm-referenced tests. Criterion-referenced tests are designed to determine at what level students are performing on various skill areas. These tests assume that development of skills follows a sequence of steps. Criterion-referenced tests try to identify how far along the skills hierarchy the student has progressed. There is no comparison against anyone else's score, only against an expected skill level. The main question that criterion-referenced tests ask is "Where is this child in the development of group skills?"

Norm-referenced tests, in contrast, are typically constructed to compare children in their abilities as to different skill areas. Although the experts who design test items may be aware of skills hierarchies, they are more concerned with how much of some skill the child has mastered, rather than at what level on the skills hierarchy the child is.

Ideally, the questions on these tests range from very simple to extremely difficult. The essential feature of norm-referenced tests is that scores on these measures can be compared to scores of children in similar groups. They answer the question "How does the child compare with other children of the same age or grade placement in the development of this skill?"

Most criterion-referenced tests are created on the state or local level. The major norm-referenced tests include the CALIFORNIA ACHIEVEMENT TESTS, the Iowa Tests of Basic Skills, the SAT, the METRO-POLITAN ACHIEVEMENT TESTS, and the TerraNova. These generally test several types of reading, language, and mathematics skills along with social studies and science, and together with study and reference skills.

Group standardized tests are designed to assess and compare the achievement of groups—they are NOT designed to provide detailed diagnostic ASSESS-MENTS of individual students. This does not mean that test information on individual students is not useful, but it does mean that using these tests to diagnose an individual student is using them for a purpose for which they were not designed. Basically, a group standardized test is simply a way of screening the achievement of many students quickly. Learning problems should not be diagnosed solely on the basis of a group standardized test result, but the results can suggest that a child be referred for more definitive, individual assessments.

A child's group test score should be considered only as a point of information. These scores must be used with other information, such as teacher comments, daily work, homework, class tests, parent observations, medical needs, and social history.

standard scores   The results of most educational tests are reported using standard scores, which are then converted into percentiles. Standard scores are translated from RAW SCORES, generally to allow for greater comparability and ease of interpretation.

Stanford Achievement Test (SAT)   A national, commercial, norm-referenced group achievement test that has been used in the United States for the past 80 years. This test provides a quick snapshot of some of the things most people expect students to learn. The test is designed to provide assessment of students' achievement in reading, mathematics, language arts, science, and social studies at appropriate levels.

See also NORM-REFERENCED TESTS.

Stanford-Binet Intelligence Scale: Fourth Edition (SB:FE or SB-IV)   One type of IQ test that can be used to assess INTELLIGENCE for individuals between the ages of two and adulthood. First developed in 1910, the test is a standard tool for many SCHOOL PSYCHOLOGISTS.

Recently revised, the test now provides multiple IQ scores (called SASs) instead of a single IQ score. In addition to being able to measure the verbal and nonverbal areas of a child's development, the Binet also provides a quantitative score, measuring the child's mathematical reasoning, and a MEMORY score, measuring the child's short-term memory. (While the Wechsler scales also have subtests that measure these areas, they do not provide IQ scores isolating these abilities.)

This test is a good choice for children who are slow at processing information because it contains only one timed subtest. However, this lack of timing can make the testing session extremely long. In addition, this test may score substantially lower than the WAIS-III for very bright individuals over age 16.

One major advantage of the Binet over other IQ tests is that it is useful for assessment of much higher and much lower abilities than most other such tests, extending down to the moderately to the severely deficient and upward to the very superior range. It remains the measure of choice among psychologists assessing possible giftedness.

stanine   An approach to grouping standard scores on tests as a means for differentiating between groups of students. "Stanine" is short for *standard nine*—a reference to the fact that stanine scores range from a low of 1 to a high of 9. For instance, a stanine score of 1, 2, or 3 is below average; 4, 5, or 6 is average; and 7, 8, or 9 is above average.

If a child achieves a stanine score that is below average in a particular area, the test reveals an area in which the child needs improvement. If the child achieves an average stanine score, the test indicates that he or she performed at about the same level as the other students who took the test. If the child achieves a stanine score above average, this means that he or she performed better in that area than other students who took the test.

Stanines are similar to percentiles in that they provide a means for assessing an individual's test performance in relation to the various levels of performance. In contrast to stanines, however, percentiles give a more detailed description of how a child compares with others who took the test by showing scores that range from 1 to 99. For example, if a student scored in the 66th percentile on a test, that student achieved a score that was higher than 66 percent of the other students who took the test. So, if 1,000 students took the test, the student in the 66th percentile scored higher than 660 students who also took the same test.

However, percentiles should not be confused with percentage correct scores. "Percentile" scores allow one student's scores to be compared with a group of students who took the test. "Percentage correct" scores simply reveal the number of items that a student answered correctly out of the total number of items.

While stanines are a fairly popular alternative to percentiles, they are often less precise or informative. Individuals whose percentile rankings are fairly close may be grouped in different stanines, while individuals whose percentiles differ broadly in the middle range may be grouped together.

Stanines and percentiles rely on measuring a student's scores against the scores of a large group of students who also took the same test. This other group of students, or the comparison group, may be composed of other students in a school district who took the test at the same time or of students from a nationally representative sample who took the test earlier.

state education agency The state board of education or other agency primarily responsible for the supervision of public elementary and secondary schools. The state education agencies are responsible for compliance to the INDIVIDUAL WITH DISABILITIES EDUCATION IMPROVEMENT ACT (IDEIA) within their individual states.

stimulant medications Drugs often used in the treatment of ATTENTION DEFICIT HYPERACTIVITY DISORDER. METHYLPHENIDATE (Ritalin) is most commonly prescribed. Other stimulant medications that are frequently prescribed include: dextroamphetamine, Dexedrine and amphetamine and dextroamphetamine (Adderall).

For more than 50 years, these drugs have been used to treat the behavior of children with hyperactive symptoms; as many as 80 percent of students with ADHD respond to these drugs. Exactly what makes these medications effective against ADHD is unknown, although experts suspect they affect the rate and balance of specific neurotransmitters in certain areas of the brain. This results in a greater ability to pay ATTENTION and stay focused, and a decrease in HYPERACTIVITY. Since these children also tend to become less impulsive, aggressive, and destructive, the drugs also help improve social acceptance.

These medications are often used in combination with behavioral and educational interventions.

Individuals who respond positively to stimulant medications generally show improvement in their academic work and in their interactions with others. This change seems to happen right away.

Several studies have found that after students with ADHD started taking stimulants, their test scores and accuracy and speed in completing homework improved. The long-term gains are less clear.

Because most stimulant medications are metabolized quickly, often several doses a day are necessary.

Stimulant medications are used by both children and adults, and are taken for as long a period a time as is helpful or necessary. Some children find that as they develop through adolescence the medication is no longer necessary; others find the medication less necessary as their situation changes, for example, in environmental or academic demands. Many find that they face the frustrations of ADHD throughout adolescence and adulthood, and some of these individuals may benefit from using stimulant medication.

Successful treatment with stimulants lies in finding the right drug at the right dosage. It is important to remember that the child with ADHD will remain impulsive and energetic even while taking stimulants, but her ability to pay attention should improve.

Treatment with stimulants for ADHD is a long-term therapy; the government estimates that 80 percent of those who need medication for ADHD in childhood will still need drugs as teenagers, and 50 percent will be helped by stimulants as adults.

Side Effects

The most common side effects include weight loss and appetite loss, together with problems in falling asleep, although these problems may fade away as a student becomes used to the drug. Some studies have found that a child's growth begins to lag, although this growth usually rebounds after the first year in those who are on low or moderate doses. Children taking dexedrine or high doses of Ritalin may experience prolonged growth lag as long as they remain on the medication, but once the drug is stopped, growth begins again. For this reason, some experts recommend "drug holidays" during vacation to allow a child's growth to catch up.

Less common side effects include stomach problems, headaches, lethargy, irritability, nausea, euphoria, DEPRESSION, nightmares, dry mouth, constipation, ANXIETY, hallucinations, nervous tics, and tremors. In children at risk for tic disorders such as TOURETTE'S SYNDROME, the medication may trigger the condition. Because individual reactions and needs change, it is very important that the use and results of the medication be monitored.

While some stimulants can be addictive if abused by teenagers or adults, low doses seem to be safe for children.

strategy instruction An important educational approach to working with students with a LEARNING DISABILITY. It is based in part on an assumption that individuals with learning disabilities have significant deficits in the area of strategy development. These deficits may be the result of underlying language disabilities and skills deficits, or of problems in acquiring executive procedures and learning strategies.

In any case, a strategy instruction approach assumes that explicit instruction in learning strategies and executive procedures is a fundamental approach to helping students with learning disabilities achieve their potential.

Strategy instruction typically involves teaching procedures for specific academic tasks, such as reading strategies like SQ3R (Survey, Question, Read, Recite, Review). Students learn to perform a sequence of specific activities geared toward a specific task and outcome, practice these procedures in a variety of contexts, and apply them independently.

Strategy instruction has proven effective, particularly in college situations where it allows students to meet course requirements independently.

Strattera See ATOMOXETINE.

structural analysis A type of word recognition that identifies structural features such as syllables, prefixes, suffixes, and roots. Other structural elements include compound words (*sunshine*) and contractions (*do not*).

A reader may use a combination of structural analysis and context clues to identify an unfamiliar word. Individuals with learning disabilities benefit from the explicit teaching of structural analysis skills in order to improve spelling and reading comprehension.

See also MORPHOLOGICAL AWARENESS.

study skills Learning strategies that help an individual organize time, materials, and information. Special educators long ago recognized the importance of teaching study skills to students with LEARNING DISABILITIES; such skills have recently become a part of many school curricula starting in the elementary grades.

While some students seem to succeed in school with only basic study skills, many learning disabled students benefit greatly from being taught ideas such as how to maintain a notebook and how to organize materials in each class. Time management is another essential study skill needed to complete long and short assignments on time as well as to schedule time for appointments, friends, and work. Note-taking and active reading strategies are also important study skills for all students, including those with learning disabilities.

stuttering A communication disorder in which the flow of speech is broken by repetitions (li-li-like this), prolongations (lllllike this), or abnormal stoppages (no sound) of sounds and syllables. There may also be unusual facial and body movements associated with the effort to speak. Known as dysphemia, stuttering is most obvious in those who do not have control over the timing and rhythm of their speech.

While experts seem to know all the characteristics of stuttering, they do not agree on the cause. Despite years of research, there are no simple answers to the cause of stuttering, but much has been learned about factors that contribute to its development. Stuttering may occur in the presence of a combination of factors, which may have different causes in different people. It may well be that what causes stuttering differs from what makes it continue or get worse. However, children who stutter are no more likely to have psychological or emotional problems than those who do not, and there is no reason to believe that emotional trauma causes stuttering.

Another common form of stuttering originates as a signal problem between the brain and nerves or muscles. In neurogenic stuttering, the brain is unable to coordinate adequately the different components of the speech mechanism. Neurogenic stuttering may also occur following a stroke or other type of brain injury.

Other forms of stuttering are classified as originating in the mind or psychogenic. Whereas at one time the major cause of stuttering was thought to be psychogenic, this type of stuttering is now known to account for only a few individuals. Although individuals who stutter may develop emotional problems such as fear of meeting new people or speaking on the telephone, these problems often result from stuttering rather than as a cause of stuttering. Psychogenic stuttering occasionally occurs in individuals who have some types of mental illness or individuals who have experienced severe mental stress or anguish.

Stuttering may be genetic, but no genes for stuttering have yet been found.

More than 3 million Americans stutter, which affects four times as many boys as girls. It is most common between ages two and six; most children outgrow the problem. Less than 1 percent of adults stutter. About 20 percent of all children go through a stage of development during which they encounter speech fluency problems severe enough to be a concern to their parents.

Symptoms and Diagnostic Path

Stuttering therapy may help prevent developmental stuttering from becoming a lifelong problem, so a speech evaluation is recommended for children who stutter for longer than six months or whose stuttering is accompanied by struggle behaviors.

Stuttering is generally diagnosed by a SPEECH LANGUAGE PATHOLOGIST, a professional trained to test and treat individuals with voice, speech, and language disorders. The diagnosis is usually based on the history of the disorder, such as when it was first noticed and under what circumstances, as well as a complete evaluation of speech and language abilities.

Treatment Options and Outlook

There are a variety of treatments available for stuttering. Any of the methods may improve stuttering to some degree, but at present there is no cure for stuttering. Developmental stuttering is often treated by educating parents about restructuring the child's speaking environment to reduce the episodes of stuttering. A speech pathologist can almost always help children improve their communication skills.

There are a variety of successful approaches for treating children. While therapy will not cure stuttering overnight, a qualified clinician can help children make significant progress toward FLUENCY. Stuttering therapy usually means changing long-standing speech behaviors, emotions, and attitudes about talking and communication in general. As a result, length and type of therapy can vary greatly depending on a person's goals.

Many of the currently popular therapy programs for persistent stuttering focus on relearning how to speak or unlearning faulty ways of speaking. The psychological side effects of stuttering that often occur, such as fear of speaking to strangers or in public, are also addressed in most of these programs.

Other forms of therapy use interventions such as medications or electronic devices. However, medications that affect brain function often have side effects that make them difficult to use for long-term treatment. Electronic devices that help an individual control fluency may be more of a bother than a help in most speaking situations and are often abandoned by individuals who stutter. Unconventional methods of stuttering therapy also exist. It is always a good policy to check the credentials, experience, and goals of the therapist and avoid working with anyone who promises a "cure" for stuttering.

Parents should provide a relaxed home environment so as to give the child opportunities to speak. Setting aside specific times when the child and parent can speak free of distractions is often helpful. Parents and family members should not criticize the child's speech or react negatively to the child's stuttering. Parents should avoid punishing the child for any disfluencies and should not ask the child to repeat stuttered words until they are spoken fluently. In addition, the family should resist encouraging the child to perform verbally for people and listen attentively to the child when he or she speaks. Listeners should wait for the child to say the intended word and should not try to complete the child's thoughts. A parent also should speak slowly and in a relaxed manner, because if the parent speaks this way, the child will often speak in the same slow, relaxed way. Family members should discuss stuttering openly if the child brings up the subject.

substitution   A reading error made when an individual replaces the written word with a different word based on structural or semantic cues.

A structural substitution is when the reader guesses a word based on its visual structure. For example, a reader reads the word *stipulate* as *stimulate* because they look similar.

A semantic substitution occurs when a reader replaces a word with a word that means the same thing. For example, a reader might read "Then they went to her house" as "Then they went to her place," replacing *house* with *place*.

Substitution is common in the ORAL READING of all students and by itself should not be considered as evidence of a reading disability. Tracking reading errors through ERROR ANALYSIS can help to determine reading patterns and problems.

support group   An organization that exists to provide support to individuals struggling with a problem, such as a LEARNING DISABILITY. Some people derive enormous satisfaction by sharing their problems and solutions with others in similar situations.

Children and Adults with Attention Deficit Hyperactivity Disorder (CHADD) is one of several national organizations with local chapters that offer help to people with learning disabilities.

Belonging to a support group can also help individuals identify which local practitioners are best qualified to diagnose and treat learning disabilities.

survival skills   This term can mean more than one thing depending on the context in which it is used. Survival skills may refer to daily self-help skills necessary to survive in life, such as feeding, dressing, and communicating. In higher education, survival skills often refer to the STUDY SKILLS necessary to be a successful learner.

syllabication   The process of dividing words into syllables. Syllabication is a popular word attack strategy taught to individuals with reading problems. Many PHONICS and structured reading programs teach syllabication.

In English, there are six types of syllables and five principles of syllabication that describe how and where to break a word apart. The six types of syllables include

1. closed: short vowel followed by a consonant (*con, pan, dis*)
2. open: ends in a single long vowel (*de, o, fi*)
3. silent "e": long vowel/consonant/silent "e" (*hive, ete, ode*)
4. R-controlled: vowel followed by an "r" (*ur, fir, cer*)
5. double vowel: any two vowels that make one sound (*poor, ear, ay*)
6. consonant "le": found at the end of a word with a consonant/le (*kle, dle, ple*)

symbol   Something that represents or stands for an idea, object, or sound. In English, the alphabet is the symbol system for language. Individuals who have difficulty processing or naming symbols will have difficulty reading, since reading is the process of interpreting symbols.

syntax   The arrangement of words in sentences, clauses, and phrases. Understanding syntax in the English language is very important because it directly affects COMPREHENSION. The following sentences, for example, contain the exact same words, but only the syntax is different—*Liz saw Bob. Bob saw Liz.* The sentences mean very different things.

Students with a LEARNING DISABILITY may have trouble understanding the rules of syntax. When speaking out loud, syntax is more flexible and fluid. Sentences in spoken language tend to be longer, and syntactical errors are often overlooked.

In spoken language, difficulties in syntax may lead to the inability to articulate a thought in a complete sentence. Many students with learning disabilities who demonstrate a solid understanding of syntax in spoken language may have considerable difficulties with syntax in written form because of the static nature of text and the rigidity of grammar. In writing, common syntactic errors include run-on sentences, incomplete sentences, subject-verb disagreement, and comma splices.

Syntactic knowledge can have a significant impact on reading and writing. Normal development of syntactic knowledge occurs in the following stages:

- holophrastic stage (10–12 months): children begin uttering one-word sentences to express ideas. For example, "milk" means "I want milk"

- two-word stage (18–24 months): children string two words together to express general ideas. For example, "Mommy sock" could mean "That sock is Mommy's" or "Mommy, the sock is over there"

- expansions (two to nine years): children begin to gradually use more descriptive and grammatically advanced sentences with subjects and verbs. For example a two-year-old may say "Car goes" for "That car goes down the road"

- later stages (nine years through adulthood): after age nine, sentence length continues to increase through early adulthood. In adolescence, average sentence length is about 10 to 12 words. Sentence structure becomes more complex, using complex subjects, interrupters, modals, and so on

Children who do not gain syntactic knowledge in the above stages may encounter problems with COMPREHENSION. Research has discovered that poor readers often have syntactic deficits. Poor readers use fewer complete sentences; they violate subject/verb agreement and use shorter sentences. In writing, they use simple sentences more often than do proficient readers.

If an individual is suspected of having problems with syntax, it is important to find out where the breakdown is occurring. There are both formal and informal syntactic ASSESSMENT procedures that can be carried out by SPEECH PATHOLOGISTS or other such professionals qualified in assessing language skills.

T

tactile The sensory system of touch, in which information is transmitted through direct physical contact via the nervous system to the brain.

tactile defensiveness Being overly sensitive to touch; withdrawing, crying, yelling, or striking out when touched.

Some experts believe that tactile defensiveness is related to disorganization in the midbrain, which is responsible for filtering incoming stimuli and—when abnormal—may not screen out all excessive tactile stimulation. As a result, a person would register even the most subtle sensations as irritating or painful, so that the person may respond to touch by grimacing or pulling away.

The central nervous system relies on different sensory nerve receptors in the skin to monitor the environment: light touch (surface), pressure (deep), temperature (hot and cold), and pain. It is quite possible for a person with tactile defensiveness to have one type of receptor that is oversensitive and the rest be normal. This explains why a person could tolerate light touch but pull away from a firm hug or prefer to run outside without a coat but be content with haircuts.

The tactile defensive individual can experience great distress in the course of daily life, constantly being bombarded by raw sensations. A person might insist on wearing only very soft clothes with large head openings or refuse to wear jewelry (especially around the neck). The slightest bump from another person may feel like a threat, and his or her defensive response may appear to be impulsive or aggressive. People with this condition may dislike group games such as tag or dodgeball, and holding hands with a partner can be physically agonizing. A person with this condition may shrink from being touched, which prevents him or her from being able to interact with friends in a normal way. Daily personal grooming, including bathing, washing hair, trimming nails, or brushing teeth can also be interpreted as uncomfortable.

tactile perception Perception through the sensory system of touch, in which direct physical contact is transmitted through the nervous system to the brain.

tardive dyskinesia A neurological syndrome characterized by repetitive, involuntary, purposeless movements caused by the long-term use of neuroleptic drugs typically prescribed for psychiatric and brain disorders. Tardive dyskinesia (TD) occurs in between 15 and 30 percent of people who receive long-term treatment with neuroleptics.

Newer atypical antipsychotic agents, including olanzapine and risperidone, appear to carry less risk of TD. The drugs that may cause TD include

- *anticholinergics:* benzhexol, biperiden (Akineton), ethopropazine, orphenadrine (Norflex, Norgesic, Orphengesic), procyclidine

- *antidepressants:* phenelzine (Nardil), fluoxetine (Prozac), sertraline (Zoloft), trazodone (Desyrel), amitriptyline (Elavil, Vanatrip), amitriptyline and perphenazine (Triavil), amoxapine (Asendin), doxepin (Sinequan), imipramine (Tofranil)

- *antiemetics:* metoclopramide (Maxolon, Reglan), prochlorperazine (Compazine)

- *antiepileptic drugs:* carbamazepine (Atretol, Epitol, Tegretol), ethosuximide (Zarontin), phenobarbital (Barbita, Luminal sodium, Solfoton), phenytoin (Dilantin)

- *antihistamines:* antihistaminic decongestants, combinations of antihistamines and sympathomimetics

- *antimalarials:* chloroquine (Aralen)
- *anti-Parkinson agents:* bromocriptine (Parlodel), levodopa (Dopar, L-Dopa, Larodopa), levodopa-carbidopa (Atamet, Sinemet)
- *anxiolytics:* alprazolam (Xanax)
- *biogenic amines:* DOPAMINE (Intropin)
- *mood stabilizers:* lithium (Cibalith-S, Eskalith, Lithane, Lithobid, Lithotabs, Lithonate)
- *oral contraceptives:* estrogens
- *stimulants:* amphetamine (Adderall), METHYL-PHENIDATE (Ritalin, Ritalin SR), caffeine

Symptoms and Diagnostic Path

Features of the disorder may include grimacing, tongue protrusion, lip smacking, puckering and pursing, and rapid eye blinking, along with rapid movements of the arms, legs, and trunk. Involuntary movements of the fingers may appear as though the patient is playing an invisible guitar or piano.

Treatment Options and Outlook

There is no standard treatment for tardive dyskinesia. The first step is to stop or lower the dose of the drug, but for patients with a severe underlying condition this may not be an option. Replacing the neuroleptic drug with substitute drugs may help some patients. Other drugs such as benzodiazepines, adrenergic antagonists, or dopamine agonists may help.

Symptoms of tardive dyskinesia may remain long after the neuroleptic drug is stopped. However, with careful management, some symptoms may improve or disappear with time.

task analysis A teaching strategy in which a learning activity is broken down into small sequential tasks. It is an effective strategy used to teach students with a LEARNING DISABILITY because it takes a large learning activity and breaks it into smaller, more easily accomplished tasks. Task analysis is also used as an ASSESSMENT tool to see precisely at what stage a skill breakdown is occurring. For example, if a student is given an assignment to define 10 vocabulary words, a task analysis might include the following steps:

1. understand, record, and remember the assignment
2. read/decode the vocabulary words
3. use a dictionary/textbook
4. paraphrase the definition
5. write the definitions

Breaking an assignment into the five steps can make a difficult and overwhelming project become more manageable.

Similarly, task analysis can be used for instruction where larger skills are broken down into subskills and each subskill taught until mastery.

See also DIRECT INSTRUCTION.

temporal lobe A part of the brain located above and behind the ears, underneath the frontal and parietal lobes. It is named for the temporal bone at the temple, just above the ear canal. The temporal lobe includes the auditory cortex located near the ear, which is the primary area for processing hearing.

temporal-sequential organization problems Children with this type of organizational problem have trouble completing long-term assignments, understanding and having a sense of time, and understanding and following directions.

Almost every task a child does involves sequence, whether that involves getting dressed, completing an assignment, or reading a book. Knowing the sequence and being able to follow it are important developmental skills.

School can be overwhelming for students who cannot recognize a step-by-step plan needed to master a concept such as memorizing the alphabet, understanding the seasons, or learning the multiplication tables. Spelling can be a particular problem for these children who cannot remember the sequence of letters, which is also required for word recognition during reading.

Concepts of time are also very difficult for these children, who have trouble mastering days of the week, months of the year, and how to tell time. The ability to manage time is also compromised, and completing a long-term assignment by the due date is quite a challenge. Because a concept of time is foreign to these children, they easily lose track of time, which can interfere with a child's ability to pace work during a test.

Test of Adolescent and Adult Language—Third Edition (TOAL-3) This test of language development helps determine areas of relative strength and weakness. The overall score may be accurate, although some of the area scores may not be valid because they are composed of only two subtest scores. In this test, the individual will

- choose a picture that depicts a dictated word
- choose which sentences with different grammar have the same meaning
- make up and repeat sentences
- write sentences using specific words
- choose words that belong together
- combine sentences

Test of Auditory Comprehension of Language—Revised (TACL-R) This developmental test assesses auditory comprehension by having children point to the correct picture from among three choices as the examiner dictates single words, words with modifiers, short sentences with different grammatical forms, and complex sentences. A child's score may be lowered if the individual is impulsive or has trouble with perceptual discrimination, even if overall language comprehension is good. This test should be used with tasks that measure the child's expressive language abilities as well.

Test of Language Competence—Expanded Edition A test of language development designed for students aged nine through 18 years, 11 months that measures more sophisticated vocabulary (semantics), sentence structure (syntax), and conversational skills. In this test, the student may be asked to

- identify multiple meanings in a sentence that could mean more than one thing
- choose inferences after related statements
- create a sentence using a picture and three words
- explain metaphors

Test of Language Development—Primary, Third Edition (TOLD-P:3) A test of language develop-

ment that measures the younger child's pictorial and oral vocabulary, understanding of sentence structure, repetition of dictated sentences, use of appropriate grammatical forms, and word discrimination and articulation. The test is appropriate for children between ages four years and eight years, 11 months.

Test of Language Development—2 Intermediate (TOLD-2 Intermediate) A test of language development that measures vocabulary and sentence structure by assessing sentence combinations, oral vocabulary, abstract relationships, the ordering of words within sentences, recognition of grammatically correct sentences, and the correcting of nonsensical sentences.

thalamus A part of the brain located above the hypothalamus; involved in the relay of information from other regions of the nervous system to the cerebral cortex. It transmits sensory information, including auditory and visual input, in addition to movement information from the CEREBELLUM and BASAL GANGLIA to the motor cortex. The thalamus is also involved in the maintenance of consciousness.

thematic maturity The sophistication of writing. Plot development, sentence structure, and cohesion based on an individual's age and grade are some elements that are considered in evaluating thematic maturity.

thinking skills The way in which an individual acquires, interprets, organizes, stores, retrieves, and applies information, also known as cognitive skills.

tics Sudden, rapid, involuntary movements associated with TOURETTE'S SYNDROME that may be either vocal, motor, or mental.

token economy A behavior therapy procedure in which tokens (such as coins or poker chips) are given for desired behavior. The tokens can then be exchanged for privileges or treats.

Tourette's syndrome (Tourette syndrome) A neurological disorder characterized by tics (rapid, sudden movements that occur involuntarily and repeatedly in a consistent fashion). To be diagnosed with Tourette's syndrome, an individual must have multiple motor tics as well as one or more vocal tics over a period of more than one year. These need not all occur simultaneously, but in general the tics may occur many times a day, usually in brief, intense groupings, nearly every day.

Common simple tics include eye blinking, shoulder jerking, picking movements, grunting, sniffing, and barking. Complex tics include facial grimacing, arm flapping, coprolalia (use of obscene words), palilalia (repeating one's own words), and echolalia (repeating another's words or phrases).

For individuals with Tourette's, tics may vary over time in frequency and severity, as well as in type and location. In some cases, symptoms may disappear for a period of weeks or even months. Although there is an involuntary quality to the tics experienced by individuals with Tourette's, most persons have some control over their symptoms, at least briefly. However, suppressing tics tends simply to postpone more severe outbursts, since the impulse to express tics is ultimately irresistible. Tics often will increase in response to stress and become less frequent with relaxation or intense focus on a task.

Up to 20 percent of children have at least a transient tic disorder at some point. Once believed to be rare, Tourette's syndrome is now known to be a more common disorder that represents the most complex and severe manifestation of the spectrum of tic disorders.

An abnormal metabolism of the neurotransmitters DOPAMINE and serotonin are linked to the disorder, which is genetically transmitted. Parents have a 50 percent chance of passing the gene on to their children. Girls with the gene have a 70 percent chance of displaying symptoms; boys with the gene have a 99 percent chance of displaying symptoms.

Symptoms and Diagnostic Path

In addition to tics, people with Tourette's syndrome also may have other syndromes, including ATTENTION DISORDER HYPERACTIVITY DISORDER, ANXIETY, mood or panic disorders, OBSESSIVE-COMPULSIVE DISORDER, behavior problems, and LEARNING DISABILITIES.

In most children, Tourette's syndrome has a fluctuating course. Anxiety, stress, and fatigue often intensify tics, which are usually significantly reduced during sleep or when the patient is focused on an activity. Psychoactive drugs, (particularly cocaine and stimulants) have a tendency to worsen tics.

In most cases, tics peak in severity between ages nine and 11, but between 5 percent and 10 percent of patients continue to have unchanged or worsening symptoms into adolescence and adulthood. In this population, the likelihood of tics continuing for decades is substantial. Patients in their seventh, eighth, and ninth decades of life may have tics that have been present since childhood. In most older patients, the tics tend to become quite stable over time, although occasionally new tics will be acquired. There is no reliable way to predict which children will have a poorer prognosis.

The single most important component of managing the condition is to obtain an accurate diagnosis. Tics occur suddenly during normal activity, unlike other movement disorders such as

- chorea: a pattern of nonrepetitive irregular movements
- stereotypy: constant, repetitive behaviors performed for no obvious reason
- dystonias: slow, constant repetitive behavior

Secondary causes of tic disorders should first be ruled out. A complete general physical examination, with specific attention to the neurologic part of the examination, is important.

The thyroid-stimulating hormone (TSH) level should be measured in most patients, since tics often occur together with hyperthyroidism. A throat culture should be checked for group A beta-hemolytic streptococcus, especially if symptoms change during ear or throat infections. However, the evidence of strep infection with a single occurrence of worsening tics is not enough to make a diagnosis of streptococcus-induced, autoimmune-caused Tourette's syndrome.

An electroencephalogram is useful only if it is difficult to differentiate tics from manifestations of epilepsy. Imaging studies are not likely to be helpful, and the importance of other studies depends on symptoms. For example, a urine drug screen for cocaine and stimulants should be considered in the case of a teenager with sudden onset of tics and inappropriate behavior symptoms. A person with a family history of liver disease associated with a Parkinsonian or hyperkinetic movement disorder should undergo tests of copper levels in the blood to rule out Wilson's disease.

The basic workup is usually appropriate in a patient with a gradual onset of symptoms, a developmental progression of tics, and a family history of tics or obsessive-compulsive disorder.

Treatment Options and Outlook

Positive reinforcement programs appear to be most helpful in managing tic disorders. Target behaviors may be categorized into two groups: skill deficiencies, or areas requiring an initial concentration to build social and academic skills, and behavior excesses, in which the goal is to help the patient decrease the frequency of these behaviors. Managing behavior excesses must be handled carefully, however, since some children who undergo BEHAVIOR MODIFICATION to directly target the Tourette's symptoms experience a worsening of symptoms.

The goal in tic control is to use the lowest dosage of medication that will bring the patient's functioning to an acceptable level. Often this will require only modest levels of tic reduction. The most common drug treatments are haloperidol (Haldol), pimozide (Orap), risperidone (Risperdal), and clonidine (Catapres). Guanfacine (Tenex) is not approved for use in children under 12 years of age. Less often, clonazepam (Klonopin) may be prescribed. For tics of mild to moderate severity, or in patients who are wary of drug side effects, an initial trial of clonidine or guanfacine may be tried. These medications are modestly effective in tic control and have a range of less specific benefits. Many children taking them may be less irritable or less impulsive, and manifestations of ADHD may improve as well.

Side effects of these drug treatments include sedation, weight gain, poor school performance, social anxiety (with school refusal), and unusual body movements, including TARDIVE DYSKINESIA, a potentially irreversible drug-caused movement disorder that may be difficult to distinguish from tics. When pimozide is used, baseline and follow-up electrocardiograms are recommended.

Most patients with Tourette's syndrome require medication for one to two years; about 15 percent of patients require long-term medication for tic control. When tics appear to be stable and adequately controlled for a period of four to six months, a slow and gradual reduction in medication should follow. With such a strategy, occasional "drug holidays" may be possible in some patients as tics lessen. If tics increase, incremental increases in medication may be needed.

Many patients with Tourette's syndrome have other conditions, that also must be treated. Treatment of ADHD with Tourette's has been controversial because of reports that stimulants hasten the onset or increase the severity of tics in some patients. This observation alone may not be a contraindication for stimulant treatment in patients with significant symptoms of ADHD. Stimulants alone may not substantially worsen the course or severity of the disorder. In some cases, it may be necessary to treat both the ADHD and the Tourette's syndrome with a stimulant in combination with either clonidine or guanfacine, or with a neuroleptic agent. A trial of clonidine or guanfacine alone may be sufficient to adequately treat both conditions. When possible, multiple drugs should not be used, especially in children.

Treatment of obsessive-compulsive disorder with antidepressants such as selective serotonin reuptake inhibitors may be effective. With these medications, there is often a significant delay between start of treatment and response, which may take as long as four to six weeks. Behavior therapy is also effective in the treatment of obsessive-compulsive disorder.

tracking   A process of using a finger or pencil to follow the eyes while reading. Tracking can be a useful strategy for an individual with visual perception difficulties because it incorporates a kinesthetic component to reading. Tracking with a pencil can be beneficial so individuals can physically break long, unfamiliar words into syllables as they read.

See also SYLLABICATION; ABILITY GROUPING.

transition plan   Movement from one place or idea to another. In the context of LEARNING DISABILITIES, a transition plan refers to the change from school to adult life. For disabled students, this may require extra effort and planning for individuals and their support/INDIVIDUALIZED EDUCATION PROGRAM (IEP) team. Transition legislation in the INDIVIDUALS WITH DISABILITIES EDUCATION IMPROVEMENT ACT states that transition services and planning be written into the IEP. The contents of a transition plan should include

- current levels of performance
- interests and aptitudes
- postschool goals
- transition activities—specific steps to be taken (e.g., career/vocational counseling)
- the designation of responsible persons to oversee the transition after high school

transposition   A reading, writing, or numeric error where letters or numbers or words are switched. For example, transposition in mathematics might involve writing or reading the number *258* for *852*, or writing *shinesun* for *sunshine*.

Methods for treating the problem of transposition could include using a multimodal strategy such as asking the student to say the letters as he or she writes the word.

traumatic brain injury   The common general term for brain injuries that impair thinking as a result of physical trauma severe enough to cause loss of consciousness or damage to the brain structure. Of all the problems that can lead to LEARNING DISABILITIES, this is the most preventable. Each year, about 2 million Americans sustain a brain injury—about one every 15 seconds. More than a million of these are sustained by children, 30,000 of whom will have permanent disabilities.

Boys are twice as likely to be injured as girls, especially between the ages of 14 and 24, followed by infants and then the elderly. Children are more likely to incur traumatic brain injury during the spring and summer. Traffic accidents account for almost half of the injuries; about 34 percent occur at home and the rest in recreation areas.

Traumatic brain injury includes both open and closed head injury, both of which can cause severe learning problems. In an open head injury, the force of impact can cause scalp injuries and skull fractures, together with blood clots and bruising. This type of injury usually affects one place in the brain, producing specific problems.

A closed head injury can cause more widespread damage as the force of impact causes the brain to smash against the opposite side of the skull, tearing nerve fibers and blood vessels. This type of *contre-coup* injury may affect the brain stem, causing physical, intellectual, emotional, and social problems. A person's entire personality may be forever changed.

In young children, abuse is the primary cause of this type of injury; 64 percent of babies under age one that are physically abused have brain injuries, usually by shaking (see SHAKEN BABY SYNDROME). In children under age 5, half of brain injuries are related to falls. Cars and biking accidents and suicide attempts are the primary causes of traumatic brain injury in school-age children and adolescents.

Traumatic brain injury is one of the conditions included in the INDIVIDUALS WITH DISABILITIES EDUCATION IMPROVEMENT ACT (IDEIA), which governs special education services for children in the United States. According to IDEIA law, traumatic brain injury is

> an acquired injury to the brain caused by an external physical force, resulting in total or partial functional disability or psychosocial impairment, that adversely affects a child's educational performance. The term applies to open or closed head injuries resulting in impairments in one or more areas, such as cognition; language; memory; attention; reasoning; abstract thinking; judgment; problem-solving; sensory, perceptual, and motor abilities; psychosocial behavior; physical functions; information processing; and speech. The term does not apply to brain injuries that are congenital or degenerative, or to brain injuries induced by birth trauma.

Because traumatic brain injury is now included under IDEIA, SPECIAL EDUCATION services can be provided if the child experiences any problems with thinking or learning skills after the accident. An INDIVIDUALIZED EDUCATION PROGRAM should be prepared to deal with the child's special needs.

Symptoms and Diagnostic Path
Individuals with traumatic brain injury may have one or more difficulties, including physical problems, thinking difficulties, and social or emotional problems.

Physical disabilities: These problems may include trouble speaking, seeing, hearing, and using the senses. Other physical symptoms may include headaches, fatigue, spasticity, seizures, and trouble with skills such as writing or drawing. Balance and walking may also be affected, and there may be partial or complete paralysis on one side of the body or both sides.

Difficulties with thinking: Because the brain has been injured, it is not surprising that the person's ability to use the brain changes. For example, children with this injury may have trouble with short-term or LONG-TERM MEMORY, or they may have trouble concentrating and only be able to focus their ATTENTION for a short time. They may think slowly. They may have trouble talking and listening to others. They may also have difficulty with reading and writing, planning, understanding the order in which events happen (called sequencing), and judgment.

Social, behavioral, or emotional problems: These difficulties may include sudden changes in mood, ANXIETY, and DEPRESSION, so that people with traumatic brain injury have trouble relating to others. They may be restless and may laugh or cry a lot. They may not have much motivation or control over their emotions.

Sometimes, certain behavior may appear long after the traumatic brain injury occurs. These behaviors may include overeating or drinking, excessive talking, restlessness, disorientation, or seizure disorders.

Some patients may experience coma after a brain injury; the degree of the coma severity is measured by the Glasgow Coma Score, or the Rancho Los Amigos Scale, which assigns a number to represent the degree to which patients can open their eyes, move, or speak. X-rays and brain scans may help if a skull fracture is suspected.

Treatment Options and Outlook

Rehabilitation should begin as soon as possible after the accident. They may include physical or occupational therapy, or speech and language therapy.

Early and ongoing help can make a big difference in how the child recovers, but as the child develops, parents and teachers may notice new problems. This is because as students grow, they are expected to use their brain in new and different ways. The damage to the brain from the earlier injury can make it hard for the student to learn new skills that come with getting older. Sometimes parents and educators may not even realize that the student's difficulty comes from the earlier injury.

Risk Factors and Preventive Measures

Traumatic brain injury can be prevented by taking appropriate safety precautions, such as insisting that children wear helmets when biking, riding a scooter, or skating, sledding, and skiing. Children also should be placed in car seats or wear seat belts, and ride in the back of the car.

tutoring   Instructing a child in a special subject or for a particular purpose. One advantage that small-group or one-on-one tutoring offers to individuals with a LEARNING DISABILITY is that it allows instruction to be individualized to meet the unique needs and learning styles of each child. Tutors can reinforce subjects that are taught in school as well as teach students how to work independently. Students often become more self-confident after working with a tutor.

Ideally, students with a learning disability should consider scheduling more than one tutoring lesson a week, since these students often need practice and repetition to master skills. Tutoring sessions should include hands-on learning and be very interactive. The tutor should guide the child through DIRECT INSTRUCTION and practice.

A parent should receive periodic reports from both the tutor and the child's teacher, and show noticeable academic improvement within a few months.

U

United States Code (USC) The code of statutes under which all federal laws are listed.

universal access/design A term originally used in architecture to denote an approach to construction that assures access to all individuals regardless of physical problems such as paralysis, eye problems, or deafness. Such an approach goes beyond assuring that there are ramps for individuals in wheelchairs, or braille symbols next to elevator buttons. Universal access is an attempt to make every aspect of a building as equally accessible for individuals with disabilities as they may be for those without.

Recently, the concept of universal access or design has been used in educational contexts; the term signifies an approach that provides equal access to appropriate education in a mainstream setting, by assuring that all of the learning needs and styles of individual students are addressed by a variety of teaching techniques.

For example, this would mean students are provided with instructional approaches that use sight, touch, and movements as well as hearing, and that testing as well as instruction allow all students to demonstrate mastery of course material. Highly specific instructional approaches assure that all students in a class are able to use their strengths to respond to course assignments.

Universal design or access represents a new way of thinking about LEARNING DISABILITIES, although there is still a great deal that is undeveloped and unproven regarding the approach.

VAKT (Visual-Auditory-Kinesthetic-Tactile) An acronym for a type of instructional method used primarily for reading that involves sight, hearing, movement, and touch. VAKT is based on the concept that individuals learn better when more than one learning method is stimulated. With this approach to teach reading, students may be asked to *see* the word (visual), *hear* the word (auditory), *write* the word on a surface or in the air using the finger (kinesthetic), and *trace* the word on a textured surface such as sandpaper or a rough board (tactile).

VAKT is not limited to reading instruction, and many special educators use some form of multisensory instruction in every lesson. The Fernald and Orton-Gillingham methods also use the VAKT technique.

See also ORTON-GILLINGHAM APPROACH.

validity An essential way of judging the effectiveness of a test by assessing the extent to which the test accurately measures what it is intended to measure. There are different types of validity according to the nature of the test.

In achievement testing, for example, "content validity" refers to the extent to which the material covered by a test represents a balanced sampling of the information that the test is meant to assess. "Criterion-related" validity refers to the extent to which performance on a specific test accurately predicts future grade performance. Finally, "construct validity" relates to the accuracy with which a test measures some abstract or theoretical idea, such as personality traits or abilities such as critical thinking or interpersonal INTELLIGENCE.

verbal apraxia A speech disorder ranging from mild to severe, in which a person has trouble speaking correctly and consistently, so that speech is labored and characterized by sound reversals, additions, and word approximations. The severity of the disorder can vary from child to child, but children with the most severe problems are unable to produce any consistent speech sounds or words.

There are two main types of speech APRAXIA: acquired apraxia of speech and developmental apraxia of speech.

Acquired apraxia of speech can affect a person at any age, although it most typically occurs in adults. It is caused by damage to the parts of the brain that are involved in speaking, from a stroke, head injury, tumor, or other illness affecting the brain. Acquired apraxia of speech involves the loss or impairment of existing speech abilities. It may occur together with muscle weakness affecting speech production (DYSARTHRIA) or language difficulties caused by damage to the nervous system (APHASIA).

Developmental apraxia of speech (DAS) occurs in children at birth, affecting more boys than girls. This speech disorder goes by several other names, including developmental verbal apraxia, developmental verbal dyspraxia, articulatory apraxia, and childhood apraxia of speech. The cause of DAS is not known, although some scientists believe that it is either related to a child's overall language development or that it is a neurological disorder affecting the brain's ability to send the proper signals to move the muscles involved in speech. However, brain imaging and other studies have not found evidence of specific brain lesions or differences in brain structure in children with DAS. These children often have family members who have a history of communication disorders or LEARNING DISABILITIES. This suggests that genetic factors may play a role in the disorder.

Symptoms and Diagnostic Path

People with either form of apraxia of speech may have a number of different speech symptoms, especially difficulty putting sounds and syllables together in the correct order to form words. Longer or more complex words are usually harder to say than shorter or simpler words. People with apraxia of speech also tend to make inconsistent mistakes when speaking. For example, they may say a difficult word correctly but then have trouble repeating it, or they may be able to say a particular sound one day and have trouble with the same sound the next day.

People with apraxia of speech often appear to be groping for the right sound or word and may try saying a word several times before they say it correctly. Another common characteristic of apraxia of speech is the incorrect use of varying rhythms, stresses, and inflections of speech used to help express meaning.

Children with developmental apraxia of speech generally can understand language much better than they are able to use language to express themselves. Some children with the disorder may also have other problems, including dysarthria; language problems such as poor vocabulary, incorrect grammar, and difficulty in clearly organizing spoken information; problems with reading, writing, spelling, or math; coordination problems; and chewing and swallowing difficulties.

The severity of both acquired and developmental apraxia of speech varies from person to person. Apraxia can be so mild that a person has trouble with very few speech sounds or only has occasional problems pronouncing words with many syllables. In the most severe cases, a person may not be able to communicate effectively with speech and may need the help of alternative or additional communication methods.

Developmental apraxia of speech is different from what is known as a developmental delay of speech, in which a child follows the "typical" path of speech development but does so more slowly than normal.

SPEECH-LANGUAGE PATHOLOGISTS diagnose and treat apraxia of speech by looking for the presence of symptoms, including those described above. Ruling out other contributing factors, such as muscle weakness or language-comprehension problems, can also help with the diagnosis.

To diagnose DAS, professionals may need to observe a child's speech over a period of time.

In formal testing for both acquired and developmental apraxia, the speech-language pathologist may ask the person to perform speech tasks such as repeating a particular word several times or repeating a list of words of increasing length. For acquired apraxia of speech, a speech-language pathologist may also examine a person's ability to converse, read, write, and perform nonspeech movements.

Brain-imaging tests such as magnetic resonance imaging (MRI) may be used to help distinguish acquired apraxia of speech from other communication disorders in people who have experienced brain damage.

Treatment Options and Outlook

In some cases, people with acquired apraxia of speech recover some or all of their speech abilities on their own ("spontaneous recovery"). Children with DAS will not outgrow the problem on their own. Speech-language therapy is often helpful for these children and for people with acquired apraxia who do not spontaneously recover all of their speech abilities.

Verbal apraxia sometimes requires years of intervention and therapy to teach the child to accurately and effectively make speech sounds. Even after motor planning for specific speech sounds or patterns is mastered, these children will often display difficulties with language skills (pronouns, grammar).

Speech-language pathologists use different approaches to treat apraxia of speech, and no single approach has been proven to be the most effective. Therapy is tailored to the individual and is designed to treat other speech or language problems that may occur together with apraxia. Each person responds differently to therapy, and some people will make more progress than others. People with apraxia of speech usually need frequent and intensive one-on-one therapy. Support and encouragement from family members and friends are also important.

In severe cases, people with acquired or developmental apraxia of speech may need to use other ways to express themselves, such as formal or informal sign language, a language notebook with pictures or written words, or an electronic communication device such as a portable computer that writes and produces speech.

verbal memory Memory for verbal information. Verbal memory is assumed to reflect functioning of the deep structures of the left temporal lobe.

Vineland Adaptive Behavior Scales, Second edition (Vineland-II) (VABS) A test of personal and social skills, assessing ADAPTIVE BEHAVIOR in four major areas: communication, daily living skills, socialization, and GROSS MOTOR SKILLS. The VABS encompasses people from birth to age 90, but is used primarily with children and adolescents from birth to age 18 years but may be used on adults suspected of having a mental handicap based on IQ. In the revised edition, updated content reflects daily living skills attuned to current cultural expectations. And more complete coverage of adult adaptive behavior improves detection of decline in older people.

The test is administered as a semistructured interview to someone who knows the child well (there are separate forms for parents and teachers). The interviewer asks general questions about the child's functioning in each area and uses the answers to rate the child. Typical interviews take about an hour.

Raw scores are converted to IQ-type standard scores for each area and for the composite adaptive behavior score. Score ranges include

- 70–80: borderline adaptive functioning
- 51–70: mildly deficient adaptive functioning
- 35–50: moderately deficient adaptive behavior
- 20–35: severely deficient adaptive behavior
- less than 20: markedly or profoundly deficient adaptive behavior

Scores above 80 are classified in about the same ranges (low average, average, above average, superior) as IQ scores.

The adaptive behavior composite score is most useful in making decisions as to whether or not the child's adaptive functioning is consistent with his or her full-scale IQ.

vision training and ADHD Some people believe that visual problems such as faulty eye movements, focus problems, and light oversensitivity of the eyes cause reading disorders. However, there are few well-designed scientific studies of this approach.

In 1972, a joint statement highly critical of the optometric approach to LEARNING DISABILITY treatment was issued by the American Academy of Pediatrics, the American Academy of Ophthalmology and Otolaryngology, and the American Association of Ophthalmology. In the absence of supporting evidence for its effectiveness, most experts warn that this approach should not be used to treat learning disabilities.

visual discrimination The ability to distinguish between visual objects, usually between those with a similar appearance, such as between the letters "p" and "q." Good visual discrimination skills are essential to early reading.

visual memory The ability to take in, store, and retrieve information presented visually. Short-term visual memory is the ability to hold visual information in short-term memory in order to process it, either moving it into LONG-TERM MEMORY or shifting focus.

Visual working memory (or nonverbal working memory) involves the ability to hold visual information in mind while considering it, reflecting on it, or in some other fashion processing it.

Long-term memory also involves visual forms, in which images are stored on a long-term basis and available for recall.

visual motor coordination The combination of visual perception with motion; the ability to see something and react with a movement.

visual motor/perceptual test A type of test that measures a child's FINE MOTOR SKILLS and perceptual ability in sensory areas. These tests include:

- Beery Developmental Test of Visual Motor Integration
- Bender Visual Motor Gestalt Test
- Detroit Test of Learning Ability–2
- Comprehensive Test of Visual Functioning
- Test of Auditory Perceptual Skills

- Learning Efficiency Test II
- Quick Neurological Screening Test
- Motor-Free Visual Perception Test

visual motor skills A subcategory of PERCEPTUAL MOTOR SKILLS involving the ability to translate information received by sight into a physical response. In education, visual motor skills are often used when copying information from a blackboard or reproducing letters or numbers. Individuals with problems in this area often have poor handwriting, and may also have more subtle and pervasive difficulties in school performance.

visual perception The ability to recognize and interpret visual information provided to the brain. Difficulties in visual perception are separate from and unrelated to impairment in the visual system that may diminish visual acuity or result in visual impairment or blindness. Visual perception involves the determination and discrimination of spatial information, as well as performance on tasks such as the discrimination of letters and words, geometric designs, and pictures.

Visual perception is an essential component of learning, especially in regard to reading development and to acquiring classroom information. Difficulties with visual perception may significantly affect an individual's ability to discriminate letters and words, and to work with mathematical information.

visual perception disabilities Students with visual perception disabilities have trouble making sense out of what they see, not because they have poor eyesight but because their brains process visual information differently.

Children with this problem have trouble organizing, recognizing, interpreting, or remembering visual images. This means that they will have trouble understanding the written and picture symbols they need in school—letters, words, numbers, math symbols, diagrams, maps, charts, and graphs.

Because this type of visual problem is subtle, it is often undiscovered until the child starts having trouble in school. VISUAL PERCEPTION problems include the ability to recognize images a person has seen before and attach meaning to them; to dis-

criminate among similar images or the words, and to separate significant figures from background details; and to recognize the same symbol in different forms (understanding, for example, that the letter "D" is the letter "D" whether it is uppercase or lowercase, in different colors or fonts). Sequences are another important visual perception skill; a child with a visual sequencing problem may not understand the difference between the words "saw" and "was."

Students with visual perception problems are usually slow to learn letters and numbers, and often make mistakes, omissions, and reversals. They often have trouble with visual memory and visualization and may be extremely slow readers.

voice recognition software A computer program that recognizes and creates text and carries out commands as the user speaks. In the past, many students with a LEARNING DISABILITY have depended on parents, teachers, tutors, or friends to transcribe their papers as they dictate. While this has been an effective writing strategy, there are some severe drawbacks to this type of dictation. It makes the student with a learning disability dependent on another person, and it is difficult for the writer to have a sense of the flow of the writing without having the draft to read and reread as each sentence is developed. With new technologies such as voice recognition, students with learning disabilities are now able to become more independent as writers, readers, and learners.

Just a few years ago speech or voice recognition technology was quite expensive and slow. It utilized *discrete speech*, which forced a user to . . . speak . . . like . . . this . . . with . . . long . . . pauses between words. Most voice recognition products now use *continuous speech*, which allows the user to speak at a natural pace.

Voice recognition or speech synthesis software allows students to speak into their computers, which turn their ORAL LANGUAGE into text. There are various programs available, but all require a significant amount of memory, the software, a microphone, and a headphone.

The obvious advantage of voice recognition for students with learning disabilities who have difficulty expressing themselves in writing is that it sidesteps the transcription process entirely. However, it is by no means a panacea for writing. Voice recognition technology has several distinct limitations. Training the software to recognize a particular voice typically involves reading passages into the computer, which may be difficult for a student who has trouble reading.

Once the initial training is complete (which can be done in less than an hour), the programs are still not accurate. The more the program is used, the better it can recognize a particular voice; however, the user must speak in a consistent voice. For example, a deep sigh into the microphone may be interpreted as a word. Correcting errors such as an unintentional sigh or a misinterpreted phrase is difficult for students with learning disabilities. Some studies have shown that voice recognition software recognized only 75 percent to 80 percent of the words spoken by college students with learning disabilities. While this may be an improvement from having to draft a composition by handwriting or typing, it still means that a student must correct up to a quarter of the document.

As the rapid pace of technology continues to gain momentum, it is likely that voice recognition will replace the use of the keyboard much as the keyboard has replaced the pencil.

Voice recognition technology will most benefit students who can speak their ideas more fluidly than they could write them. By using their more sophisticated vocabulary and syntax, students' written compositions can be a better reflection of their abilities. If a student has severe spelling difficulties, voice recognition allows him or her to bypass spelling nearly entirely. Students who are fast processors and lose their ideas before they get them out on paper will find voice recognition valuable.

Wechsler Adult Intelligence Scale—Third Edition (WAIS-III) One of the most widely used IQ tests in the country, designed for older teenagers and adults (from ages 16 through 74 years, 11 months). First introduced in 1939, it was written by David Wechsler and has been updated to reduce bias in testing and scoring. This version is a harder edition of the WECHSLER INTELLIGENCE SCALE FOR CHILDREN—III (WISC-III). Although the WAIS–III will score about four points higher than the WISC-III, the test of choice for 16 year olds is still the WISC-III because it offers a larger number of valid subtest items to which the teenager can respond.

The WISC-III and the STANFORD-BINET INTELLIGENCE TEST are the two most commonly used IQ tests in U.S. schools. There are many other tests used to assess overall intelligence, academic achievement, and specific LEARNING DISABILITIES.

Wechsler Individual Achievement Test (WIAT) This achievement test measures achievement in all areas that are specified in the federal law's definition of LEARNING DISABILITIES—oral expression, listening and READING COMPREHENSION, basic reading skills, written expression, mathematics calculation, and mathematical reasoning. The test is designed for students between ages 5 years and 19 years, 11 months. The test includes the following areas:

- oral expression: children describe scenes, give directions, and explain steps in a process while looking at pictures
- listening comprehension: examiner presents word and children identify the picture; examiners present passages and children respond orally to questions
- reading comprehension: children read passages and respond to oral questions

- basic reading skills: children read words on a list in 10 seconds
- written expression: children write spelling words and a short passage
- mathematics calculation: children complete math problems
- mathematics reasoning: children use math reasoning in response to practical questions

Wechsler Intelligence Scale for Children—III (WISC-III) The IQ test of choice for most situations, appropriate for children between the ages of six years and 16 years, 11 months. This test does a good job of measuring the ability to process visual and verbal information, allowing the child to demonstrate strengths and weaknesses in several areas. These include:

- interpretation and problem solving with words or visual images
- speed of information processing
- planning and organization
- attention
- short-term and long-term memory

See also WECHSLER PRESCHOOL AND PRIMARY SCALE OF INTELLIGENCE—REVISED; WECHSLER ADULT INTELLIGENCE SCALE—THIRD EDITION.

Wechsler Preschool and Primary Scale of Intelligence—Revised (WPPSI-R) A simpler version of the WECHSLER INTELLIGENCE SCALE FOR CHILDREN—III (WISC-III) that is designed for young children from ages three years through seven years, three months. While six- and seven-year-olds usually score higher on the WISC-III, those who are below average intellectually have more of an opportunity to demonstrate their range of problem-solving skills on this test than on the WISC-III. The latest revision of this test (the WPPSI-III) will be published soon.

See also WECHSLER ADULT INTELLIGENCE SCALE—THIRD EDITION.

Wernicke's aphasia   See APHASIA.

Wernicke's area   A part of the brain located in the temporal lobe near the primary auditory cortex that is critical to language comprehension, especially at the level of the meaning of individual words (rather than SYNTAX, which is regulated by BROCA'S AREA).

Damage to this part of the brain results in Wernicke's aphasia, which makes individuals unable to understand words while listening, and unable to produce meaningful sentences.

whole language approach   An educational philosophy characterized by the belief that language learning is a natural outgrowth of a child-centered process that integrates speaking, listening, reading, and writing. The whole language approach emphasizes the fact that reading is closely linked to spoken language. As a result, students of this approach are exposed to language-rich classrooms to help make them better readers and writers.

The way American schools teach children to read and write for many years has been affected by the influence of two opposite schools of thought. A conventional curriculum tends to rely on PHONICS and basic readers. This traditional theory of learning, which was popularized during the 19th century, is based on the idea that children learn a complex skill such as reading by first making sense of letters and then progressing to the understanding of sounds, words, and sentences. Proponents of this theory believe that children learn to read by learning to decode (see DECODING) the language; understanding follows after they break the code and master the parts. Traditional American education begins with reading lessons that focus on phonics (sounding out first letters, then combinations of letters), tightly controlled vocabulary, and

short basic reading passages, followed by exercises, each with only one correct answer.

Whole language represents a completely different philosophy about teaching, learning, and the role of language in the classroom, emphasizing the idea that children should use language in ways that relate to their own lives and cultures. In the whole language classroom, the final answer is not as important as the process. Children are encouraged to decode words by their context.

Whole language advocates point out that the average first grader has already acquired a vocabulary of 10,000 words and inherently understands many of the rules of grammar without being formally taught. The common techniques of whole language teaching, which include daily journal and letter writing plus reading much real literature, represent that philosophy in action.

The popularity of the whole language approach has been so dramatic that some teachers complain they cannot find basic readers anymore. In addition, many new teachers say their university professors no longer discuss how to teach phonics.

Critics of the whole language approach believe it overemphasizes understanding at the expense of accuracy. The whole language movement had a significant impact on reading and writing instruction in the 1980s and 1990s, when the appeal of whole language instruction influenced many schools to revise their curricula. As a result of this movement, a vigorous debate emerged amongst educators over how children learn language. Many special educators felt that whole language was flawed by its neglect of explicit language skills such as phonics, spelling, and grammar. Since a language-rich classroom does not help many students, especially those with LEARNING DISABILITIES, learn to read and spell, a "back to basics" movement in education began to move back to explicit skill instruction.

On the other hand, advocates of the whole language approach say that an overemphasis on rules and rote learning is stifling and leads children to see reading and writing as boring and difficult chores, rather than as an interesting way of gathering information.

Research strongly indicates that students will be the most successful if a balanced approach is used, teaching phonics in a systematic fashion within the context of real stories. Today, many classrooms use this combination approach utilizing elements of both whole language and phonics, spelling and grammar.

Williams syndrome A rare, congenital disorder characterized by physical and developmental problems, including an impulsive and outgoing personality, limited spatial skills and motor control, and intellectual disability (such as developmental delay, LEARNING DISABILITIES, MENTAL RETARDATION, or ATTENTION DEFICIT DISORDER). Most individuals with Williams syndrome have a deletion of genetic material on chromosome 7, which probably causes the physical and developmental problems characteristic of the disease.

Symptoms and Diagnostic Path

Symptoms vary among patients but may include "elfin" facial features, heart and blood vessel problems, high blood calcium levels (hypercalcemia), low birth weight, slow weight gain, feeding problems, irritability during infancy, dental and kidney abnormalities, sensitive hearing, and musculoskeletal problems. Although individuals with Williams syndrome may be competent in areas such as language, music, and interpersonal relations, they usually have a below-average IQ and are often considered to be mildly to moderately mentally retarded.

Treatment Options and Outlook

There is neither a cure for Williams syndrome nor a standard treatment. Patients need regular monitoring for potential medical problems by a physician familiar with the disorder. The prognosis varies; some patients may be able to master self-help skills, complete academic or vocational school, and live in supervised homes or on their own, while others may not progress to this level.

Woodcock-Johnson, Third Edition (WJ-III) The updated version of an individually administered ASSESSMENT system that educators and psychologists have found useful in assessing INTELLIGENCE and achievement. The WJ-III, which is designed for people from two years through 90+ years, includes two forms

- WJ-III Tests of Achievement (WJ-III ACH)
- WJ-III Tests of Cognitive Abilities (WJ-III COG)

The highly flexible system assesses the widest array of cognitive and achievement abilities among major available test systems and allows for administration of the entire battery or selected subtests. The WJ-III is the first major cognitive or achievement battery to assume that the person giving it has access to a computer: Those administering the tests can only score the WJ-III with specialized software included in each test kit.

If the complete battery is administered, the WJ-III provides assessments in the following individual subtests:

- verbal comprehension
- visual-auditory learning
- spatial relations
- sound blending
- concept formation
- visual matching
- numbers reversed
- incomplete words
- auditory work memory
- general information
- retrieval fluency
- picture recognition
- auditory attention
- analysis-synthesis
- decision speed
- memory for words
- rapid picture naming
- planning
- pair cancellation
- letter-word identification
- reading fluency
- story recall
- understanding directions
- calculation
- math fluency
- spelling

- writing fluency
- passage comprehension
- applied problems
- writing samples
- story recall—delayed
- word attack
- picture vocabulary
- oral comprehension
- editing
- reading vocabulary
- quantitative concepts
- academic knowledge
- spelling of sounds
- sound awareness
- punctuation and capitals

Depending on which individual subtests are administered, the WJ-III groups results into the following cognitive clusters:

- verbal ability
- thinking ability
- cognitive efficiency
- comprehensive knowledge
- long-term retrieval
- visual-spatial thinking
- auditory processing
- fluid reasoning
- processing speed
- short-term memory
- phonemic awareness
- phonemic awareness III
- working memory
- broad attention
- cognitive fluency
- executive processes
- knowledge

The WJ-III also groups individual tests into the following achievement clusters:

- oral language
- oral expression
- listening comprehension
- total achievement
- broad reading
- broad math
- broad written language
- basic reading skills
- reading comprehension
- mathematics calculation skills
- mathematics reasoning
- basic writing skills
- written expression
- academic skills
- academic fluency
- academic applications
- academic knowledge
- phoneme/grapheme knowledge

Given the large number of areas tested, the WJ-III can provide extensive information on a wide range of cognitive and academic strengths and weaknesses. The WJ-III provides a very reliable and valid means of determining "discrepancies between potential and achievement" required by federal law for determination of LEARNING DISABILITIES.

word attack skills   The ability to read a word using phonetic, structural, or context cues. Word attack skills using phonetic cues require a child to understand the sound-symbol relationship. Phonetic word attack skills can be assessed by asking a child to read nonsense words (such as "thrump").

Word attack skills using structural cues require individuals to identify prefixes, suffixes, and roots, or to break up a word by syllables. These skills are assessed by asking a child to divide a word into syllables (such as *com/pre/hend*) or break a word into meaningful word parts (such as *un/happy*).

Good readers use contextual cues when they rely on the context of a sentence to decode (see DECODING) a word. Poor word attack skills are one of the most common reading problems among children with a LEARNING DISABILITY; therefore, poor word attack skills are often improved by using PHONICS-based word attack instruction.

word deafness   See AUDITORY PROCESSING DISORDER.

word-finding deficits   See SOUND/LETTER/WORD RETRIEVAL.

word prediction   A type of software that supports word processing by predicting what word the user will write next—based on SYNTAX, the first letters typed, and frequency of use. A list of words appears in a window on the computer screen. If the list contains the intended word, the user can select the word by entering the number next to the word, point and click, or scroll down the list until the correct word is selected. The word is then automatically inserted into the text and the next word will be predicted even before a letter has been typed. If the intended word is not shown in the prediction list after the first letter is typed, the program continually revises the list after each letter is typed. If the intended word is not in the prediction program, the user can add words to the dictionary.

Different word prediction programs vary slightly. Many are now available with synthesized speech to read the word list aloud, which is useful for students who have difficulty distinguishing between words that look similar. Some word prediction programs are more sophisticated and offer a more extensive dictionary.

However, while this program can be useful for creating sophisticated writing, it also can be more confusing to the user by offering too many word choices.

With regard to spelling, word prediction programs can be either liberating or limiting. For students who can write the first several letters of a word with relative accuracy, it can be very helpful in predicting longer, more difficult words. On the other hand, word prediction does not recognize phonetic similarities; therefore, it can be quite limiting for students who do not have strong sound-symbol skills. For example, if a student using word prediction is attempting to write *philosophically* and first types in *fil . . .*, the program will not include words that started with *phil-*. Word prediction

assumes that students have the ability to interrupt the flow of writing to sound out the beginning of a word. This can cause problems for students who find sounding out words laborious and disruptive to the writing process.

Word prediction programs offer several advantages. For some students with poor typing skills, the program can minimize the number of keystrokes and help students who have problems choosing the right words. Since the programs use syntax to predict words, the predicted list may act as a necessary prompt to locate the suitable word. Not only is this useful for word retrieval, it also can help students who misuse words due to syntactical errors.

On the other hand, some students with LEARNING DISABILITIES may find word prediction programs frustrating. For students who do not want to interrupt the logical flow of their writing, word prediction may be distracting by requiring the student to stop and choose words, especially if the individual has good typing skills. If a student has trouble recognizing words, word prediction will not be very useful unless it is used in conjunction with synthesized speech.

word processing   Using a computer program as a writing tool. Word processing offers many advantages for children with a LEARNING DISABILITY. First, editing is considerably easier on a word processor, making it possible for individuals to focus on creating meaning rather than the mechanics of writing. Also, the use of a word processor allows individuals to create neat and legible documents rather than messier versions written out conventionally on paper.

The significance of creating more professional-looking compositions has proven to motivate individuals to create longer written pieces.

In addition, word processors make writing more visible. For many students with learning disabilities, reading their own handwriting is difficult and frustrating. In addition, instructors can better read student writing in class when it is projected on a screen. Because word processors make editing and spelling considerably easy to repair, it allows individuals to concentrate on generating meaning rather than mechanics. This liberation from the "nuts and bolts" aspect of writing can lead to better compositions.

In addition to physical writing problems, students with visual problems often find word processors make writing easier. Digital text can be made large and colored for easier understanding. Individuals with short-term memory weaknesses can also be empowered by a word processor because the time lapse between having an idea and getting it on paper or on screen is dramatically diminished. The burden of arranging a sentence and spelling words in a fixed way on paper is eliminated when one can write with a word processor and easily revise the idea once it is expressed.

word recognition An ability to apply any number of strategies to recognize and understand a word. Word recognition strategies include:

- configuration—using visual cues such as the shape and size of the word
- context analysis—using surrounding information (including pictures) to predict a word
- SIGHT WORDS—instant recognition of a word without further analysis
- phonemic analysis—"sounding out" a word
- SYLLABICATION—dividing a word into syllables
- structural analysis—using morphological information such as prefixes, suffixes, and roots

See also WORD ATTACK SKILLS.

word retrieval See SOUND/LETTER/WORD RETRIEVAL.

writing process A particular approach to writing instruction that has become common in school systems and colleges during the past 25 years. There are many different meanings of the phrase "writing process," but most refer to the concept that writing is part of a thinking process involving many different mental activities over a period of time. Effective instruction in writing teaches students how to generate, organize, and revise their writing, rather than focusing solely on written language structures.

In its early years of development, the process theory of writing instruction focused largely on individual expression and the facilitation of the development of a student's "voice." This approach to the writing process was in many ways a reaction to traditional methods of writing instruction, which focused mainly on structural and mechanical elements such as grammar, punctuation, and following paragraph and essay models.

In the early 1980s, Linda Flower and John Hayes developed a theoretical model of writing as a thought process involving a number of different mental activities, including planning, generating, organizing, translating, reviewing, and editing. In their model, any given activity might interrupt any other one at any stage. The Flower/Hayes model continues to be useful, especially for understanding the writing problems of students with LEARNING DISABILITIES and ATTENTION DISORDER. However, the primary contemporary model emphasizes the ways in which writing is a social practice, and focuses on collaborative approaches to developing writing skills and producing written work.

In practical terms, effective writing instruction involves understanding that writing involves different activities of generating, organizing, drafting, and revising, and that incorporates collaborative activities in helping students develop a sense of voice, audience, and using writing as a communication tool.

A process approach to writing is particularly vital for students with learning disabilities, in that it enables them to take the different cognitive tasks involved in writing and spread them over a series of steps and periods of time. For example, a student with DYSLEXIA may benefit from putting off any attention to editing and spelling until late in the process, instead focusing mainly on generating ideas and language first.

Likewise, a student with attention deficit disorder may do better by taking a highly specific approach to planning a paper and mapping out the steps that will be involved, using a checklist to monitor completion of each step.

written expression, disorders of A disorder resulting from problems in poor writing skills, which are significantly below what would be considered normal for the student's age, INTELLIGENCE, and education. These poor writing skills cause problems with the student's academic success or other important areas of life. Writing is a complex task integrating COGNITION, LANGUAGE, and MOTOR SKILLS. Some children have difficulty in one aspect of the process, such as producing legible handwriting or SPELLING (this is called dysgraphia); others have difficulty organizing and sequencing their ideas. Problems in one area can delay the acquisition of skills in the other areas.

Strategizing, organizing, marshaling intention into movement, flexibility, and constant monitoring are crucial in writing and editing an essay, a book report, or piece of narrative writing. Working MEMORY is also crucial to the writing process.

Many of these processes that are called upon when a child writes are in the domain of what is called EXECUTIVE FUNCTIONING. Executive functioning refers to a cluster of mental control abilities, including skills such as the capacity to plan ahead, choose and implement strategies, and organize one's thinking and actions. Executive functions also include abilities such as maintaining awareness of what one is doing and staying on task, controlling one's impulses, and monitoring the quality of one's own performance and making adjustments if necessary. Executive functioning is performed by the advanced parts of the brain—the frontal lobes and the prefrontal cortex. Brain imaging has shown that the frontal lobes may be divided into 17 or more subregions, each responsible for a slightly different kind of work. So, a problem anywhere in this area will affect the way a child approaches and performs any task.

In addition, writing requires more memory than just about anything else a student is asked to do in school. Writers need to simultaneously retrieve spelling, punctuation, capitalization, letter formation rules, vocabulary and content information, transitions and connections, and all the other ingredients of written output.

The writing problem for some children is language-based and may coexist with DYSLEXIA; for others, it is caused by a motor outflow difficulty. Still others experience a severe problem with organizing thoughts, formulating ideas, and coming up with the energy and attention to complete the task. Any one of these problems will create resistance, frustration, and anger.

About 5 percent of students in the United States are believed to have written expression disorder, and boys are diagnosed much more often than girls. Other disabilities linked with the disorder of written expression include reading disorder, EXPRESSIVE LANGUAGE DISORDER, mathematics disorder, and developmental coordination disorder.

Symptoms and Diagnostic Path

Symptoms of a disorder of written expression may include written sentences and paragraphs that are inadequately formed; many errors in spelling, punctuation, and grammar; and extremely poor handwriting. These students also typically reverse or rotate the letters of the alphabet or write so poorly that the letters are unrecognizable. There may be a random mixture of cursive and printed letters. Students with this disorder often have poor SELF-ESTEEM, social problems, and a higher dropout rate. If a student has trouble self-monitoring, is unable to regulate a flow of ideas, and cannot pace himself or herself, than the process becomes so stressful that eventually, the student simply shuts down and refuses to even attempt the task.

A specific problem with handwriting alone—characterized by poorly formed letters, problems with the spatial organization of the letters and words on the page, and heavy line pressure—is called dysgraphia. Dysgraphia is a graphomotor problem, caused by a difficulty between motor memory and its connection to the fingers. A sequence of visualization and precise small muscle movements must be used to translate the thought of a word into letters that come together to make that word and that are grouped with other words to make sentences. This disorder typically appears when a child is first introduced to writing, as they make inappropriately sized and spaced letters.

Dysgraphia is also sometimes used to categorize more general writing problems, although in many cases these issues may be more clearly attributable to a more pervasive learning problem, such as ATTENTION DEFICIT HYPERACTIVITY DISORDER or a specific reading disability. Dysgraphia may be suspected if the child has bad or illegible handwriting or an awkward or cramped pencil grip. There may be inconsistency with the way letters and words look, problems with writing within the margins or line spacing, and inconsistent spacing between words.

A disorder of written expression is usually noticed in fourth or fifth grade, when writing skills become an important part of schoolwork. Because of a child's immature motor skills, the problem is not usually diagnosed before age eight.

Because standardized group testing is not accurate enough to diagnose this disorder, special psychoeducational tests must be individually administered to the child to uncover this problem. There are many tests that can be administered to determine which areas of the writing process are causing problems. However, most evaluators on a child study team in a school system will rely on the following battery of tests:

Written tests The WOODCOCK-JOHNSON Psychoeducational Battery—Revised is a test for ages three to 80 that yields samples of dictation and writing. The WECHSLER INDIVIDUAL ACHIEVEMENT TEST (WIAT-II) is a tool that measures achievement skills and helps diagnose learning disabilities for preschool-age children through adults. Tests of Written Language—3 is a written language assessment tool used with students from ages 7.5 to 17. This test measures expressive skills in written language, such as punctuation, capitalization, and spelling, and the ability to write logical and coherent sentences and paragraphs.

Tests of sustained attention These computerized tests include the Connor Continuous Performance Tests and the Tests of Variable Attention. Both examine attention over a long period (14 to 22.5 minutes) and measure discrete aspects of attention.

Tests of executive functions The WISC-IV, the newest version of the well-known intelligence test, has some subtests that reveal executive function deficits. More comprehensive tests of executive function typically administered and interpreted by neuropsychologists include: the Wisconsin Card Sort, Tower of Hanoi, Tower of London, Trails A & B, and the Stroop Color and Word Test.

Executive motor skills Another set of tests evaluates a student's executive motor (physical) skills. While almost all educational and learning tasks involve analysis, planning, monitoring, and possible adjustments of strategy (all of which are executive functions controlled by the brain), many tasks related to writing must be translated into physical acts. Tests that measure these executive motor skills include the Luria Test of Praxis, Fine Motor Coordination, Purdue Pegboard or the Grooved Pegboard, and the Hallstead-Reitan Finger Tapping Test.

Treatment Options and Outlook

Most early and significant LEARNING DISORDERS in the area of written expression will be expressed by the second or third grade (the graphomotor difficulties may be noticed earlier), so it is important to intervene early.

Although there is no proven effective treatment for the disorder of written expression, educators try to help in many ways. The treatment process depends on the areas of difficulty that are affecting the child's written expression.

Emphasis on the rehearsed, systematic remedial teaching of writing and a heavy emphasis on student practice of writing may help with difficulties with spelling and the mechanics of writing such as capitalization and punctuation. Checklists that outline all the steps involved in a writing process may help. For example, a student could be taught several different ways to create an outline and use a checklist to make sure all the steps in creating an outline have been used.

Some teachers may allow students with a disorder in written expression to use other methods, such as an oral report, to assess their understanding of a subject instead of asking them to write a paper or take a written test. Computer SPELL-CHECKING systems, grammar checks, and other programs also may help.

Handwriting problems (dysgraphia) may be treated with therapy for physical (motor) disorders to help control writing movements. Many children with dysgraphia benefit from explicit instruction in the skills required for handwriting. If the child is having trouble recalling the shape of letters (encoding) and neatly getting them onto paper, a repetitive multisensory approach will help. This is effective in younger children, who might enjoy sculpting letters in the air, drawing letters in sand or whipped cream, or using graph paper or a paper with raised lines to recognize where to place and how to space letters. A special pencil can encourage proper pencil grip, and helping a child align the arms and body in order to write can be beneficial. There are also slant boards that help the child work at a vertical surface, which promotes the development of proper hand and wrist position and keeps the paper from sliding. Along with a foot stool, this will help keep the child's body from collapsing or the child's head from getting too close to the paper. Special paper and slant boards are usually available in teacher supply stores. Computers also may help students with dysgraphia.

Both therapy for dysgraphia and the remediation of poor mechanics of writing should take place two or three times a week and must be written into an INDIVIDUAL EDUCATION PROGRAM (IEP). Along with special services, an IEP should list a number of ACCOMMODATIONS or modifications to the school's program.

Even if untreated, the disorder of written expression will gradually improve. However, even when good help is available, the student tends to have chronic problems with writing skills.

written language Printed text. Production of written language requires many subskills such as handwriting or typing, SPELLING, grammar, organizing, planning, and revising. Related skills such as fluent spoken language, reading, and vocabulary are also important in competent writers. Individuals with a LEARNING DISABILITY often have trouble with one or more of the skills necessary to communicate effectively using written language.

zone of proximal development   The gap between the level of a student's independent function and how he or she may perform learning tasks with help. This term was coined by Russian psychologist Lev Vygotsky (1896–1934) and refers to the fact that it is crucial to provide help before a child gets frustrated. Failure can be avoided when teachers are aware of a student's zone of proximal development and provide just enough support to enable students to achieve a goal that would not have been possible independently.

This concept may play a key role in educational approaches, in that it represents a way of thinking about what is involved in meeting students' needs, and of understanding teaching and learning as a dynamic and developmental process, rather than as a static juxtaposition of instruction and learning readiness.

This theory allows a teacher to see a student's learning problems not as impediments but rather as a starting point for a process of development that challenges students within the scope of what they are able to master successfully with appropriate instruction. An approach to teaching that incorporates this concept must also mean that a teacher begins to teach a child at his or her current level, rather than at arbitrary curricular standards.

APPENDIXES

I. National Organizations

II. Government Sources of Information and Help

III. Assistive Technology Resources

IV. Hotlines

V. Commercial Technology Resources

VI. Books of Interest to People with Learning Disabilities

APPENDIX I
NATIONAL ORGANIZATIONS

AMERICANS WITH DISABILITIES ACT (ADA) RESOURCES

ADA Homepage
U.S. Department of Justice
http://www.usdoj.gov/crt/ada/adahom1.htm

Online page that offers information on the Americans with Disabilities Act.

ANGELMAN SYNDROME

Angelman Syndrome Foundation, Inc.
3015 East New York Street
Suite A2265
Aurora, IL 60504
(800) 432-6435 or (630) 978-4245
http://www.angelman.org

Foundation provides information on diagnosis, treatment, management, and offers support and advocacy through education, information exchange, and research. The group also offers local contacts and a newsletter.

APHASIA

Aphasia Hope Foundation
2436 West 137th Street
Leawood, KS 66224
(913) 402-8306; (866) 449-5804
http://www.aphasiahope.org

This nonprofit organization promotes research into the cure and prevention of aphasia and provides patients access to the best possible treatments, both physical and emotional, for living with this disease. The foundation maintains an electronic bulletin board and a Web-based forum for posting questions to aphasia professionals and caregivers, provides information on ongoing research and legislation focusing on aphasia, and offers an outlet through which persons with aphasia can share their stories.

National Aphasia Association
29 John Street
Suite 1103
New York, NY 10038
(800) 922-4622
http://www.aphasia.org

A nonprofit organization that promotes research and offers rehabilitation, education, and support services. The mission of the NAA is to reconnect people with aphasia into the community by educating the public about aphasia, promoting the development and use of community resources, and advocating on behalf of those who are left, literally, without a voice. Professional/consumer newsletter, directory, fact sheets, brochures/pamphlets, and online publications are available.

APRAXIA

Apraxia-KIDS
http://www.apraxia-kids.org

Beginning as a listserv for parents of children with apraxia of speech, KIDS grew to become a forum for parents, therapists, and professionals all over the world.

Childhood Apraxia of Speech Association of North America (CASANA)
1151 Freeport Road, #243
Pittsburgh, PA 15238
(412) 767-6589
Apraxia-KIDS information/referral helpline: (412) 343-7102
http://www.apraxia-kids.org

The national nonprofit organization representing the needs of children with apraxia and their families provides credible, reliable, and comprehensive information on apraxia of speech in children. Guided by a distinguished professional advisory board of the top experts in childhood apraxia of speech, information and resources are based on the current prevailing professional literature and expert opinion.

ASPERGER SYNDROME

Asperger Syndrome Coalition of the United States
P.O. Box 49267
Jacksonville Beach, FL 32240-9267

A national nonprofit support and advocacy organization for Asperger disorder and related disorders committed to providing the most up-to-date and comprehensive information on Asperger disorder and related conditions.

Asperger's Disorder Home Page
Web site only
http://www.aspergers.com

Web site offering list of U.S. specialists, bibliography, and links.

ASSISTIVE TECHNOLOGY

See Appendix III.

ATAXIA

The National Ataxia Foundation
2600 Fernbrook Lane
Suite 119
Minneapolis, MN 55477
(763) 553-0020
http://www.ataxia.org

Nonprofit organization with 45 chapters that supports research and offers information and educational programs.

ATTENTION DEFICIT HYPERACTIVITY DISORDER

Attention Deficit Disorder Association
P.O. Box 543
Pottstown, PA 19464

(484) 945-2101
http://www.add.org

The mission of ADDA is to provide information, resources, and networking to adults with ADHD and to the professionals who work with them. Bringing together scientific perspectives and the human experience, the information and resources provided to individuals and families affected by ADHD and professionals in the field focuses on diagnoses, treatments, strategies, and techniques for helping adults with ADHD lead better lives. ADDA currently provides an annual national conference; *FOCUS*, the quarterly publication; written tools, such as "Guiding Principles for Coaching Individuals with Attention Deficit Hyperactivity Disorder"; audiotapes and videotapes on a wide range of adult ADHD topics; ADHD teleclasses; networking opportunities for adults with ADHD as well as for the professionals who work with them; and advocacy in the field of adult ADHD.

Attention Deficit Information Network, Inc.
475 Hillside Avenue
Needham, MA 02194
(781) 455-9895
http://www.addinfonetwork.com

A nonprofit organization offering information to families of children and adults with Attention Deficit Disorder (ADD), and to professionals, through a network of AD-IN chapters. AD-IN was founded in 1988 by several parent support group leaders. Today it acts as a community resource for information on training programs and speakers available to those who work with individuals with ADD. The organization also presents conferences and workshops for parents and professionals on current issues, research, and treatments for ADD and makes an annual, post-secondary scholarship award.

Camps for Children and Adults with Attention Deficit Disorder
499 NW 70th Avenue
Suite 101
Plantation, FL 33317
(954) 587-3700

Children and Adults with Attention Deficit Disorder (CHADD)
8181 Professional Place
Suite 201
Landover, MD 20785

(301) 306-7070
http://www.chadd.org

A nonprofit organization founded in 1987 in response to the frustration and sense of isolation experienced by parents and their children with ADHD. At that time, there were very few places for support or information, and people misunderstood ADHD. Many clinicians and educators knew little about the disability, and individuals with ADHD were often mistakenly labeled a behavior problem, unmotivated, or not intelligent enough. From one parent support group in Florida, the organization grew dramatically to become the leading nonprofit organization for children and adults with ADHD. Today the organization continues to be run by volunteers, with the support of a small national staff, and offers education, advocacy, and support.

National Attention Deficit Disorder Association
P.O. Box 1303
Northbrook, IL 60065-1303
E-mail: mail@add.org
http://www.add.org

notMYkid.org
33 West Indian School Road
Phoenix, AZ 85013-3205
(602) 652-0163
http://www.notmykid.org

One ADD Place
Web site only
http://www.oneaddplace.com

Web site virtual neighborhood offering information on ADD/ADHD, including articles, products and services, and information on seminars, workshops, and links to other ADD-related Web sites.

AUTISM

Autism Network International
P.O. Box 35448
Syracuse, NY 13235
(315) 476-2462
http://ani.autistics.us

Self-help group dedicated to supporting people with autism, offering peer support, tips, problem solving, and information and referrals.

Autism Research Institute
4182 Adams Avenue
San Diego, CA 92116

(619) 281-7165
http://www.autism.com/ari/contents.html

Research organization investigating autism, offering information to families by mail or phone.

Autism Society of America
7910 Woodmont Avenue
Suite 300
Bethesda, MD 20814-3015
(800) 3AUTISM, ext. 150; (301) 657-0881
http://www.autism-society.org

A nonprofit organization that seeks to promote life-long access and opportunities for persons within the autism spectrum and their families, to be fully included, participating members of their communities through advocacy, public awareness, education, and research related to autism.

Autism Society of America Foundation (ASAF)
7910 Woodmont Avenue
Suite 300
Bethesda, MD 20814
(800) 3AUTISM, ext. 127; (301) 657-0881, ext. 127
http://www.autism-society.org/foundation/
    foundation.html

A fundraising organization founded in 1996 by the Autism Society of America, the largest and oldest organization representing people with autism. ASAF was established to raise and allocate funds for research to address the many unanswered questions about autism. The ASAF has implemented action on several autism research priorities, developing up-to-date statistics; developing a national registry of individuals and families with autism who are willing to participate in research studies; and implementing a system to identify potential donors of autism brain tissue for research purposes and to facilitate the donation process. In addition, the foundation contributes money for applied and biomedical research in the causes of and treatment approaches to autism. Founded in 1965 by a small group of parents, the society is the leading source of information and referral on autism and the largest collective voice representing the autism community for more than 33 years. Today, members are connected through a volunteer network in 50 states.

Cure Autism Now
5455 Wilshire Boulevard
Suite 715
Los Angeles, CA 90036

(323) 549-0500; (888) 828-8476
http://www.cureautismnow.org

A nonprofit research organization dedicated to accelerating and funding critical biological research for effective treatments, prevention, and a cure for autism and related disorders. The organization offers a professional/consumer newsletter, a directory, fact sheets, brochures/pamphlets, and online publications.

Families for Early Autism Treatment
P.O. Box 255722
Sacramento, CA 95865
http://www.feat.org

Nonprofit organization of parents and professionals offering support and information.

National Alliance for Autism Research
99 Wall Street, Research Park
Princeton, NJ 08540
(609) 430-9160; (888) 777-NAAR
http://www.naar.org

Organization dedicated to the prevention, treatment, and cure of autism spectrum disorders through biomedical research. NAAR also conducts conferences for parents and scientific working groups on issues of importance to autism research, provides fellowships to promising young scientists, and distributes educational materials. Since 1997, NAAR has committed more than $20.9 million to directly fund 211 autism research projects. Fellowships are available.

BRAIN INJURY/RESEARCH

Brain Injury Association of America
8201 Greensboro Drive
Suite 611
McLean, VA 22102
761-0750; (800) 444-6443
http://www.biausa.org

The mission of the Brain Injury Association of America is to create a better future through brain injury prevention, research, education, and advocacy. The helpline offers information about brain injury to persons with brain injury, their families, professionals, and other interested callers. Educational materials are available: consumer newsletter, brochures/pamphlets, professional/consumer directory, fact sheets, and online publications. Information is available in Spanish.

Children's Brain Tumor Foundation
274 Madison Avenue
Suite 1301
New York, NY 10016
(212) 448-9494; (866) 228-HOPE
http://www.cbtf.org

Group that seeks to improve treatment and outlook for children with brain and spinal cord tumors through research and treatment, education and support.

Dana Alliance for Brain Initiatives, The
745 Fifth Avenue, Suite 900
New York, NY 10151
http://www.dana.org

The Dana Alliance, a nonprofit organization of 150 neuroscientists, was formed to help provide information about the personal and public benefits of brain research.

National Brain Tumor Foundation
22 Battery Street
Suite 612
San Francisco, CA 94111
(415) 834-9970; (800) 934-2873
http://www.braintumor.org

Foundation that offers resources and support, plus research. Affected patients can receive referrals to a network of support groups.

CAMPS

Courage Camps
3915 Golden Valley Road
Golden Valley, MN 55422
(763) 520-0504
http://www.couragecamps.org

Web site offering information on safe camps for children and adults with a range of disabilities.

Directory of Summer Camps for Children with Learning Disabilities and ADHD
http://www.mysummercamps.com/camps/Special_
    Needs_Camps/Learning_Disabilit ies_and_ADHD

Kids Camps
Web site only
http://www.kidscamps.com

Web site offering all types of special needs camps around the country.

CEREBRAL PALSY

United Cerebral Palsy Association
1660 L Street NW
Suite 700
Washington, DC 20036
(202) 973-7197; (800) 872-5827
http://www.ucpa.org

Nonprofit group providing referral services, advocacy, research, and information.

COMMUNICATION

(See also Stuttering)

American Speech-Language-Hearing Association (ASHA)
10801 Rockville Pike
Rockville, MD 20852
(800) 638-8255 (voice) or (301) 897-5700 (TTY)
http://www.asha.org

The professional, scientific, and credentialing association for more than 99,000 speech-language pathologists, audiologists, and speech, language, and hearing scientists in the United States. The organization provides information and referrals to the public on speech, language, communication, and hearing disorders.

DEAFNESS/HARD OF HEARING

Alexander Graham Bell Association for the Deaf, Inc.
3417 Volta Place NW
Washington, DC 20007
(202) 337-5221 (Voice/TT); (800) 337-5220
http://www.agbell.org

The association is a support network and advocate for listening, learning, talking, and living independently with hearing loss. Through publications, outreach, training, scholarships, and financial aid, AG Bell promotes the use of spoken language and hearing technology. Headquartered in Washington, D.C., with chapters located in the United States and Canada and a network of international affiliates, AG Bell's global presence provides its members and the public with the support they need.

American Association of the Deaf-Blind
814 Thayer Avenue
Suite 302
Silver Spring, MD 20910
(301) 495-4403; (301) 495-4402 (TTY)
http://www.aadb.org

A national consumer organization of, for, and by people who have dual hearing and vision loss, to ensure all deaf-blind persons achieve their maximum potential through increased independence, productivity, and integration into the community. The association holds a biennial conference.

American Society for Deaf Children
P.O. Box 3355
Gettysburg, PA 17325
(717) 334-7922 (TTY); (800) 942-2732 (Voice/TTY)
http://www.deafchildren.org

A national organization of families and professionals committed to educating, empowering, and supporting parents and families of children who are deaf or hard-of-hearing. The ASDC helps families find meaningful communication options, particularly through the competent use of sign language, in their home, school, and community.

BEGINNINGS for Parents of Children Who Are Deaf or Hard of Hearing, Inc.
P.O. Box 17646
Raleigh, NC 27619
(919) 850-2746; (800) 541-4327 (in-state only);
   (919) 850-2746 (TTY)
http://www.ncbegin.org

BEGINNINGS provides support and information to parents and professionals dealing with deaf and hard-of-hearing issues in children. It also provides impartial information on communication options, placement, and educational programs; workshops for professional personnel who work with children who are deaf and hard-of-hearing; and advocacy and support for young people. The group offers a professional/consumer newsletter, fact sheets, brochures, a parent manual, and reports. Some Spanish materials are available.

Better Hearing Institute (BHI)
515 King Street
Suite 420
Alexandria, VA 22314
(703) 684-3391; (800) EAR-WELL (327-9355)
http://www.betterhearing.org

A nonprofit organization with a mission to educate the public and medical profession on hearing loss, its treatment, and prevention. BHI maintains a "Hearing Helpline" service that provides information on hearing loss, sources of assistance, and other available hearing help to callers anywhere in the United States and Canada.

Laurent Clerc National Deaf Education Center and Clearinghouse
Gallaudet University
800 Florida Avenue NE
Washington, DC 20002-3695
(202) 651-5051 (Voice); (202) 651-5052 (TT)
http://clerccenter.gallaudet.edu

National Institute on Deafness and Other Communication Disorders
31 Center Drive
Bethesda, MD 20892-3456
(800) 241-1044 (Voice); (800) 241-1055 (TT)
http://www.nidcd.nih.gov

The clearinghouse is a national resource center for health information on hearing, balance, smell, taste, voice, speech, and language for health professionals, patients, industry, and the public. The clearinghouse collects and disseminates information through its e-mail and information hotline service; the Combined Health Information Database (CHID), a searchable health information database at http://chid.nih.gov; and publications on the normal and disordered processes of human communication. Professional/line publications, and reports are available. Some Spanish materials are available.

Self Help for Hard of Hearing People (SHHH)
7910 Woodmont Avenue
Suite 1200
Bethesda, MD 20814
(301) 657-2248 (Voice); (301) 657-2249 (TT)
http://www.hearingloss.org

The nation's foremost consumer organization representing people with hearing loss. SHHH's national support network includes an office in the Washington, D.C., area, 13 state organizations, and 250 local chapters. The SHHH mission is to open the world of communication to people with hearing loss through information, education, advocacy, and support. SHHH provides information to consumers, professionals, and family members through a Web site, an award-winning publication (*Hearing Loss*), and hearing-accessible national and regional conventions. SHHH affects accessibility, public policy, research, public awareness, and service delivery related to hearing loss on a national and global level.

DEVELOPMENTAL DISABILITIES
(See also Down syndrome)

American Association on Mental Retardation
444 North Capitol Street NW
Suite 846
Washington, DC 20001
(202) 387-1968; (800) 424-3688
http://www.aamr.org

National organization providing information, services, and support, plus advocacy.

Arc (formerly Association for Retarded Citizens)
1010 Wayne Avenue
Suite 650
Silver Spring, MD 20910
(301) 565-3842
http://www.thearc.org

Volunteer organization committed to the welfare of all children and adults with mental retardation, offering information, books, and an annual conference.

Association of University Centers on Disabilities (AUCD)
10 Wayne Avenue
Suite 920
Silver Spring, MD 20910
(301) 588-8252
http://www.aucd.org

The national association representing University Centers for Excellence in Developmental Disabilities (UCEDDs), Maternal and Child Health Leadership Education in Neurodevelopmental Disabilities (LEND) Programs, and Developmental Disabilities Research Centers (DDRCs). The mission of AUCD is to help member centers by advancing policy and practice for and with people with developmental and other disabilities, their families, and communities. The association holds an annual meeting and publishes a newsletter/bulletin and reports, professional/consumer directory, fact sheets, brochures/pamphlets, and online publications.

Council for Exceptional Children (CEC)
1110 North Glebe Road
Suite 300
Arlington, VA 22201
(703) 620-3660; (800) 224-6830;
  (866) 915-5000 (TTY)
http://www.cec.sped.org

CEC is the largest international professional organization dedicated to improving the educational success of individuals with disabilities. The organization advocates for appropriate government policies, sets professional standards, provides continual professional development, advocates for newly and historically underserved individuals with exceptionalities, and helps professionals obtain conditions and resources necessary for effective professional practice. Professional journal, brochures, and newsletter are available.

Clearinghouse on Disability Information
Office of Special Education and Rehabilitative Services (OSERS)
Communication and Media Support Services (CMSS)
U.S. Department of Education
550 12th Street SW
Room 5133
Washington, DC 20004
(202) 245-7303; (202) 205-5637 (TTY)
http://www.ed.gov/about/offices/list/osers/codi.html

The clearinghouse provides information by conducting research and providing documents in response to inquiries. Information provided includes areas in which federal funding is available for disability-related programs. Clearinghouse staff also will refer requests to other sources of disability-related information, when necessary. Information provided may be useful to disabled individuals and their families, schools and universities, teachers and school administrators, and organizations who have persons with disabilities as clients.

Developmental Delay Resources
4401 East West Highway
Suite 207
Bethesda, MD 20814
(301) 652-2263
http://www.devdelay.org

National nonprofit membership organization providing information and networking opportunities to parents and professionals working with children who have developmental delays.

National Association of State Directors of Special Education, Inc. (NASDSE)
1800 Diagonal Road
Suite 320
Alexandria, VA 22314
(703) 519-3800; (703) 519-7008 (TTY)
http://www.nasdse.org

A nonprofit organization established to promote and support education programs and related services for children and youths with disabilities in the United States. NASDSE provides services to state agencies to facilitate their efforts to maximize educational outcomes for individuals with disabilities. The group holds an annual meeting and publishes a quarterly newspaper as well as miscellaneous reports released throughout the year. Most new reports are available for downloading from the NASDSE Web site.

National Institute for People with Disabilities
460 West 34th Street
New York, NY 10001
(212) 273-6100
http://www.yai.org

Nonprofit agency serving children and adults with developmental disabilities in New York, including information and referrals.

Office of Special Education and Rehabilitative Services, Office of Special Education Programs (OSEP)
550 12th Street SW
Room 4109
Washington, DC 20202-2550
(202) 245-7426
http://www.ed.gov/about/offices/list/osers/index.html?src=oc

Group dedicated to improving results for infants, toddlers, children, and youths with disabilities from birth through age 21, providing leadership and financial support to assist states and local districts. The Individuals with Disabilities Education Act authorizes formula grants to states and discretionary grants to institutions of higher education and other nonprofit organizations to support research, demonstrations, technical assistance and dissemination, technology and personnel development, and parent-training and information centers. Organization offers professional and consumer fact sheets, brochures/pamphlets, online publications, and reports are available. Some Spanish materials are available.

Voice of the Retarded
5005 Newport Drive
Suite 108
Rolling Meadows, IL 60008
(847) 253-6020
http://www.vor.net

Organization that provides support, information, and advocacy, with a large collection of research files.

DISABILITIES

American Association of People with Disabilities
1629 K Street NW
Suite 503
Washington, DC 20006
(202) 457-0046; (800) 840-8844
http://www.aapd-dc.org

Organization offering support and information, and supporting full implementation and enforcement of disability nondiscrimination laws.

Association for the Severely Handicapped
29 West Susquehanna Avenue
Suite 210
Baltimore, MD 21204
(410) 828-8274
http://www.tash.org

An international advocacy association of people with disabilities, their families and others; with 38 chapters throughout the world. It actively promotes the full inclusion and participation of those with disabilities and seeks to eliminate physical and social obstacles that interfere with quality of life.

Association on Higher Education and Disability (AHEAD)
P.O. Box 540666
Waltham, MA 02454
(781) 788-0003
http://www.ahead.org

An international, multicultural organization of professionals committed to full participation in higher education for persons with disabilities. The association promotes education, communication, and training through numerous training programs, workshops, publications, and conferences. AHEAD was founded in 1977 to address the need and concern for upgrading the quality of services and support available to those with disabilities in higher education.

Children's Defense Fund
Haley Farm
P.O. Box 840
Clinton, TN 37717
(865) 457-6466
http://www.childrensdefense.org

A nonprofit research and advocacy organization that provides a strong voice for children who cannot speak for themselves, including children with disabilities.

The organization has regional offices throughout the country.

Commission on Mental and Physical Disability Law–American Bar Association
740 15th Street NW
Washington, DC 20005
(202) 662-1000
http://www.abanet.org/disability/home.html

This ABA affiliated group is committed to justice for those with physical disabilities, and maintains resources and references for helping the disabled community.

Disability Rights Advocates
449 15th Street
Suite 303
Oakland, CA 94612
(510) 451-8644
http://www.dralegal.org

Nonprofit civil rights organization for people with disabilities.

Disability Rights Education and Defense Fund, Inc.
2212 Sixth Street
Berkeley, CA 94710
(510) 644-2555 (Voice/TDD)
http://www.dredf.org

A national law and policy center dedicated to protecting and helping people with disabilities through legislation, litigation, advocacy, technical help, and education.

Disability Rights Section, Civil Rights Division, U.S. Department of Justice
950 Pennsylvania Avenue NW
Disability Rights Section
New York Avenue
Washington, DC 20530
(800) 514-0301; (800) 514-0383 (TTY)
http://www.ada.gov

The Disability Rights Section (DRS) is part of the Civil Rights Division of the U.S. Department of Justice. DRS focuses on all disabilities and is especially knowledgeable about the interpretation of the Americans with Disabilities Act of 1990. The organization offers an information line for all inquiries and assistance to state and local government entities, private sector business professionals, and the general public. Professional and consumer newsletter/bulletin, fact sheets, brochures/

pamphlets, and online publications are available. Some materials in Spanish and other languages are available.

Family Resource Center on Disabilities
20 East Jackson Boulevard
Room 300
Chicago, IL 60604
(800) 952-4199; (312) 939-3513
http://www.frcd.org

Coalition of parents, professionals, and volunteers dedicated to improving services for all children with disabilities.

National Association of Protection and Advocacy Systems
900 Second Street NE
Suite 211
Washington, DC 20002
(202) 408-9514
http://www.napas.org

A national membership organization for the federally mandated nationwide network of disability rights agencies, protection and advocacy systems, and client assistance programs.

National Center on Secondary Education and Transition (NCSET)
University of Minnesota Institute on Community
   Integration
6 Pattee Hall
150 Pillsbury Drive SE
Minneapolis, MN 55455
(612) 624-2097
http://www.ncset.org

NCSET comprises six organizations that work with national, state, and local agencies and organizations to improve secondary education and transition for youth with disabilities and their families.

National Clearinghouse on Women and Girls with Disabilities
114 East 32nd Street
New York, NY 10016
(212) 725-1803

Clearinghouse that provides catalog of manuals, supplements, videos, and directories, many of which deal with sexual issues faced by women and girls with disabilities.

National Dissemination Center for Children with Disabilities (NICHCY)
P.O. Box 1492
Washington, DC 20013-1492

(202) 884-8200; (800) 695-0285
http://www.nichcy.org

A national information and referral center that provides information on disabilities and disability-related issues to families, educators, and other professionals. NICHCY's special focus is children ages 0 to 22. Services include providing personalized responses to specific questions, including in Spanish. NICHCY also makes available a wide variety of publications, including fact sheets on specific disabilities, state resource sheets, parent guides, bibliographies, and the issue papers "News Digest" and "Transition Summary." Most publications can be printed off the Internet. NICHCY can put people in touch with disability organizations, parent groups, and professional associations at the state and national level and provide an information search of the center's databases and library for unique needs and concerns. Also offered are professional/consumer fact sheets, brochures/pamphlets, online publications, and reports. Materials also are available in Spanish, on disk, and as camera-ready originals.

National Information Center for Children and Youth with Disabilities
1875 Connecticut Avenue
8th floor
Washington, DC 20009
(800) 695-0285
http://www.nichcy.org

This national information and referral center provides information on disabilities and disability-related issues for families, educators, and other professionals with a special focus on children from birth to age 22. The association provides information on specific disabilities, early intervention, special education and related services, individualized education programs, family issues, disability organizations, professional associations, education rights, and transition to adult life, among other topics. The group also offers referrals, information service, and materials in English and Spanish.

Information clearinghouse that provides free information on disabilities and related issues, focusing on children and youth (birth to age 25). Free services include: personal responses, referrals, technical assistance, and information searches.

National Institute on Disability and Rehabilitation Research (NIDRR)
400 Maryland Avenue SW
Washington, DC 20202
(202) 205-8134; (202) 205-4475 (TTY)

http://www.ed.gov/about/offices/list/osers/nidrr/index.html?src=mc

A component of the Office of Special Education and Rehabilitative Services of the U.S. Department of Education, NIDRR provides support for a comprehensive program of national and international research into all aspects of the rehabilitation of people with disabilities and their successful integration into education, work, and community life. Grants are to institutions of higher education and qualified organizations. The fellowship program provides grants to individuals with advanced rehabilitation credentials. Online directory of projects, brochures/pamphlets, and reports are available.

National Library Service for the Blind and Physically Handicapped
Library of Congress
1291 Taylor Street NW
Washington, DC 20011
(202) 707-5100
http://www.loc.gov.NLS

Voice mail system. Operators provide information on audiocassette, large print, and braille books and magazines. Callers with learning disabilities must meet certain guidelines to use these services.

National Organization on Disability
910 16th Street NW
Suite 600
Washington, DC 20006
(202) 293-5960
http://www.nod.org

National disability network group concerned with all disabilities of all ages.

Sibling Support Project of the ARC
6512 23rd Avenue NW
Suite 213
Seattle, WA 98117
(206) 297-6368
http://www.thearc.org/siblingsupport

National program dedicated to interests of brothers and sisters of those with special developmental needs.

World Institute on Disability
510 16th Street
Suite 100
Oakland, CA 94612
(510) 763-4100
http://www.wid.org

Nonprofit public policy center dedicated to independence and inclusion of people with disabilities.

DOWN SYNDROME

(See also Developmental Disabilities)

National Down Syndrome Congress
1370 Center Drive
Suite 102
Atlanta, GA 30338
(800) 232-6372
http://www.ndsccenter.org

National advocacy organization for Down syndrome, offering research, education, and resources.

National Down Syndrome Society
666 Broadway
New York, NY 10012
(800) 221-4602; (212) 460-9330
http://www.ndss.org

National organization that sponsors research and offers support, resources, information, and advocacy.

DYSLEXIA

Davis Dyslexia Correction Center
1601 Bayshore Highway
Suite 260
Burlingame, CA 94010
(650) 692-8990; (800) 729-8990
http://www.davisdyslexia.com

Davis Dsylexia is based in the United States. Affiliated organizations have been established in France, Germany, Holland, Switzerland, Mexico, and the United Kingdom.

Dyslexia Research Institute
5746 Centerville Road
Tallahassee, FL 32309
(850) 893-2216
http://www.dyslexia-add.org

The goal of the Dyslexia Research Institute is to expand the knowledge of parents and professionals in the area of dyslexia and attention deficit disorders. Direct instruction is provided through a full multisensoral curriculum for both adults and children. The institute provides instruction through informational seminars, teacher training, and advocacy/consultation. Research papers are available.

Hello Friend/Ennis William Cosby Foundation
P.O. Box 4061
Santa Monica, CA 90411
http://www.hellofriend.org

Foundation dedicated to dyslexia resources and information for parents, students, and educators.

The International Dyslexia Association (IDA) (formerly The Orton Dyslexia Society)
Chester Building
8600 LaSalle Road
Suite 382
Baltimore, MD 21286-2044
(800) ABC-D123 (for general information);
     (410) 296-0232 (for detailed information)
http://www.interdys.org

With 11,000 members in 45 branches around the world, IDA offers an international network that brings professionals in the field of dyslexia and parents together for a common purpose. The group offers informational meetings and support groups, referrals, journals, and publications regarding dyslexia.

Recording for the Blind and Dyslexic, Inc.
20 Roszel Road
Princeton, NJ 08540
(609) 452-0606; (866) 732-3585
http://www.rfbd.org

Operators provide information on more than 80,000 recorded textbooks and other classroom materials, from fourth grade through postgraduate levels, available for loan. Callers with learning disabilities are eligible to participate but must complete the certification requirements.

EDUCATION

Association of Educational Therapists
1804 West Burbank Boulevard
Burbank, CA 91506
(800) 286-4267
http://www.aetonline.org

National membership organization that provides referrals to local educational therapists.

Association on Higher Education and Disability
P.O. Box 21192
Columbus, OH 43221
(614) 488-4972
http://www.ahead.org

An international, multicultural organization of professionals committed to full participation in higher education for persons with disabilities. The association promotes education, communication, and training through numerous training programs, workshops, publications, and conferences. AHEAD was founded in 1977 to address the need and concern for upgrading the quality of services and support available to those with disabilities in higher education.

George Washington University HEATH Resource Center
2121 K Street NW
Suite 220
Washington, DC 20037
(202) 973-0904; (800) 544-3284
http://www.health.gwu.edu

HEATH (Higher Education and Adult Training for People with Handicaps) is a national clearinghouse that provides free information on postsecondary education and related issues for individuals with learning disabilities.

Independent Educational Consultant Association
3251 Old Lee Highway
Suite 510
Fairfax, VA 22030
(703) 591-4850
http://www.educationalconsulting.org

A nonprofit, international professional association representing full-time, experienced, independent educational consultants. Chartered in 1976. IECA sponsors professional training institutes, workshops, and conferences, publishes a directory of qualified consultants, offers information to students and their families regarding school selection issues, and works to ensure that those in the profession adhere to the highest ethical and business standards. IECA has developed a strict set of ethical guidelines that govern the actions of consultants in their relationships with students and families, schools and colleges, and with colleagues. These include a responsibility to understand each student's special strengths, values, and needs, while striving to include all family members in the educational planning process. An IECA member does not accept any compensation from educational institutions for placement of a child. IECA also established the Independent Educational Consultants Association Foundation, which supports projects that will benefit those involved in the process of making educational choices, including students, families, educational consultants, and other professionals.

National Association for the Education of Young Children (NAEYC)
1509 16th Street NW
Washington, DC 20036-1426
(202) 232-8777; (800) 424-2460
http://www.naeyc.org

National membership organization that focuses on children from birth to age eight. Sponsors an annual conference, publishes a bimonthly journal, and has a catalog of books, brochures, videos, and posters.

National Association of Private Special Education Centers
1522 K Street NW
Suite 1032
Washington, DC 20005
(202) 408-3338
http://www.napsec.org

Referral services for those interested in private special education in the United States, including publications and conferences.

National Center on Educational Outcomes
University of Minnesota
350 Elliott Hall
75 East River Road
Minneapolis, MN 55455
(612) 626-1530
http://www.umn.edu/NCEO

Provides national leadership in the participation of students with disabilities and limited English proficient (LEP) students in national and state assessments, standards-setting efforts, and graduation requirements.

National Center on Accelerating Student Learning
http://kc.vanderbilt.edu/CASL

Designed to accelerate learning for students with disabilities in the early grades and thereby to provide a solid foundation for strong achievement in the intermediate grades and beyond. CASL is a five-year collaborative research effort supported by the U.S. Department of Education's Office of Special Education Programs (OSEP). Participating institutions are the University of Maryland, Teachers College of Columbia University, and Vanderbilt University.

National Head Start Association
1651 Prince Street
Alexandria, VA 22314
(703) 739-0875
http://www.nhsa.org

A not-for-profit membership organization representing Head Start programs in America. NHSA provides a national forum for the continued enhancement of Head Start services for poor children from birth to age five years, and their families. It is the only national organization dedicated exclusively to the concerns of the Head Start community.

Parent Advocacy Coalition for Educational Rights
8161 Normandale Boulevard
Minneapolis, MN 55437
(952) 838-9000
http://www.pacer.org

Parent-to-parent organization with lots of resources for parents of children with disabilities, including training programs for parents and youth, technical assistance, and advocacy.

FETAL ALCOHOL SYNDROME

National Organization on Fetal Alcohol Syndrome
900 17th Street NW
Suite 910
Washington, DC 20006
(202) 785-4585; (800) 66NOFAS
http://www.nofas.org

Nonprofit organization founded in 1990 to address alcohol use during pregnancy, the leading known preventable cause of mental retardation and birth defects. NOFAS recognizes the importance of health education in order to reduce the number of alcohol-exposed births and fulfills its mission by implementing innovative ideas in prevention, education, intervention, and advocacy.

FRAGILE X SYNDROME

National Fragile X Foundation
P.O. Box 190488
San Francisco, CA 94119
(925) 938-9300; (800) 688-8765
http://www.nfxf.org

Nonprofit organization that provides advocacy, consultation, information, research, newsletters, referrals, and education.

LEAD POISONING

The Environmental Protection Agency Safe Drinking Water Hotline
(800) 426-4791
http://www.epa.gov/safewater/hotline

For information on laboratories certified to test for lead in water.

The National Center for Healthy Housing
10227 Wincopin Circle
Suite 100
Columbia, MD 21044
(410) 992-0712
http://www.centerforhealthyhousing.org

For information about lead in housing.

The National Lead Information Center
(800) 424-LEAD (5323)
http://www.epa.gov/lead/nlic.htm

Materials about lead poisoning are available in Spanish and English.

LEARNING DISABILITIES

Association for Children and Adults with Learning Disabilities
4900 Girard Road
Pittsburgh, PA 15227
(412) 881-2253
http://www.acldonline.org

AC-ACLD has been providing direct services to individuals with Specific Learning Disabilities since 1966. Its mission is to enhance the quality of life for children and adults with Specific Learning Disabilities and related neurobiological disorders by facilitating self-sufficiency and financial independence.

Council for Exceptional Children and the Division for Learning Disabilities
1920 Association Drive
Reston, VA 22091-1589
(800) 328-0272; (703) 620-3660
Council for Exceptional Children: www.cec.sped.org
Division for Learning Disabilities: www.dldcec.org

An international, professional association with more than 52,000 educator members. Their principal purpose is to advance the education of all exceptional children and youth—those with disabilities and those who are gifted. DLD is the division of the CEC that focuses on the special needs of individuals with learning disabilities. This membership organization has 17 specialized divisions including the Division of Learning Disabilities, which is dedicated to the field of learning disabilities. CEC conducts an annual conference, publishes a newsletter and magazines.

Council for Learning Disabilities
P.O. Box 4014
Leesburg, VA 20177
(517) 258-1010
www.cldinternational.org

The CLD is an international organization of and for professionals who establish standards of excellence and promote innovative strategies for research and practice through collaboration and advocacy.

Learning Disabilities Association of America
4156 Library Road
Pittsburgh, PA 15234
(412) 341-1515; (888) 300-6710
http://www.ldanatl.org

National nonprofit membership organization dedicated to enhancing the quality of life for everyone with a learning disability and their families, and offers advocacy, education, research, and services. LDA was formed in 1964 by a group of concerned parents on behalf of children with learning disabilities; it is the only national organization devoted to defining and finding solutions for the broad spectrum of these problems.

Learning Resources Network
P.O. Box 9
River Falls, WI 54022
(715) 426-9777; (800) 678-5376
http://www.lern.org

Organization providing information and support about learning disabilities and those who teach adult education.

LD On-Line
Web site only
http://www.ldonline.org

A to Z database on all aspects of learning disabilities and children.

National Center for Learning Disabilities
381 Park Avenue South
Suite 1401
New York, NY 10016
(888) 575-7373 (general information);
   (212) 545-7510 (detailed information)
http://www.ld.org

Develops training and educational materials for parents and practitioners including *Every Child Is Learning*, a training program to help preschool teachers and parents recognize the early warning signs of learning disabilities. NCLD seeks to raise public awareness and understanding, furnish national information and referrals, and arrange educational programs and legislative advocacy. NCLD provides educational tools to heighten understanding of learning disabilities, including the annual publication called *Their World*, quarterly newsletters, informative articles, specific state-by-state resource listings, and informative videos regarding learning disabilities.

Nonverbal Learning Disorders Association
2446 Albany Avenue
West Hartford, CT 06117
(860) 570-0217
http://www.nlda.org

A nonprofit corporation dedicated to research, education, and advocacy for nonverbal learning disorders.

Schwab Foundation for Learning
1650 South Amphlett Boulevard
Suite 300
San Mateo, CA 94402
(800) 230-0988; (650) 655-2410
www.schwablearning.org

Group that provides services to parents and educators to help students with learning differences succeed. Services include a lending library and *Bridges to Reading*, a step-by-step guide to understanding, identifying, and addressing reading problems.

LOWE SYNDROME

Lowe Syndrome Association
18919 Voss Road
Dallas, TX 75287
(612) 869-5693
http://www.lowesyndrome.org

Voluntary health organization of parents, professionals, and others to provide information and support, and to support research and treatments.

MENTAL RETARDATION

(See Developmental Disabilities and Down Syndrome)

PRADER-WILLI SYNDROME ORGANIZATIONS

Prader-Willi Syndrome Association
5700 Midnight Pass Road
Suite 6
Sarasota, FL 34242
(941) 312-0400; (800) 926-4797
http://www.pwsausa.org

A nonprofit organization that provides a newsletter and other publications, an annual national conference, and chapters throughout the country to provide family support and advocacy.

PROFESSIONAL ORGANIZATIONS

National Association of School Psychologists (NASP)
4340 East West Highway
Suite 402
Bethesda, MD 20814
(301) 657-0270
http://www.naspweb.org

Professional organization for school psychologists that promotes educationally and psychologically healthy environments for all children. NASP supports research and training, advocacy, program evaluation, and caring professional service. NASP is the largest association of school psychologists in the world.

National Association of Social Workers (NASW)
750 First Street NE
Suite 700
Washington, DC 20002
(202) 408-8600
http://www.naswdc.org

NASW is the largest membership organization of professional social workers in the world. The group works to enhance the professional growth and development of its members, to create and maintain professional standards, and to advance sound social policies.

RETT SYNDROME

International Rett Syndrome Association
9121 Piscataway Road
Suite 2B
Clinton, MD 20735
(301) 856-3334; (800) 818-7388
http://www.rettsyndrome.org

A support group for parents of children with Rett syndrome; founded by parents in early 1984. IRSA is a partnership of parents and professionals dedicated to better understanding Rett syndrome. Members include parents, relatives, doctors, therapists, researchers, and friends interested in providing a better future for girls with Rett syndrome. IRSA supports medical research to determine the cause and find a cure for Rett syndrome; increases public awareness of the condition; and provides information and support to families of affected children.

Rett Syndrome Research Foundation (RSRF)
4600 Devitt Drive
Cincinnati OH 45246
(513) 874-3020
http://www.rsrf.org

A nonprofit foundation created in 1999 by six parents of girls with Rett syndrome that is dedicated to finding a treatment and cure, promoting research and offering information, advocacy, referrals to support groups, genetic counseling, and other services.

National Spasmodic Dysphonia Association, Inc. (NSDA)
One East Wacker Drive
Suite 2430
Chicago, IL, 60601
(800) 795-NSDA (6732)
http://www.dysphonia.org

Association that increases public awareness about spasmodic dysphonia and promotes the care, welfare, and rehabilitation of those who have the disease through education and support of research. NSDA promotes education about spasmodic dysphonia in the medical community and general public. Professional/consumer brochures, fact sheets, books, and audiovisuals are available.

SPECIAL EDUCATION

Center for Special Education Finance
American Institutes for Research
1791 Arastradero Road

Palo Alto, CA 94304-1337
(650) 843-8136
http://www.dssc.org/frc/TAGuide/tad/csef.htm

Provides information and research on issues regarding special education spending. Publishes newsletter, policy papers, state analysis series, briefs, and reference documents.

Council of Educators for Students with Disabilities (CESD)
9801 Anderson Mill Road
Suite 230
Austin, TX 78750
(512) 219-5043
http://www.504idea.org

Provides information and training to assist educators in complying with federal laws protecting students with disabilities, including IDEIA '97 and Section 504 of the Rehabilitation Act of 1973.

Disability Resources, Inc.
http://www.disabilityresources.org

A nonprofit organization that offers alphabetical listings by disability and/or state of local and national resources.

Edlaw, Inc.
1310 Minor Avenue, #207
Seattle, WA 98101
http://www.edlaw.net/frames.html

Source for information on special education law; download laws, regulations, and more.

Information Center on Disabilities and Gifted Education
110 North Glebe Road
Arlington, VA 22201-5705
(888) 915-5000
http://www.ericec.org

Information on learning disabilities, parenting, and teaching.

SPEECH PROBLEMS

National Black Association for Speech-Language and Hearing
P.O. Box 61328
Charleston, SC 29419
(843) 574-6441
http://www.nbaslh.org

A nonprofit organization dedicated to promoting the sharing of information about communication impairments and differences among African Americans; professional development of speech-language pathologists, audiologists, and students; and advocacy of quality service delivery to the black community. Professional journal and newsletter/bulletin are available.

National Center for Voice and Speech (NCVS)

The Denver Center for the Performing Arts
1245 Champa Street
Denver, CO, 80204
(303) 446-4834
http://www.ncvs.org

An interdisciplinary team of investigators and healthcare professionals dedicated to studying the powers, limitations, and enhancement of human voice and speech. There are two performance sites: the Denver Center for the Performing Arts and the University of Iowa. NCVS research focuses on a better understanding of neurophysiological, biomechanic, anatomic, aerodynamic, and acoustic processes involved in speech and voice production. The organization also is dedicated to training scientists interested in careers in communications research, continuing education for clinicians, and the dissemination of information to the general public. NCVS research and dissemination is supported by the National Institute on Deafness and Other Communication Disorders. Professional/consumer brochures/pamphlets, online publications, professional monographs/books, and professional reports are available. Some Spanish and French materials are available.

STUTTERING

(See also Communication)

National Center for Stuttering

200 East 33rd Street
Suite 17C
New York, NY 10016
(800) 221-2483
http://www.stuttering.com

Center that offers information, a hotline, treatment, continuing education, and research.

National Stuttering Association (NSA)

119 West 40th Street, 14th Floor
New York, NY, 10018
(212) 944-4050; (800) 937-8888
http://www.westutter.org

A national network of support groups created to meet the needs of children and adults who stutter. NSA offers information and support, provides referrals to specialists, serves as an advocate for the stuttering community, and raises the consciousness of the general public about the disorder. Professional and consumer fact sheets, brochures/pamphlets, and books are available.

Speak Easy International Foundation, Inc.

233 Concord Drive
Paramus, NJ 07652
(201) 262-0895
http://www.speak-easy.org

The foundation seeks to motivate, instill confidence, enhance self-image, and reinforce fluency in people who stutter; serve as an advocacy group; encourage family and friends of people who stutter to become cognizant of the speech dysfluent individual's plight and problems; educate the public; and help its members attain a viable status in society. The foundation holds an annual symposium and retreat; brochures/pamphlets are available.

Stuttering Foundation of America

3100 Walnut Grove Road
Suite 603
Memphis, TN 38111
(901) 452-7343; (800) 992-9392
http://www.stutteringhelp.org; http://www.tarta-
    mudez.org (Spanish)

Foundation provides help and support to individuals who stutter, their families, and professionals who serve them by providing comprehensive, up-to-date, accurate information on stuttering in the forms of videotapes, books, brochures, workshops, and conferences. SFA also supports stuttering research. Foundation offers professional/consumer newsletter/bulletin, fact sheets, brochures/pamphlets, online publications, monographs/books, computer software/assistance education, audiovisuals, reports, and videotapes. Some materials are available in Spanish, French, and Italian. The foundation also provides information through its Spanish-language Web site.

TOURETTE'S SYNDROME

Tourette Syndrome Association, Inc.

42-40 Bell Boulevard
Suite 205
Bayside, NY 11361
(718) 224-2999; (800) 237-0717
http://www.tsa-usa.org
Organization offers information, resources on
    Tourette's syndrome.

VESTIBULAR DISORDERS

Vestibular Disorders Association
P.O. Box 13305
Portland, OR 97213-0305
(503) 229-7705; (800) 837-8428
http://www.vestibular.org

A nonprofit organization that provides information to people with vestibular disorders, such as labyrinthitis, benign paroxysmal positional vertigo, Ménière's disease, and perilymph fistula. The organization offers a consumer newsletter/bulletin, directory, fact sheets, brochures/pamphlets, online publications, monographs/books, and videotapes. Some Spanish materials are available.

WILLIAMS SYNDROME

Williams Syndrome Association
P.O. Box 297
Clawson, MI 48017-0297
248-244-2229; 800-806-1871
http://www.williams-syndrome.org

APPENDIX II
GOVERNMENT SOURCES OF INFORMATION AND HELP

Americans with Disabilities Act (ADA) Hotline
(800) 949-4232

The ADA Hotline provides technical assistance, information on services, and outreach regarding the Americans with Disabilities Act (ADA). Operators are equipped with a listing of learning disabilities associations and can answer questions about how ADA protects individuals with learning disabilities. An answering machine is available during non-business hours, and follow-up calls are placed the next working day.

Comprehensive Regional Assistance Centers
(800) USA-LEARN; (800) 437-0833 (TTY)
http://www.ccnetwork.org

Sponsored by the U.S. Department of Education, the 15 Comprehensive Centers are part of an emerging network of organizations that support and assist states, districts, and schools in meeting the needs of children served under the Improving America's Schools Act (1994).

Department of Education
400 Maryland Avenue SW
Washington, DC 20202
(800) USA-LEARN
http://www.ed.gov

Department administers more than 200 programs involving education.

National Mental Health Information Center
P.O. Box 42577
Washington, DC 20015
(800) 789-2647
http://www.mentalhealth.org

Substance Abuse and Mental Health Services Administration group that provides information and resources on mental health including database of community resources, extensive catalog, events, and more.

National Institute of Child Health and Human Development (NICHD)
P.O. Box 3006
Rockville, MD 20847
(800) 370-2943
http://www.nichd.nih.gov

Institute that supports research into the health of children and offers information on a wide variety of topics relevant to children and maternal health.

National Institute of Mental Health (NIMH)
6001 Executive Boulevard MSC 9663
Room 8184
Bethesda, MD 20892
(301) 443-4513; (866) 615-6464
http://www.nimh.nih.gov

Foremost mental health research organization in the world.

National State Policy Database
http://www.nasdse.org/national_state_policy_
database.htm

Contains special education regulations for 30 states. To access information on the site enter search terms on the main page. This site is under development.

Office for Civil Rights
U.S. Department of Education, OCR
330 C Street SW
Suite 5000
Washington, DC 20202-1100
(202) 205-5413
http://www.ed.gov/offices/OCR

Agency ensures equal access to education, and enforces civil rights. To file a formal civil rights complaint (a Section 504 complaint), contact this office or the regional office servicing your area.

Office of Special Education and Rehabilitation Services
Switzer Building
330 C Street SW
Suite 3006
Washington, DC 20202
(202) 205-5465
http://www.ed.gov/offices/OSERS

Office supports programs that help in educating children with special needs and also supports research. OSERS includes the Office of Special Education Programs, Rehabilitation Services Administration, and the National Institute on Disability and Rehabilitation Research.

Office of Special Education Programs
Switzer Building
330 C Street SW
Suite 3086
Washington, DC 20202
(202) 205-5507

The OESP administers programs relating to education of all children, youth, and adults with disabilities, through age 22.

Rehabilitation Services Administration
Switzer Building
330 C Street SW
Suite 3026
Washington, DC 20202
(202) 205-5482
http://www.ed.gov/offices/OSERS/RSA/rsa.html

RSA guides programs that help those with physical or mental disabilities get hired by providing counseling, health services, job training, and other support.

National Institute on Disability and Rehabilitative Research
Switzer Building
330 C Street SW
Suite 3060 MES
Washington, DC 20202
(202) 205-8134
http://www.ed.gov/offices/OSERS/NIDRR/nidrr.html

NIDRR conducts research and administers ADA technical assistance centers.

Office of Educational Research and Improvement
555 New Jersey Avenue NW
Washington, DC 20208
(202) 219-1385
http://www.ed.gov/offices/OERI

Provides support for educational research and statistics and offers a variety of services. Its agencies include the National Center for Educational Statistics; the National Institute on Early Childhood Development and Education; National Institute on the Education of At Risk Students; National Institute on Student Achievement, Curriculum, and Assessment.

APPENDIX III
ASSISTIVE TECHNOLOGY RESOURCES

ABLEDATA Web site National Institute on Disability and Rehabilitative Research
8630 Fenton Street
Suite 930
Silver Spring, MD 20910
(800) 277-0216; (301) 608-8998
http://www.abledata.com

Electronic database of information on assistive technology and rehabilitation equipment in the United States, including more than 23,000 products.

Adaptive Computing Technology Center
Web site only
http://www.missouri.edu/adaptive

Web site that provides information on technology that combines adaptive devices with standard computer equipment.

Alliance for Technology Access
1304 Southpoint Boulevard
Suite 240
Petaluma, CA 94954
(707) 778-3011
http://www.ataccess.org

Network of community-based resource centers around the country offering information and support to children and adults with disabilities on standard assistive and information technology.

Apple Computer's Worldwide Disability Solutions Group
Web site only
http://www.apple.com/accessibility

Web site that offers help for people with disabilities who want to use a Macintosh computer, including links to organizations and manufacturers and software programs.

Assistive Technology Industry Association
401 North Michigan Avenue
Chicago, IL 60611
(312) 321-5172; (877) 687-2842
http://www.atia.org

A not-for-profit membership of organizations manufacturing or selling technology-based assistive devices for people with disabilities, or providing services associated with or required by people with disabilities. Among its primary goals is the establishment and continuation of an assistive device technology conference on an annual basis.

Center for Applied Special Technology
40 Harvard Mills Square
Suite 3
Wakefield, MA 01880
(781) 245-2212
http://www.cast.org

Nonprofit organization whose mission is to expand opportunities for people with disabilities through innovative multimedia computer technology.

Center for Electronic Studying
5265 University of Oregon
Eugene, OR 97403-5265
(541) 346-2544
http://www.ces.uoregon.edu

Center investigating ways in which computer technology can be used to enhance students' efforts to study and learn content-area material. Funded by the U.S. Department of Education, the Center has launched three projects blending portable computer technology with instruction on computer-based study strategies.

Closing the Gap
P.O. Box 68
526 Main Street
Henderson, MN 56044

(507) 248-3294
http://www.closingthegap.com

Internationally recognized source for information on the use of microcomputer-related technology by and for exceptional individuals. Publishes newsletter, resource directory and holds annual international conference each fall in Minneapolis, Minnesota.

DREAMMS for Kids
Web site only
http://www.dreamms.org

Nonprofit parent-professional agency that offers information and research in assistive technology. Services include newsletters, Tech Paks, and special programs aimed at kids and computers.

Equal Access to Software and Information
Web site only
http://www.rit.edu/~easi

EASI offers information and guidance in access-to-information technologies by individuals with disabilities.

National Center to Improve Practice
http://www2.edc.org/NCIP

Promotes the effective use of technology to enhance educational outcomes for students with sensory, cognitive, physical, and social/emotional disabilities. Funded by the U.S. Department of Education.

Rehabilitation Engineering and Assistive Technology Society of North America
1700 North Moore Street
Suite 1540
Arlington, VA 22209

(703) 524-6686
http://www.resna.org

Resource for those interested in assistive technology.

RESNA Technical Assistance Project
1700 North Moore Street
Suite 1540
Arlington, VA 22209-1903
(703) 524-6686
http://www.resna.org/taproject

Information and consultation to assistive technology programs in states and territories funded under the Technology-Related Assistance for Individuals with Disabilities Act Amendments of 1994 (PL 103-218).

UNLV Assistive Technology Curriculum Project
Department of Special Education
University of Nevada, Las Vegas
4505 Maryland Parkway
Box 3014
Las Vegas, NV 89154-3014
(702) 895-1106
http://www.dinF.NE.jp/doc/english/Us_Eu/conf/csun
    _98/csun_98_114.htm

This project has integrated knowledge of the ADA, assistive technology, and disability issues into a university curriculum.

APPENDIX IV
HOTLINES

American Association for Vocational and Instructional Materials
(800) 228-4689

An operator is available from 8 A.M. to 5 P.M. EST, Monday through Friday, to provide information on educational materials (software, videos, manuals), including a listing of Category L modules that deal with teaching students with special needs. Products are available for purchase.

Equal Employment Opportunity Commission
(800) 669-3362

Voice mail directs calls from 7 A.M. to 5:30 P.M. EST, Monday through Friday. Operators accept orders for publications, fact sheets, posters, and a resource directory for people with disabilities, including learning disabilities. They do not answer questions relating to employment but can give referrals to local EEOC offices.

ERIC Clearinghouse on Adult, Career, and Vocational Education Center for Employment, Education & Training
(800) 848-4815

A 24-hour voice mail service that provides information on ERIC digests, annotated bibliographies, and assorted publications, some with information on learning disabilities. ERIC does not answer specific questions on disabilities, local programs, or jobs.

Federal Student Aid Information Center Hotline
(800) 4-FEDAID; (433-3243)

Provides information from 9 A.M. to 8 P.M. EST, Monday through Friday, on eligibility, benefits, applications, and other questions about student aid. Voice mail directs calls during business hours.

GED Hotline
(800) 629-9433

A 24-hour operator service provides information on local GED classes and testing services; offers an accommodations guide for people taking the GED who have a learning disability.

The International Dyslexia Association
(410) 296-0232

A 24-hour voice mail service to receive information requests: 1-800-ABC-0123 (1-800-222-3123)

From 8:30 A.M. to 4:30 P.M. EST, Monday through Friday, staff provide information on appropriate materials on dyslexia, referrals for testing and tutors, branches of IDA, and workshops and conferences.

Job Accommodation Network
(800) 526-7324

A free consulting service from 8 A.M. to 8 P.M. EST, Monday through Thursday, and 8 A.M. to 5 P.M. EST on Friday to provide information on: equipment, methods, and modifications with which persons with disabilities can improve their work environment. All information is specific to the disability, including learning disabilities.

Learning Resources Network
(800) 678-5376

An operator service from 8 A.M. to 5 P.M. EST, Monday through Friday, to provide information to practitioners of adult continuing education, give consulting information, take orders for publications, and provide phone numbers of associations and organizations that deal with learning disabilities.

National Center for Research in Vocational Education
(800) 762-4093

An operator is available from 8 A.M. to 5 P.M. Pacific Time, Monday through Friday, to provide information on products, electronic services, and vocational education. A catalog and newsletter are also available. The Office of Student Services produces materials on learning disabilities and a subcatalog for special populations.

National Clearinghouse on Postsecondary Education for Individuals with Disabilities
HEATH Resource Center
(800) 544-3284

Information specialists available from 9 A.M. to 5 P.M. EST, Monday through Friday, to provide resource papers, directories, information on national organizations, and a resource directory for people with learning disabilities.

National Library of Education at the U.S. Office of Educational Research and Improvement
(800) 424-1616

An operator is available from 9 A.M. to 4 P.M. EST, Monday through Friday, to provide statistical information on education and schools, publications, references to other agencies, and references to a specialist on learning disabilities.

National Library Services for the Blind and Physically Handicapped
(800) 424-8567

A voice mail system directs calls from 8 A.M. to 4:30 P.M. EST, Monday through Friday; operators provide information on audiocassette, large print, and braille books and magazines for recreational reading. Callers with learning disabilities must meet certain guidelines to use these services.

National Literacy Hotline
(800) 228-8813

A 24-hour bilingual (Spanish/English) operator service to provide information on literacy/education classes, GED testing services, volunteer organizations, and learning disabilities.

Recording for the Blind and Dyslexic, Inc.
(800) 221-4792

Operators are available from 8:30 A.M. to 7 P.M., Monday through Friday, to provide information on more than 80,000 recorded textbooks (in four-track cassette or computer disk) and other classroom materials, from fourth grade through postgraduate levels, available on loan. There is an application and certification process and one-time fee ($37.50). Callers with learning disabilities are eligible to participate but must complete the certification requirements.

APPENDIX V
COMMERCIAL TECHNOLOGY RESOURCES

Each of these Web sites has a variety of products and information about assistive technology:

Able Generation
http://www.ablegeneration.com

Pediatric therapeutic furniture for children with special needs.

Adaptive and Assistive Technology@Rehab Tool.com
http://www.rehabtool.com

Offers a variety of high-tech assistive and adaptive technology products, augmentative and alternative communication devices, computer access equipment, multilingual speech synthesis and voice recognition software.

Adaptive Technology Consulting, Inc.
http://www.adaptivetech.net

Provides, installs, and trains in the use of equipment for the blind, visually impaired, and individuals with reading difficulties.

Apple Computer Disability Resources
http://www.apple.com/disability

Innovative products and programs designed to help individuals with disabilities lead independent lives.

Assistive Technology, Inc.
http://www.assistivetech.com

Provides innovative solutions to help people with learning, communication, and access difficulties lead more independent and productive lives.

Don Johnston
http://www.donjohnston.com

Computer products designed to provide a means for people with special needs to discover their potential and experience success.

Freedom Scientific
11800 31st Court North
St. Petersburg, FL 33716-1805
(800) 444-4443
http://www.freedomscientific.com

A nonprofit organization whose goal is to deliver information access through technology. From reading machines to talking GPS-based personal locators, Freedom Scientific has solutions to make its users successful in the real world.

Super School Software
1857 Josie Avenue
Long Beach, CA 90815-3432
(562) 594-8580
http://www.superschoolsoftware.com

Software and IEP Writer.

APPENDIX VI
BOOKS OF INTEREST TO PEOPLE WITH LEARNING DISABILITIES

BOOKS FOR CHILDREN AND TEENS WITH LEARNING DISABILITIES

Fisher, G., and R. Cummings. *The Survival Guide for Kids with LD*. Minneapolis: Free Spirit Publishing, 1990.

Gehret, J. *Learning Disabilities and the Don't-Give-Up-Kid*. Fairport, N.Y.: Verbal Images Press, 1990.

Landau, E. *Dyslexia*. New York: Franklin Watts, 1991.

Levine, M. *Keeping a Head in School: A Student's Book about Learning Abilities and Learning Disorders*. Cambridge, Mass.: Educators Publishing Services, 1990.

BOOKS FOR COLLEGE-BOUND STUDENTS WITH LEARNING DISABILITIES

Kravets, Marybeth, and Imy F. Wax. *The K&W Guide to Colleges for the Learning Disabled*. 3rd ed., 1995.

An analysis of more than 200 U.S. colleges offering programs and services specifically geared to students with learning disabilities. Available for $28 plus $3.00 shipping and handling, from Educators Publishing Service, Inc., 31 Smith Place, Cambridge, MA 02130; (800) 225-5750.

Mangrum, Charles T., II, and Stephen S. Strichart, eds. *Peterson's Colleges with Programs for Students with Learning Disabilities*. 4th ed., 1994.

A comprehensive guide to more than 800 colleges and universities in the United States and Canada, including two-year, four-year, and graduate programs. Available for $31.95, plus $6.75 shipping and handling, from Peterson's Guides, P.O. Box 2123, Princeton, NJ 08543; (800) 338-3282.

Nadeau, Kathleen G. *The Survival Guide for College Students with ADD or LD*. Washington, D.C.: Magination Press, 1994.

BOOKS FOR ADULTS WITH LEARNING DISABILITIES

Adelman, P., and C. Wren. *Learning Disabilities, Graduate School, and Careers: The Student's Perspective*. Lake Forest, Ill.: Learning Opportunities Program, Barat College, 1990.

Cordoni, B. *Living with a Learning Disability*. Carbondale: Southern Illinois University Press, 1987.

Hallowell, Edward M., and John J. Ratey. *Driven to Distraction: Recognizing and Coping with Attention Deficit Disorder from Childhood through Adulthood*. New York: Touchstone, 1995.

Kravets, M., and I. Wax. *The K&W Guide: Colleges and the Learning Disabled Student*. New York: HarperCollins, 1992.

Mangrum, C., and S. Strichart, eds. *Colleges with Programs for Students with Learning Disabilities*. Princeton, N.J.: Peterson's Guides, 1992.

BOOKS FOR PARENTS

Adams, M. J. et al. *Phonemic Awareness in Young Children: A Classroom Curriculum*. Baltimore: Brookes Publishing, 1997.

Attwood, Tony. *Asperger's Syndrome: A Guide for Parents and Professionals*. London: Taylor & Francis Group, 1997.

Barkley, Russell. *Taking Charge of ADHD: The Complete, Authoritative Guide for Parents*. New York. Guilford Press, 2000.

Blackburn, Lynn Bennett. *Growing up with Epilepsy: A Practical Guide for Parents*. New York: Demos Medical Publications, 2003.

Directory of Facilities and Services for the Learning Disabled, 17th ed. Novato, Calif.: Academic Therapy, 1998.

Forehand, Rex, and Nicholas Long. *Parenting the Strong-Willed Child—Revised and Updated Edition: The Clinically Proven Five-Week Program for Parents of Two- to Six-Year Olds.* New York: McGraw-Hill, 2002.

Greene, L. *Learning Disabilities and Your Child: A Survival Handbook.* New York: Fawcett Columbine, 1987.

Hallowell, Edward M., and John J. Ratey. *Driven to Distraction: Recognizing and Coping with Attention Deficit Disorder from Childhood through Adulthood.* New York: Touchstone, 1995.

Klass, Perri, and Eileen Costello. *Quirky Kids: Understanding and Helping Your Child Who Doesn't Fit In—When to Worry and When Not to Worry.* New York: Ballantine, 2003.

Mackenzie, L. *The Complete Learning Disabilities Directory.* Lakeville, Conn.: GreyHouse, 1997.

Novick, B., and M. Arnold. *Why Is My Child Having Trouble in School?* New York: Villard Books, 1991.

Pierangelo, Roger, and Rochelle Crane. *The Special Education Yellow Pages.* Upper Saddle River, N.J.: Prentice Hall, 2000.

Powers, Michael, with Janet Poland. *Asperger Syndrome and Your Child: A Parent's Guide.* New York: HarperResource, 2003.

Seligman, Martin E. *The Optimistic Child: Proven Program to Safeguard Children from Depression and Build Lifelong Resilience.* New York: Harper, 1996.

Shaywitz, Sally. *Overcoming Dyslexia: A New and Complete Science-Based Program for Overcoming Reading Problems at Any Level.* New York: Knopf, 2003.

Siegel, Bryna. *The World of the Autistic Child: Understanding and Treating Autistic Spectrum Disorders.* London: Oxford University Press, 1998.

Silver, L. *The Misunderstood Child: A Guide for Parents of Children with Learning Disabilities.* 3rd ed. New York: Time Books, 1998.

———. *Dr. Silver's Advice to Parents on Attention-Deficit Hyperactivity Disorder.* Washington, D.C.: American Psychiatric Press, 1993.

Smith, S. *No Easy Answers.* Rev. ed. New York: Bantam Books, 1995.

Spear-Swerling, Louise, and Robert Sternberg. *Off Track: When Poor Readers Become Learning Disabled.* Boulder, Colo.: Westview Press, 1997.

Spence, Sue, Vanessa Cobham, Ann Wignall, and Ronald M. Rapee. *Helping Your Anxious Child: A Step-By-Step Guide for Parents.* Oakland, Calif.: New Harbinger Publications, 2000.

Thompson, Sue. *Source for Nonverbal Learning Disorders.* East Moline, Ill.: LinguiSystems, 1997.

Twatchman-Cullen, Diane, and Jennifer Twachtman-Reilly. *How Well Does Your IEP Measure Up? Quality Indicators for Effective Service Delivery.* Higganum, Conn.: Starfish Specialty Publications, 2002.

Vail, P. *Smart Kids with School Problems.* New York: E. P. Dutton, 1987.

Weiss, E. *Mothers Talk about Learning Disabilities.* New York: Prentice Hall, 1989.

BOOKS AND PAMPHLETS FOR TEACHERS AND SPECIALISTS

Adelman, P., and C. Wren. *Learning Disabilities, Graduate School, and Careers.* Lake Forest, Ill.: Learning Opportunities Program, Barat College, 1990.

Silver, L. *ADHD: Attention Deficit-Hyperactivity Disorder, Booklet for Teachers.* Summit, N.J.: CIBA-GEIGY, 1989.

Smith, S. *Success Against the Odds: Strategies and Insights from the Learning Disabled.* Los Angeles: Jeremy Tarcher, 1991.

RELATED PAMPHLETS AVAILABLE FROM THE NATIONAL INSTITUTES OF HEALTH

Facts about Dyslexia
National Institute of Child Health and Human Development
Building 31, Room 2A32
9000 Rockville Pike
Bethesda, MD 20892
(301) 496-5133

Developmental Speech and Language Disorders—Hope through Research
National Institute on Deafness and Other Communicative Disorders
P.O. Box 37777
Washington, DC 20013; (800) 241-1044

GLOSSARY

abstraction The ability to relate ideas or understand concepts at a higher level than the literal or concrete meaning.

adaptive physical education A special physical education program developed to fit the limits and disabilities of persons with handicaps.

afferent Movement of impulses toward the brain.

amphetamines A group of drugs used to stimulate the cerebral cortex of the brain that are sometimes used to treat hyperactivity.

anosmia Absense of sense of smell.

articulation The production of speech sounds resulting from the movements of the lips, jaw, and tongue as they modify air flow.

association Ability to relate concepts presented through the senses (visual, auditory, tactile, or kinesthetic).

basal ganglia Size of brain where extrapyramidal system originates; includes caudate nucleus, globus pallidus, and putamen; thalamus, subthalamus, substantia nigra, and red nucleus sometimes included.

basic skill area Subjects such as reading, writing, spelling, mathematics.

bilateral Refers to using both sides of the body or the arms or leg (extremities) on both sides of the body.

body image The concept and awareness of a person's own body as it relates to space, movement, and other objects.

brain stem Composed of midbrain, pons, and medulla; contains reticular activating system and other key centers.

cognition The process of recognizing, interpreting, judging, reasoning, and knowing. Perception is considered a part of cognition by some psychologists, but not by others.

cognitive The process of knowing in the broadest sense, including perception, memory, and judgment.

cognitive ability Intellectual ability; thinking and reasoning skills.

cognitive deficit A perceptual, memory, or conceptual problem that interferes with learning.

cognitive retraining Developing or relearning the processes involved in thinking.

cognitive style A person's typical approach to learning activities and problem solving.

compensation The process by which a person is taught how to cope with learning problems by focusing on personal strengths, and how to work around abilities that may be weak.

conceptualization The process of forming a general idea from what is observed, such as seeing peas, beans and tomatoes and recognizing that they are all vegetables.

conceptual disorder Disturbances in thinking, reasoning, generalizing, or memorizing.

confidential file A file maintained by the school that contains evaluations of whether a child is handicapped, as well as any other information related to special education placement. Parents have the right to inspect the file and have copies of any information contained in it.

configuration The visual shape or form of words; may be used as a cue in word-attack skills.

congenital A condition existing at birth or before birth but that does not imply an inherited problem.

coordination The harmonious functioning of muscles in the body to perform complex movements.

coping skills The ability to deal with problems and difficulties by attempting to overcome them or accept them.

cross-categorical   A system in which a teacher addresses more than one handicapping condition within one instructional period.

cross dominance   A condition also known as mixed dominance in which the preferred eye, hand, or foot are not on the same side of the body. For example, a child may be right-footed but left-handed.

cumulative file   A general file maintained by a school for every student. Parents have a right to inspect the file and have copies of any information contained in it.

decoding   The process of getting meaning from written or spoken symbols.

developmental lag   A delay in some aspect of physical or mental development.

directionality   The ability to know right from left, up from down, forward from backward, and direction and orientation.

discrimination   The ability to discern fine differences among stimuli, whether visual, auditory, tactile, and so on.

disinhibition   A lack of restraint in responding to a situation. A child who is disinhibited reacts impulsively and often inappropriately.

distractibility   Shifting of attention from a task to other stimuli.

echolalia   Repetition of words or phrases.

emotional lability   Exhibiting rapid and drastic changes in emotions (such as laughing, crying, anger) without apparent reason.

frustration tolerance   The ability to deal with frustrating events in daily life without becoming angry or aggressive.

insertions   The addition of letters or numbers that do not belong in a word or numeral, such as "wheare" for "where."

inversions   Mistakes in reading, spelling, or math that involve confusion of up-down directionality of letters or numbers, such as *m* for *w* or *6* for *9*.

itinerant teacher   A special education teacher who is shared by more than one school.

kinesthetic   Pertaining to the muscles.

kinesthetic method   A way of teaching words by using the muscles. For example, a student might trace a word with a finger in sand while saying aloud the word or its letters.

laterality   The tendency to use the hand, foot, eye, and ear on the left or right side of the body.

motor   Term that refers to the origin or execution of muscular activity.

perseveration   Repeating words, motions, or tasks. A child who perseverates often has trouble shifting from one task to another, and continues working on an old task long after classmates have moved on.

prefrontal area   Brain location of processes of foresight, abstract thinking, and judgment.

premorbid   A term to describe the patient's condition before an injury.

psychomotor   A term that relates to the motor effects of psychological processes. Psychomotor tests are tests of motor skill which depend upon sensory or perceptual motor coordination.

readiness   The acquisition of skills considered prerequisite for academic learning.

registration   A very brief sensory/memory function by which information enters the memory system. It is then entered into short-term memory or decays and is lost. Registration is very resistant to impairments.

reversals   Trouble in reading or reproducing letters by themselves, letters as contained in words, or words in sentences in their proper order. The term also may refer to a reversal of mathematical concepts (adding for subtracting, or multiplying for dividing).

sensorimotor   The relationship between sensation and movement.

strabismus   Weakness of eye muscles allowing eyes to cross.

subdural   Beneath the tough membrane (dura) covering the brain and spinal cord.

syntax   Grammar, sentence structure, and word order in oral or written language.

syndrome   A set of symptoms that indicates a specific disorder.

tactile   The ability to receive and interpret stimuli through contact with the skin.

unilateral   Pertaining to only one side.

ventricles   Four natural cavities in the brain that are filled with cerebrospinal fluid

BIBLIOGRAPHY

Agner, K. D. "Diagnosis and treatment of Bipolar Disorder in Children and Adolescents," *Journal of Clinical Psychiatry* 65 Suppl 15 (2004): 30–34.

Ahn, M. S., and J. A. Frazier. "Diagnostic and Treatment Issues in Childhood-Onset Bipolar Disorder," *Essential Psychopharmacology* 6, no. 1 (2004): 25–44.

Akshoomoff, N. K., and E. Courchesne Pierce. "The Neurobiological Basis of Autism from a Developmental Perspective," *Development and Psychopathology* 14 (2002): 613–634.

Alerian, A. J. "Use of Selective Serotonin Reuptake Inhibitors in Childhood Depression," *Lancet* 364, no. 9435 (August 2004): 660–661.

Aman, M. G. "Management of Hyperactivity and Other Acting-Out Problems in Patients with Autism Spectrum Disorder," *Semin Pediatric Neurology* 11, no. 3 (September 2004): 225–228.

American Academy of Pediatrics. "The Pediatrician's Role in the Diagnosis and Management of Autistic Spectrum Disorder in Children," *Pediatrics* 107 (2001): 1,221–1,226.

American Educational Research Association, American Psychological Association, and National Council on Measurement in Education. *Standards for Educational and Psychological Testing.* Washington, D.C.: American Psychological Association, 1999.

American Academy of Pediatrics Committee on Children with Disabilities. "The Pediatrician's Role in the Diagnosis and Management of Autistic Spectrum Disorder in Children," *Pediatrics* 107, no. 5 (2001): 1,221–1,226.

American Psychiatric Association. *Diagnostic and Statistical Manual of Mental Disorders—Fourth Edition, Text Revision: DSM-IV-TR.* Washington, D.C.: American Psychiatric Association, 2000.

Anderson, Elizabeth, and Pauline Emmons. *Unlocking the Mysteries of Sensory Dysfunction.* Arlington, Tex.: Future Horizons, 1996.

Anderson, M. "Annotation: Conceptions of Intelligence," *Journal of Child Psychology and Psychiatry* 42, no. 3 (March 2001): 287–298.

Armstrong, Thomas. *The Myth of the A.D.D. Child: 50 Ways to Improve Your Child's Behavior and Attention Span without Drugs, Labels, or Coercion.* New York: Plume, 1997.

Arnold, L. E. "Treatment Alternatives for Attention-Deficit/Hyperactivity Disorder," in P. J. Jensen, and J. Cooper, eds. *Attention-Deficit/ Hyperactivity Disorder: State of the Science and Best Practices.* Kingston, N.J.: Civic Research Institute, 2002.

Autism Society of America. "Biomedical and Dietary Treatments" (Fact sheet). Bethesda, Md.: Autism Society of America. Available online. URL: http://www.autism-society.org/site/PageServer?pagename=BiomedicalDietaryTreatments.

Baird, G., T. Charman, S. Baron-Cohen, et al. "A Screening Instrument for Autism at 18 Months of Age: A 6-Year Follow-up Study," *Journal of the American Academy of Child and Adolescent Psychiatry* 39 (2000): 694–702.

Ball, S., et al. "Early Screening for Dyslexia—A Collaborative Pilot Project," *International Journal of Language and Communication* Disorders 36 (2001): 75–76.

Barkley, R. A. *Attention Deficit Hyperactivity Disorder: A Handbook for Diagnosis and Treatment.* 2nd ed. New York: Guilford Press, 1998.

———. *Taking Charge of ADHD: The Complete, Authoritative Guide for Parents.* New York: Guilford Press, 2000.

Batshaw, Mark L., and Yvonne Perret. *Children with Disabilities: A Medical Primer.* Atlanta: Paul L. Brookes, 1992.

Baumgaertel, A. "Alternative and Controversial Treatments for Attention-Deficit/Hyperactivity Disorder," *Pediatric Clinics of North America* 46 (1999): 977–992.

Behrmann, M., et al. "The Eye Movements of Pure Alexic Patients during Reading and Nonreading Tasks," *Neuropsychologia* 39, no. 9 (2001): 983–1,002.

Berenbaum, S. A. "Cognitive Function in Congenital Adrenal Hyperplasia," *Endocrinology and Metabolism Clinics of North America* 30, no. 1 (March 2001): 173–192.

Berument, S. K., M. Rutter, C. Lord, A. Pickles, and A. Bailey. "Autism Screening Questionnaire: Diagnostic Validity," *British Journal of Psychiatry* 175 (1999): 444–451.

Birmaher, B., N. D. Ryan, D. E. Williamson, et al. "Childhood and Adolescent Depression: A Review of the Past 10 Years. Part 1," *Journal of the American Academy of Child and Adolescent Psychiatry* 35, no. 11 (1996): 1,427–1,439.

Bishop, D. V. "Genetic Influences on Language Impairment and Literacy Problems in Children: Same or Different?" *Journal of Child Psychology and Psychiatry* 42, no. 2 (February 2001): 189–198.

Block, Mary Ann. *No More Ritalin: Treating ADHD without Drugs.* New York: Kensington Publishing Co., 1997.

Boone, K. B., et al. "Neuropsychological Profiles of Adults with Klinefelter Syndrome," *Journal of the International Neuropsychological Society* 7, no. 4 (May 2001): 446–456.

Bos, Candace S., and Sharon Vaughn. *Strategies for Teaching Students with Learning and Behavior Problems.* Needham Heights, Mass.: Allyn & Bacon, 1997.

Boyles, Nancy S., and Darlene Contadino. *Parenting a Child with Attention Deficit Hyperactivity Disorder.* Los Angeles: Lowell House, 1996.

———. *The Learning Differences Sourcebook.* New York: NTC Contemporary, 1998.

Bradley, W., et al., eds. *Neurology in Clinical Practice: Principles of Diagnosis and Management.* Vol. 1. 2nd ed. Boston: Butterworth-Heinemann, 1996.

Brent, D. A., M. Oquendo, B. Birmaher, et al. "Familial Transmission of Mood Disorders: Convergence and Divergence with Transmission of Suicidal Behavior," *Journal of the American Academy of Child & Adolescent Psychiatry* 43, no. 10 (October 2004): 1,259–1,266.

Brent D. A. "Antidepressants and Pediatric Depression—The Risk of Doing Nothing," *New England Journal of Medicine* 14, no. 351 (October 2004): 1,598–1,601.

Briskman, J., F. Happe, and U. Frith. "Exploring the Cognitive Phenotype of Autism: Weak 'Central Coherence' in Parents and Siblings of Children with Autism: II. Real-Life Skills and Preferences," *Journal of Child Psychology and Psychiatry* 42, no. 3 (March 2001): 309–316.

Brook, U., and D. Geva. "Knowledge and Attitudes of High School Pupils Towards Peers' Attention Deficit and Learning Disabilities," *Patient Education and Counseling* 43, no. 1 (April 2001): 31–36.

Brown, J., P. Cohen, J. G. Johnson, et al. "Childhood Abuse and Neglect: Specificity of Effects on Adolescent and Young Adult Depression and Suicidality," *Journal of the American Academy of Child and Adolescent Psychiatry* 38, no. 12 (1999): 1,490–1,496.

Brown, W. E., et al. "Preliminary Evidence of Widespread Morphological Variations of the Brain in Dyslexia," *Neurology* 56, no. 6 (March 27, 2001): 781–783.

Burke, Jeffrey D., R. Loeber, and B. Birmaher. "Oppositional Defiant Disorder and Conduct Disorder: A Review of the Past 10 Years. Part II," *Journal of the American Academy of Child and Adolescent Psychiatry* 41, no. 11 (November 2002): 1,275–1,293.

Butler, F. M., et al. "Teaching Mathematics to Students with Mild-to-Moderate Mental Retardation: A Review of the Literature," *Mental Retardation* 39, no. 1 (February 2001): 20–31.

Butterworth, B., M. Cappelletti, and M. Kopelman. "Category Specificity in Reading and Writing: The Case of Number Words," *Nature Neuroscience* 4, no. 8 (August 2001): 784–786.

Cahall, Jeanne S. *Stages of Reading Development.* 2nd ed. New York: Harcourt Brace, 1996.

Campbell, Linda. *Teaching and Learning through Multiple Intelligences.* Needham Heights, Mass.: Allyn & Bacon, 1996.

Catts, H. "Estimating the Risk of Future Reading Difficulties in Kindergarten Children: A Research-Based Model and Its Clinical Implementation," *Language Speech and Hearing Services in Schools* 32 (2001): 38–50.

———. "The Relationship Between Speech-Language Impairments and Reading Disabilities," *Journal of Speech & Hearing Research* 36, no. 5 (1993): 948–958.

Chabot, R. J., and G. Serfontein. "Quantitative Electroencephalographic Profiles of Children with Attention Deficit Disorder," *Biological Psychiatry* 40 (1996): 951–963.

Chabot, R. J., F. di Michele, L. Prichep, and E. R. John. "The Clinical Role of Computerized EEG in the Evaluation and Treatment of Learning and Attention Disorders in Children and Adolescents," *Journal of Neuropsychiatry and Clinical Neuroscience* 13, no. 2 (Spring 2001): 171–186. Review.

CHADD. "Children and Adults with Attention-Deficit/Hyperactivity Disorder," Fact Sheet #5. Available online. URL: http://www.chadd.org/fs/fs5.htm.

Comings, David E. *Tourette Syndrome and Human Behavior.* Duarte, Calif.: Hope Press, 1990.

Committee for Education and the Workforce. "Final IDEA Bill." Available online. URL: http://edworkforce.house.gov/issues/108th/education/idea/conferencereport/confrept.htm. Downloaded April 2005.

Committee on Children with Disabilities, American Academy of Pediatrics. "Technical Report: The Pediatrician's Role in the Diagnosis and Management of Autistic Spectrum Disorder in Children," *Pediatrics* 107, no. 5 (2001): 1–18.

Como, P. G. "Neuropsychological Function in Tourette Syndrome," *Advances in Neurology* 85 (2001): 103–111.

Connor, D. F., and R. J. Steingard. "New Formulations of Stimulants for Attention-Deficit Hyperactivity Disorder: Therapeutic Potential," *CNS Drugs* 18, no. 14 (2004): 1,011–1,030.

Council for Exceptional Children. Summary of Significant Issues in IDEA 2004. Available online. URL: http://www.cec.sped.org/pp/IDEA_120204.pdf. Accessed May 31, 2005.

Courchesne E., R. Carper, and N. Akshoomoff. "Evidence of Brain Overgrowth in the First Year of Life in Autism," *Journal of the American Medical Association* 290, no. 3 (2003): 337–344.

Daly, E., E. J. MacDermott, and A. Green. "Diagnostic Review of 66 Children with Learning Disability Attending a Single Center," *Irish Medical Journal* 94, no. 6 (June 2001): 184–185.

Davis, B., D. Krug, and R. S. Dean. "Neuropsychological Clusters within Intelligence Levels for Learning Disabled Children," *International Journal of Neuroscience* 106, nos. 3–4 (2001): 239–251.

Davis, Ronald D., and Eldon M. Braun. *The Gift of Dyslexia: Why Some of the Smartest People Can't Read and How They Can Learn.* New York: Perigee, 1997.

Dery, M., J. Toupin, R. Pauze, and P. Verlaan. "Frequency of Mental Health Disorders in a Sample of Elementary School Students Receiving Special Educational Services for Behavioural Difficulties," *Canadian Journal of Psychiatry* 49, no. 11 (November 2004): 769–775.

Doyle, A. E., et al. "Separating Attention Deficit Hyperactivity Disorder and Learning Disabilities in Girls: A Familial Risk Analysis," *American Journal of Psychiatry* 158, no. 10 (October 2001): 1,666–1,672.

Dugdale, A. "Rationale for Psychostimulants in ADHD," *British Medical Journal* 8, no. 330 (January 2005): 95.

Education Commission of the States. "Policy Brief on Early Childhood Assessment." Available online. URL: http://64.233.187.104/search?q=cache:5fkbudDJJykJ:www.ecs.org/clearinghouse/43/19/4319.doc+early+childhood+assessment&hl=en&ie=UTF-8. Posted March 2003.

Ehlers, S., C. Gillberg, and L. Wing. "A Screening Questionnaire for Asperger Syndrome and Other High-Functioning Autism Spectrum Disorders in School-Age Children," *Journal of Autism and Developmental Disorders* 29, no. 2 (1999): 129–141.

Eli Lilly. "Strattera." Available online. URL: http://www.strattera.com.

———. "Lilly Announces Important Liver Safety Update to Strattera Label." Available online. URL: http://newsroom.lilly.com/ReleaseDetail.cfm?ReleaseID=150719. Posted December 17, 2004

El-Sayed, E., J. O. Larsson, H. E. Persson, et. al. "Altered Cortical Activity in Children with Attention-Deficit/Hyperactivity Disorder during Attentional Load Task," *Journal of the American Academy of Child and Adolescent Psychiatry* 41 (2002): 811–819.

Ewing-Cobbs, L., J. M. Fletcher, and H. S. Levin. "Traumatic Brain Injury," in B. P. Rourke, ed. *Syndrome of Nonverbal Learning Disabilities: Neurodevelopmental Manifestations.* New York: Guilford Press, 1995, pp. 433–459.

Food and Drug Administration. "Strattera." Available online. URL: http://www.fda.gov/cder/consumerinfo/druginfo/strattera.HTM. Posted March 6, 2003.

Filipek, P. A., P. J. Accardo, G. T. Baranek, et al. "The Screening and Diagnosis of Autism Spectrum Disorders," *Journal of Autism and Developmental Disorders* 29, no. 2 (1999): 439–484.

Filipek, P. A., P. J. Accardo, S. Ashwal, et al. "Practice Parameter: Screening and Diagnosis of Autism," *Neurology* 55 (2000): 468–479.

Fischman, J. "New Reading Programs Spell Help for Frustrated Kids," *U.S. News & World Reports* 16, no. 130 (April 16, 2001): 48–50.

Flanagan, O., and S. O. Nuallain. "A Study Looking at the Effectiveness of Developmental Screening in Identifying Learning Disabilities in Early Childhood," *Irish Medical Journal* 95, no. 5 (May 2001): 148–150.

Foley, D. L., A. Pickles, H. M. Maes, et al., "Course and Short-term Outcomes of Separation Anxiety Disorder in a Community Sample of Twins," *Journal of the American Academy of Child and Adolescent Psychiatry* 43, no. 9 (September 2004): 1,107–1,114.

Fuchs, T., N. Birbaumer, W. Lutzenberger, J. H. Gruzelier, et al. "Neurofeedback Treatment for Attention-Deficit/Hyperactivity Disorder in Children: A Comparison with Methylphenidate," *Applied Psychophysiology and Biofeedback* 28 (2003): 1–12.

Gaddes, William H., and Dorothy Edgell. *Learning Disabilities and Brain Function: A Neuropsychological Approach.* New York: Springer-Verlag, 1994.

Gardener, Howard. *Multiple Intelligences.* New York: Basic Books, 1993.

———. *Leading Minds: Anatomy of Success.* New York: Basic Books, 1995.

Gates, B., R. Newell, and J. Wray. "Behavior Modification and Gentle Teaching Workshops: Management of Children with Learning Disabilities Exhibiting Challenging Behaviour and Implications for Learning Disability Nursing," *Journal of Advanced Nursing* 34, no. 1 (April 2001): 86–95.

Goldman, L. R., and S. H. Koduru. "Chemicals in the Environment and Developmental Toxicity to Children: A Public Health and Policy Perspective," *Environmental Health Research* 108, Supplement 3 (2000): 443–448.

Goodley, D., and M. Rapley. "How Do You Understand 'Learning Difficulties'? Towards a Social Theory of Impairment," *Mental Retardation* 39, no. 3 (June 2001): 229–232.

Gross, D., L. Fogg, C. Garvey, and W. Julion. "Behavior Problems in Young Children: An Analysis of Cross-Informant Agreements and Disagreements," *Resident Nursing Health* 27, no. 6 (December 2004): 413–425.

Gross-Tsur, V., et al. "Cognition, Attention, and Behavior in Prader-Willi Syndrome," *Journal of Child Neurology* 16, no. 4 (April 2001): 288–290.

Hagberg, B. A. "Rett Syndrome: Clinical Peculiarities, Diagnostic Approach, and Possible Cause," *Pediatric Neurology* 5, no. 2 (1989): 75–83.

Hall, D. A., G. W. Humphreys, and A. C. Cooper. "Neuropsychological Evidence for Case-Specific Reading: Multi-Letter Units in Visual Word Recognition," *The Quarterly Journal of Experimental Psychology* 54, no. 2 (May 2001): 439–467.

Hallowell, Edward M., and John J. Ratey. *Driven to Distraction: Recognizing and Coping with Attention Deficit Disorder from Childhood through Adulthood.* New York: Simon & Schuster, 1995.

Harnadek, M. C. S., and B. P. Rourke. "Principal Identifying Features of the Syndrome of Nonverbal Learning Disabilities in Children," *Journal of Learning Disabilities* 27 (1994): 54.

Hasselbring, T. S., and C. H. Glaser. "Use of Computer Technology to Help Students with Special Needs," *Future Child* 10, no. 2 (Winter 2000): 102–122.

Hayes, D. "Recent Developments in Antidepressant Therapy in Special Populations," *American Journal of Managed Care* 10, no. 6 (July 2004): S179–S185.

Hviid, A., M. Stellfeld, J. Wohlfahrt, and M. Melbye. "Association between Thimerosal-Containing Vaccine and Autism," *Journal of the American Medical Association* 290, no. 13 (2003): 1,763–1,766.

Izard, C., et al. "Emotion Knowledge as a Predictor of Social Behavior and Academic Competence in Children at Risk," *Psychological Science* 12, no. 1 (January 2001): 18–23.

Jenkins, R. "Use of Psychotropic Medication in People with a Learning Disability," *British Journal of Nursing* 9, no. 13 (July 13–26, 2001): 844–850.

Kamhi, A. G., M. M. Allen, and H. W. Catts. "The Role of the Speech-Language Pathologist in Improving Decoding Skills," *Seminars in Speech and Language* 22, no. 3 (2001): 175–184.

Kelly, Kate, and Peggy Ramundo. *You Mean I'm Not Lazy, Stupid or Crazy?! A Self-Help Book for Adults with Attention Deficit Disorder.* New York: Fireside, 1996.

Kher, U. "Deconstructing Dyslexia. Blame It on the Written Word," *Time* (March 26, 2001), p. 56.

Kirkendall, D. T., S. E. Jordan, and W. E. Garrett. "Heading and Head Injuries in Soccer," *Sports Medicine* 31, no. 5 (2001): 369–386.

Klein, D. F. "SSRIs in Children and Suicide," *Science* 305, no. 5689 (September 3, 2004): 1,401.

Klin, A., Sparrow, et al. "Asperger Syndrome," in B. P. Rourke, ed. *Syndrome of Nonverbal Learning Disabilities: Neurodevelopmental Manifestations.* New York: Guilford Press, 1995.

Korvatska E., J. Van de Water, T. F. Anders, and M. E. Gershwin. "Genetic and Immunologic Considerations in Autism," *Neurobiology of Disease* 9 (2002): 107–125.

Kranowitz, Carol Stock. *The Out-of-Sync Child: Recognizing and Coping With Sensory Integration Dysfunction.* New York: Perigee, 1998.

Kratochvil, C. J., L. L. Greenhill, J. S. March, et al. "The Role of Stimulants in the Treatment of Preschool Children with Attention-Deficit Hyperactivity Disorder," *CNS Drugs* 18, no. 14 (2004): 957–966.

Kurtz, S. M. "Treating ADHD in Schools," *School Nurse News* 21, no. 5 (November 2004): 29–33.

Laforce, R., Jr., S. Hayward, L. V. Cox. "Impaired Skill Learning in Children with Heavy Prenatal Alcohol Exposure," *Journal of the International Neuropsychology Society* 7, no. 1 (2001): 112–114.

Lannetti, D. W. "Extending Coverage of the Americans with Disabilities Act to Individuals with Attention Deficit Hyperactivity Disorder: A Demonstration of Inadequate Legislative Guidance," *Tort & Insurance Law Journal* 35, no. 1 (Fall 1999): 155–173.

Law, J. "Prevalence and Natural History of Primary Speech and Language Delay: Findings from a Systematic Review of the Literature," *International Journal of Language & Communication Disorders* 35 (2000): 150–188.

Lerner, J. W. *Learning Disabilities: Theories, Diagnosis, and Teaching Strategies.* 8th ed. Boston, Mass.: Houghton Mifflin, 2002.

Levelt, W. J. "Defining Dyslexia," *Science* 292, no. 5520 (May 2001): 1,300–1,301.

Lewinsohn, P. M., D. N. Klein, and J. R. Seely. "Bipolar Disorders in a Community Sample of Older Adolescents: Prevalence, Phenomenology, Comorbidity, and Course," *Journal of the American Academy of Child and Adolescent Psychiatry* 34, no. 4 (1995): 454–463.

Lewinsohn, P. M., P. Rohde, and J. R. Seely. "Major Depressive Disorder in Older Adolescents: Prevalence, Risk factors, and Clinical Implications," *Clinical Psychology Review* 18, no. 7 (1998): 765–794.

Little, L. "Peer Victimization of Children with Asperger Spectrum Disorders," *Journal of the American Academy of Child and Adolescent Psychiatry* 40, no. 9 (September 2001): 995–996.

Loeber, R., J. Burke, B. Lahey, et al. "Oppositional Defiant and Conduct Disorder: A Review of the Past 10 Years, Part I," *Journal of the American Academy of Child and Adolescent Psychiatry* 39, no. 12 (December 2000): 1,468–1,484.

Loo, S. K. "EEG and Neurofeedback Findings in ADHD," *ADHD Report* 11 (2003): 1–6.

Loo, S. K., C. Hopfer, P. D. Teale, and M. L. Reite. "EEG Correlates of Methylphenidate Response in ADHD: Association with Cognitive and Behavioral Measures," *Journal of Clinical Neurophysiology* 21, no. 6 (November–December 2004): 457–464.

Lord, C., S. Risi, L. Lambrecht, et al. "The Autism Diagnostic Observation Schedule-Generic: A Standard Measure of Social and Communication Deficits Associated with the Spectrum of Autism," *Journal of Autism and Developmental Disorders* 30, no. 3 (2000): 205–230.

Louters, L. L. "Don't Overlook Childhood Depression," *Journal of the American Academy of Physicians' Assistants* 17, no. 9 (September 2004): 18–24.

Lovaas, O. I. "Behavioral Treatment and Normal Educational and Intellectual Functioning in Young Autistic Children," *Journal of Consulting and Clinical Psychology* 55 (1987): 3–9.

Malhotra, S., and N. Gupta. "Childhood Disintegrative Disorder," *Journal of Autism and Developmental Disorders* 29, no. 6 (1999): 491–498.

Martin, C. S., C. J. Romig, and L. Kirisci. "DSM-IV Learning Disorders in 10- to 12-Year-Old Boys with and without a Parental History of Substance Use Disorders," *Prevention Science* 1, no. 2 (June 2000): 107–113.

Mather, D. S. "Does Dyslexia Develop from Learning the Alphabet in the Wrong Hemisphere? A Cognitive Neuroscience Analysis," *Brain Language* 76, no. 3 (March 2001): 282–316.

McArthur, G. M., and J. H. Hogben. "Auditory Backward Recognition Masking in Children with a Specific Language Impairment and Children with a Specific Reading Disability," *Journal of the Acoustical Society of America* 109, no. 3 (March 2001): 1,092–1,100.

McCann, B. S., and P. Roy-Byrne. "Attention-Deficit/Hyperactivity Disorder and Learning Disabilities in Adults," *Seminars in Clinical Neuropsychiatry* 5, no. 3 (July 2000): 191–197.

McDougle, C. J., K. A. Stigler, and D. J. Posey. "Treatment of Aggression in Children and Adolescents with Autism and Conduct Disorder," *Journal of Clinical Psychiatry* 64, Supplement 4 (2003): 16–25.

McDougle, C. J. "Methylphenidate an Effective Treatment for ADHD?" *Journal of Autism and Developmental Disorders* 34, no. 5 (October 2004): 593–594.

McEachin, J. J., T. Smith, and O. I. Lovaas. "Long-term Outcome for Children with Autism Who Received Early Intensive Behavioral Treatment," *American Journal on Mental Retardation* 97 (1993): 359–372.

Mercer, C. D., and A. R. Mercer. *Teaching Students with Learning Problems.* 6th ed. New York: Prentice Hall College, 2001.

Merikangas, K. R., and N. C. Low. "The Epidemiology of Mood Disorders," *Current Psychiatry Reports* 6, no. 6 (December 2004): 411–421.

Monastra, V. J., D. M. Monastra, and S. George. "The Effects of Stimulant Therapy, EEG Biofeedback and Parenting Style on the Primary Symptoms of Attention-Deficit/Hyperactivity Disorder," *Applied Psychophysiology and Biofeedback* 27 (2001): 231–249.

Monroe, S. M., P. Rohde, J. R. Seeley, et al. "Life Events and Depression in Adolescence: Relationship Loss as a Prospective Risk Factor for First Onset of Major Depressive Disorder," *Journal of Abnormal Psychology* 108, no. 4 (1999): 606–614.

Mooney, Jonathan, and David Cole. *Learning Outside the Lines: Two Ivy League Students with Learning Disabilities and ADHD Give You the Tools for Academic Success and Educational Revolution.* New York: Simon & Schuster, 2000.

Motsch, S., and H. Muhlendyck. "Frequency of Reading Disability Caused by Ocular Problems in 9- and 10-Year-Old Children in a Small Town," *Strabismus* 8, no. 4 (December 2000): 283–285.

MTA Cooperative Group. "A 14-month Randomized Clinical Trial of Treatment Strategies for Attention Deficit Hyperactivity Disorder," *Archives of General Psychiatry* 56, no. 12 (1999).

Mulrine, A. "Are Boys the Weaker Sex?" *U.S. News & World Reports* 131, no. 4 (July 30, 2001): 40–47.

Murphy, Kevin R., and Suzanne Levert. *Out of the Fog: Treatment Options and Coping Strategies for Adult Attention Deficit Disorder.* New York: Hyperion, 1995.

Murray, M. L., C. S. de Vries, and I. C. Wong. "A Drug Utilisation Study of Antidepressants in Children and Adolescents Using the General Practice Research Database," *Archives of Disease in Childhood* 89, no. 12 (December 2004): 1,098–1,102.

Nagle, R. J. "Issues in Preschool Assessment," in B. Bracken, ed., *The Psychoeducational Assessment of Preschool Children.* Boston: Allyn and Bacon, 2000.

National Association of School Psychologists. "IDEA information." Available online. URL: http://www.nasponline.org/advocacy/IDEAinformation.html. Accessed May 31, 2005.

———. "NASP's Legislative Updates." Available online. URL: http://nasponline.org/advocacy/index.html#legupdates. Accessed May 31, 2005.

———. "U.S. Senate Report 108-105." Available online. URL: http://www.nasponline.org/advocacy/IDEACommittee.pdf. Accessed May 31, 2005.

———. "U.S. House of Representatives Committee Report 108-77: "Improving Education Results for Children with Disabilities Act of 2003." Available online. URL: http://www.nasponline.

org/advocacy/IDEAHouseReport.pdf. Accessed May 31, 2005.

National Dissemination Center for Children with Disabilities. "Asperger's Disorder." Available online. URL: http://www.nichcy.org/resources/asperger.asp. Posted April 1, 2004.

———. "Autistic Disorder." Available online. URL: http://www.nichcy.org/resources/autism.asp. Posted April 1, 2004.

———. "Childhood Disintegrative Disorder." Available online. URL: http://www.nichcy.org/resources/disintegrative.asp." Posted April 2, 2004.

———. "PDD-NOS." Available online. URL: http://www.nichcy.org/resources/pddnos.asp. Posted April 1, 2004.

National Mental Health Association. "Children's Mental Health Statistics." Available online. URL: http://www.nmha.org/children/prevent/stats.cfm.

Neville, B. G. "Mental Health Services for People with Learning Disabilities. Medical Needs Are Important Too," *British Medical Journal* 322, no. 7281 (February 3, 2001): 302.

Newman, T. B. "A Black-Box Warning for Antidepressants in Children?" *New England Journal of Medicine* 351, no. 16 (October 14, 2004): 1,595–1,598.

Nyden, A., et al. "Neurocognitive Stability in Asperger Syndrome, ADHD, and Reading and Writing Disorder: A Pilot Study," *Developmental Medical Child Neurology* 43, no. 3 (March 2001): 165–171.

Paulesu, E., et al. "Dyslexia: Cultural Diversity and Biological Unity," *Science* 291, no. 5511 (March 16, 2000): 2,165–2,167.

Pelham, W. E., T. Wheeler, and A. Chronis. "Empirically Supported Psychosocial Treatments for Attention Deficit Hyperactivity Disorder," *Journal of Clinical Child Psychology* 27 (1998): 190–205.

Pelletier, P. M., S. A. Ahmad, and B. P. Rourke. "Classification Rules for Basic Phonological Processing Disabilities and Nonverbal Learning Disabilities: Formulation and External Validity," *Child Neuropsychology* 7 (2001): 84–98.

Pennington, B. F. *Diagnosing Learning Disorders: A Neuropsychological Framework.* New York: Guilford Press, 1991.

———. *The Development of Psychopathology: Nature and Nurture.* New York: Guilford Press, 2002.

Petti, V. L., S. L. Voelker, D. L. Shore, and S. E. Hayman-Abello. "Perception of Nonverbal Emotion Cues by Children with Nonverbal Learning Disabilities," *Journal of Developmental and Physical Disabilities* 15 (2003): 23–26.

Percy, A. K. "Research in Rett Syndrome: Past, Present, and Future," *Journal of Child Neurology* 3 (1988): 572–575.

President's Commission on Excellence in Special Education. "A New Era: Revitalizing Special Education for Children and Their Families." Available online. URL: http://www.ed.gov/inits/commissionsboards/whspecialeducation/reports/index.html.

Powers, M. D., ed. *Children with Autism: A Parent's Guide, Second Edition.* Bethesda, Md.: Woodbine House, 2000.

Ramus, F. "Dyslexia. Talk of Two Theories," *Nature* 412, no. 6845 (July 26, 2001): 393–395.

Rashid, F. L., M. K. Morris, and R. Morris. "Naming and Verbal Memory Skills in Adults with Attention Deficit Hyperactivity Disorder and Reading Disability," *Journal of Clinical Psychology* 57, no. 6 (June 2001): 829–838.

Research Units on Pediatric Psychopharmacology Network. "Risperidone in Children with Autism and Serious Behavioral Problems," *New England Journal of Medicine* 347, no. 5 (2002): 314–321.

Richek, M. A., et al. *Reading Problems: Assessment and Teaching Strategies.* Boston: Allyn & Bacon, 2001.

Rickards, H. "An International Perspective on Tourette Syndrome," *Developmental Medical Child Neurology* 43, no. 6 (June 2001): 428–429.

Ricker, J. H., F. G. Hillary, and J. DeLuca. "Functionally Activated Brain Imaging (O-15 PET and fMRI) in the Study of Learning and Memory after Traumatic Brain Injury," *Journal of Head Trauma Rehabilitation* 16, no. 2 (April 2001): 191–205.

Robbins, D. I., D. Fein, M. I. Barton, and J. A. Green. "The Modified Checklist for Autism in Toddlers: An Initial Study Investigating the Early Detection of Autism and Pervasive Developmental Disorders," *Journal of Autism and Developmental Disorders* 31, no. 2 (2001): 149–151.

Rourke, Byron P., ed. *Syndrome of Nonverbal Learning Disabilities.* New York: Guilford Press, 1995.

Russell, J., and E. L. Hill. "Action-Monitoring and Intention Reporting in Children with Autism," *Journal of Child Psychology and Psychiatry* 43, no. 3 (March 2000): 317–328.

Sakurai, Y., Y. Ichikawa, and T. Mannen. "Pure Alexia from a Posterior Occipital Lesion," *Neurology* 58, no. 6 (March 27, 2001): 778–781.

Schaffer, D., P. Fisher, M. K. Dulkan, et al. "The NIMH Diagnostic Interview Schedule for Children Version 2.3 (DISC-2.3): Description, Acceptability, Prevalence Rates and Performance in the MECA Study," *Journal of the American Academy of Child and Adolescent Psychiatry* 35, no. 7 (1996): 865–877.

Smith, Corrine, and Lisa Strick. *Learning Disabilities: A to Z.* New York: Simon & Schuster, 1997.

Snowling, M. J. "From Language to Reading and Dyslexia," *Dyslexia* 7, no. 1 (January–March 2001): 37–46.

Spear-Swerling, L., and R. J. Sternberg. *Off-track: When Poor Readers Become Learning Disabled.* Boulder, Colo.: Westview, 1996.

Spencer, T., J. Biederman, and T. Wilens. "Attention-Deficit/Hyperactivity Disorder and Comorbidity," *Pediatric Clinics of North America* 46, no. 5 (1999): 915–927.

Stein, David B. *Ritalin Is Not the Answer: A Drug-Free, Practical Program for Children Diagnosed With ADD or ADHD.* San Francisco: Jossey-Bass, 1999.

Stein, M. T., M. D. Levine, and M. I. Reiff. "School Underachievement in the Fifth Grade," *Journal of Developmental and Behavioral Pediatrics* 22, no. 2 (April 2001): S117–S121.

Stein, M. T., et al. "A School-Aged Child with Delayed Reading Skills," *Journal of Developmental and Behavioral Pediatrics* 22, no. 2 (April 2001): S111–S115.

Stevens, Laura J., and William G. Crook. *12 Effective Ways to Help Your ADD/ADHD Child: Drug-Free Alternatives for Attention-Deficit Disorders.* New York: Penguin Putnam, 2000.

Stone, W. L., E. E. Coonrod, and O. Y. Ousley. "Brief Report: Screening Tool for Autism in Two-Year-Olds (STAT): Development and Preliminary Data," *Journal of Autism and Developmental Disorders* 30, no. 6 (2000): 607–612.

Strichart, Stephen S., and Charles T. Mangrum II, eds. *Peterson's Colleges With Programs for Students with Learning Disabilities or Attention Deficit Disorders (Peterson's Colleges with Programs for Students).* Boston: Peterson's Guides, 2000.

Sudderth, David, and Joseph Kandel. *Adult ADD: The Complete Handbook: Everything You Need to Know About How to Cope and Live Well with ADD/ADHD.* Roseville, Calif.: Prima, 1997.

Swanson, H. L., and C. Sachse-Lee. "Mathematical Problem Solving and Working Memory in Children with Learning Disabilities: Both Executive and Phonological Processes are Important," *Journal of Experimental Child Psychology* 79, no. 3 (July 2001): 294–321.

Swanson, J. M., and K. McBurnett. "Effect of Stimulant Medication on Children with Attention Deficit Disorder: A review of Reviews," *Exceptional Children* 60 (1993): 154–162.

Tadevosyan-Leyfer, O., M. Dowd, R. Mankoski, B. Winklosky, et al. "A principal components analysis of the autism diagnostic interview-revised," *Journal of the American Academy of Child and Adolescent Psychiatry* 42, no. 7 (2003): 864–872.

Tan, M., and R. Appleton. "Attention Deficit and Hyperactivity Disorder, Methylphenidate, and Epilepsy," *Archives of Disabled Children* 90, no. 1 (January 2005): 57–59.

Taylor, K. E., A. J. Richardson, and J. F. Stein. "Could Platelet Activating Factor Play a Role in Developmental Dyslexia?" *Prostaglandins, Leukotrienes, and Essential Fatty Acids* 64, no. 3 (March 2001): 173–180.

Thompson, S. "Nonverbal Learning Disorders." LDOnline. Available online. URL: http://www.ldonline.org/ld_indepth/general_info/nld.html. Posted 1996.

———. "Nonverbal Learning Disorders Revisited in 1997." LDOnline. Available online. URL: http://www.ldonline.org/ld_indepth/general_info/nld.html. Posted 1997.

Timimi S. "Rethinking Childhood Depression," *British Medical Journal* 329, no. 7479 (December 11, 2004): 1,394–1,396.

Townes, B. D. "Adult Outcome of Verbal Learning Disability: An Optimistic Note," *Seminars in Clinical Neuropsychiatry* 5, no. 3 (July 2000): 210–211.

Turkington, Carol A. *Making the Antidepressant Decision.* New York: McGraw-Hill, 2001.

U.S. Department of Health and Human Services, Substance Abuse and Mental Health Services Administration (SAMHSA) National Mental Health Information Service, Center for Mental Health Services. "Children's Mental Health Facts: Children and Adolescents with Anxiety Disorders." Available online. URL: http://www.mentalhealth.org/publications/allpubs/CA-0007/default.asp.

Vellutino, F. R., J. M. Fletcher, M. J. Snowling, and D. M. Scanlon. "Specific Reading Disability (Dyslexia): What Have We Learned in the Past Four Decades?" *Journal of Child Psychology and Psychiatry* 45, no. 1 (2004): 2–40.

Vicari, S., S. Bellucci, and G. A. Carlesimo. "Procedural Learning Deficit in Children with Williams Syndrome," *Neuropsychologia* 39, no. 7 (2000): 665–677.

Vitiello, B., and P. Jensen. "Medication Development and Testing in Children and Adolescents," *Archives of General Psychiatry* 54 (1997): 871–876.

Volkmar, F. R. "Childhood Disintegrative Disorder: Issues for DSM-IV," *Journal of Autism and Developmental Disorders* 22 (1999): 625–642.

Volkmar, F., A. Klin, W. Marans, and D. Cohen. "Childhood Disintegrative Disorder," in D. Cohen and F. Volkmar, eds., *Handbook of Autism and Pervasive Developmental Disorders.* New York: Wiley, 1997.

Volkmar, F. R., C. Lord, A. Bailey, R. T. Schultz, and A. Klin. "Autism and Pervasive Developmental Disorders," *Journal of Child Psychology and Psychiatry* 45, no. 1 (2004): 135–170.

Weissman, M. M., S. Wolk, R. B. Goldstein, et al. "Depressed Adolescents Grown Up," *Journal of the American Medical Association* 281 (1999): 1,701–1,713.

Willcutt, E. G., et al. "A Comparison of the Cognitive Deficits in Reading Disability and Attention-Deficit/Hyperactivity Disorder," *Journal of Abnormal Psychology* 110, no. 1 (February 2001): 157–172.

Winner, B. J. "Disability and the ADA: Learning Impairment as a Disability," *Journal of Law and Medical Ethics* 28, no. 4 (Winter 2000): 410–411.

Wolf, L. E. "College Students with ADHD and Other Hidden Disabilities, Outcomes and Interventions," *Annals of the New York Academy of Science* 931 (June 2001): 385–395.

Wong, I. C., F. M. Besag, P. J. Santosh, and M. L. Murray. "Use of Selective Serotonin Reuptake Inhibitors in Children and Adolescents," *Drug Safety* 27, no. 13 (2004): 991–1,000.

Zalsman, G., O. Pumeranz, G. Peretz, et. al. "Attention Patterns in Children with Attention Deficit Disorder with or without Hyperactivity," *Scientific World Journal* 3 (November 13, 2003): 1,093–1,107.

Zero to Three. *New Visions for the Developmental Assessment of Infants and Young Children.* Washington, D.C.: Zero to Three, 1996.

Zito, J. M., D. J. Safer, S. dosReis, et al. "Trends in the Prescribing of Psychotropic Medications to Preschoolers," *Journal of the American Medical Association* 283 (2000): 1,025–1,030.

INDEX

A

ability grouping **1**
ability tests **1–2,** 8–9
academic classes **2**
academic skills disorders **2**
acalculia **2–3,** 7, 80, 106
accessibility 3, 9, **233**
accommodations **3–4,** 9, 42, 139, 214
    attention deficit hyperactivity disorder 28–29, 30
    college programs 60, 61, 139
    dyspraxia 84
    nonverbal learning disabilities 166
    Rehabilitation Act of 1973 3, 142, 195–196
    Scholastic Aptitude Test 202
accuracy of tests **4,** 167
achievement **4.** *See also* discrepancy between potential and achievement
achievement tests **4,** 16, 134, 167, 220
    California Achievement Test **55,** 167, 220
    Kaufman Test of Educational Achievement **121**
    Metropolitan Achievement Test **153,** 167, 220
    Stanford Achievement Test 167, 219, **220**
    Wechsler Individual Achievement Test **239,** 246
ACID (arithmetic, coding, information, and digit span) profile **4**
acoustic cortex **4**
active reading **4–5,** 147, 219
active-working memory **149**

adaptive behavior **5–6,** 8, 150, 236
Adderall **74–75,** 221
ADHD Rating Scale 6, 44
Administration on Developmental Disabilities **6**
advocacy skills 203
affect **6**
agnosia **6–7,** 123
    finger **102,** 106, 176
agraphia 3, **7,** 13, 106
alcohol use **7–8**
    and bipolar disorder 45
    fetal exposure 7, 22, 91–92, 100–101, 128, 129, 150
alexia 7, **8**
alternative educational setting, interim **119**
American Association on Mental Retardation adaptive behavior scales 6, **8**
American College Test 1, **8–9,** 14, 61, 219
American Psychological Association 187, 188, 189
Americans with Disabilities Act 5, **9,** 42, 139, 250
    and ability tests 1–2
    accommodations requirements 3, 9, 139
    attention deficit hyperactivity disorder 30
    college admission 59, 60
    Down syndrome 79
amphetamine **74–75,** 221, 277
analogy **9,** 202
anarithmia (acalculia) **2–3,** 7, 80, 106
Angelman syndrome **9–11,** 250
angular gyrus **11**
anomia **11,** 83

anosmia 277
anoxia **11**
antecedent event **11,** 44
anticonvulsant drugs 41, 47–48, 93
antidepressant drugs 41, 47, 72, 102–103
antipsychotic drugs 41, 48
antisocial behavior **11–12,** 66, 67, 172
anxiety **12,** 87, 96, 154, 222
    attention deficit hyperactivity disorder 24, 25
    autistic spectrum disorders 15, 16, 36, 39, 41
    nonverbal learning disabilities 165, 166
    obsessive-compulsive disorder 169
    perfectionism 179
aphasia 7, **13,** 62, 80, 250
    and alexia 8
    anomia 11, 13, 83
    Broca's 13, **52,** 163
    conduction 13, 14
    dysnomia 83
    expressive 52, 97
    fluent 13, **102**
    frontal lobe 13, 104
    global 13, **107**
    Landau-Kleffner syndrome 123
    nonfluent 13, **163**
    Wernicke's 13, 240
aphasoid **13**
aphemia **13**
apraxia **13–14,** 62, 97, 106
    constructional **67**
    and kinesthetic intelligence 159

apraxia *(continued)*
  national organizations
      250–251
  Rett syndrome 198
  speech 13–14, 72, 234–235
aptitude **14**
  and achievement
      discrepancy. *See*
      discrepancy between
      potential and achievement
arcuate fasciculus **14**
arithmetic and mathematics **14,**
    131, 132, **147–148**
  acalculia **2–3,** 7, 80, 106
  assessment 4, 8, 90, 121
  calculations 14, 132
  developmental disorder 2,
      72, 132, 133
  dyscalculia 2, 14, 72, **80–81,**
      106, 128, 176
  logical intelligence 159
  problem solving 186
  reasoning 14, 132
arousal **14,** 20
articulation **14–15,** 217, 277
  communication disorder 62,
      63
  developmental disorder 62,
      72, 132, 138
      expressive language 73
      speech and language 74
Asperger's syndrome **15–16,** 38,
    179, 180, 198, 251
assessment **16–17, 94–95,**
    134–135, 137
  accuracy of tests **4,** 167
  behavioral rating scales. *See*
      behavioral rating scales
  bias 45, 95, 167
  criterion-referenced tests
      69–70, 168, 219
  diagnostic tests 75, 76
  differential diagnosis 76
  early childhood **85**
  educational evaluation **86,**
      113–114
  emotional and behavioral
      87–88, 89
  error analysis **94**

family history **99**
grade equivalent scores **107**
holistic **111**
intelligence tests. *See*
    intelligence tests
minimum competency
    testing **155**
miscue analysis **155**
multicultural **157**
multifactored **158**
needs **161**
neurological **161**
neuropsychological 16, **162**
norm-referenced tests 70,
    166–168, 190, 219–220
outcomes assessment **175**
performance 16, 69–70
personality **179**
portfolio 16–17, **184**
pretests **186**
psychological **187**
readiness **190–191**
reading 191–192
reflex tests **195**
reliability of tests **196**
standardized tests 16, 75,
    219–220
task analysis 227
validity of tests **234**
assistive technology **17–19,** 65,
    135–136, 216
  attention deficit hyperactivity
      disorder 29
  cerebral palsy 57
  resources **269–270, 273**
  screen reader programs 18,
      121–122, 202, 218
  spell checker programs 18,
      218–219
  voice recognition software
      18, **237–238**
  word prediction software
      18, **243**
  word processing software
      18, **243–244**
Assistive Technology Act of 2004
    19
astereognosis **19**
ataxia 11, **19,** 251
atomoxetine **19–20,** 25

attention **20–31, 113,** 130, 133
  Angelman syndrome 10, 11
  and anxiety 12
  and arousal 14, 20
  attention deficit hyperactivity
      disorder **20–30.** *See also*
      attention deficit
      hyperactivity disorder
  auditory integration training
      32
  and auditory sequencing 35
  autism 36
  cognitive ability 59
  concentration **65**
  distractibility 78
  and memory 149
  selective **202**
  sustained **30–31,** 246
attention deficit hyperactivity
    disorder 6, **20–30,** 131, 133
  accommodations 28–29, 30,
      142
  active-working memory 149
  antisocial personality
      disorder 11, 12
  and anxiety 12
  arousal regulation 14
  assessment 4, 16, 22–25, 30,
      134
      ADHD rating scale **6,**
          44
      behavioral rating scales
          6, 44, 57, 67
  auditory processing disorder
      34
  autistic spectrum disorders
      15, 39
  basal ganglia 21, 43
  communication disorder 62
  comorbid conditions 64
  conduct disorder 66
  corpus callosum 69
  depression 24, 25, 64, 71
  diet 28, **76,** 99–100, 148
  differential diagnosis 12, 23,
      45, 50, 51, **76**
  dopamine 21–22, 78
  electroencephalogram
      activity 87
  environmental toxins 22, 91

executive functions 96
experiential learning 96
fetal alcohol exposure 22,
101
frontal lobe problems 104
genetic factors 21, 106
hyperkinesis 111
impulsive behavior 20, 23,
24, 25, 30, 113
Individuals with Disabilities
Education Improvement
Act 115
inhibition and disinhibition
78, 117
minimal brain dysfunction
154–155
multiple disabilities 158
national organizations
251–252
neurotransmitters 21–22,
78, 163
and obsessive-compulsive
disorder 64, 169
and oppositional defiant
disorder 22, 25, 172
and perfectionism 178
phenylketonuria 181
Rehabilitation Act of 1973
28–29, 142, 196
reticular activating system
197–198
self-regulation problems
204, 205
support groups 224
and Tourette's syndrome 22,
229, 230
treatment 25–28, 29, 30, 86,
221–222
atomoxetine 19–20, 25
auditory integration
training 32
dextroamphetamine/am
phetamine 74–75
fluoxetine 102–103
methylphenidate 20,
25–26, 153–154
pemoline 26, 177
vision training 236
attributions 31
external 97, 144
internal 119–120, 144
and locus of control 144
atypical learner 31
audiologist 31, 34, 214
audiology 31
auditory integration training
32–33, 35, 37
auditory processing 31, 32,
33–35, 55, 130
comprehension 64
discrimination 31–32,
33–34, 102, 116–117
memory 33, 35, 117
autism 35–42, 128, 179, 180,
198–199
Asperger's syndrome 15–16,
38, 179, 180, 198, 251
auditory integration training
32, 37
auditory processing disorder
34
childhood disintegrative
disorder 38, 57, 58, 198
communication skills 39, 40,
62
differential diagnosis 9
discrete trial teaching 37, 77
eligibility for services 95
epilepsy 92
Grandin as person with
107
national organizations
252–253
Rett syndrome 38, 180,
198–199, 264
automatization 42
auxiliary aids and services 42

B

background knowledge 43
back-to-basics movement 43
basal ganglia 14, 21, 38, 43, 277
basal reader 43
basic skills 43–44, 277
behavior
adaptive 5–6, 8, 150, 236
antecedent event 11, 44
antisocial 11–12, 66, 67, 172
clinical observation 58
disinhibition 77–78
emotional and behavioral
disorder 87–89
oppositional 171–172
perseveration 179, 278
reinforcement 44, 161, 184,
230
rule-governed 200
self-regulation 204–205
behavioral modification 44–45,
68–69, 90, 99
attention deficit hyperactivity
disorder 26–28, 29
autistic spectrum disorders
16, 40
fragile X syndrome 104
obsessive-compulsive
disorder 170
parent skills training 176
reinforcement 44, 161, 184,
230
social skills training 210
token economy 228
Tourette's syndrome 230
behavioral psychology 11, 44
behavioral rating scales 6, 44, 57
Connors Rating Scales 44,
67, 89
distraction measurement 78
emotional-behavioral tests 89
behavioral unit 11, 44
Bender Visual-Motor Gestalt Test
45, 157
bias 45, 95, 167
bilateral motor coordination 45,
277
bilingual approach 45, 90
biofeedback 87
bipolar disorder 39, 45–49
birth
anoxic brain damage 11
low birth weight 49
premature 207
black mold, toxic 90, 92, 156
blending of sounds 49, 117, 192,
211
blindness, legal criteria 141
borderline intellectual
functioning 49–50
borderline personality disorder
50, 64

botulinum toxin therapy in
  spasmodic dysphonia 212–213
brain **50–52**
  acoustic cortex **4**
  angular gyrus **11**
  anoxic damage **11**
  arcuate fasciculus 14
  basal ganglia 14, 21, 38, **43,**
    277
  cerebellum 19, **55**
  cerebral cortex **55–56**
  contralateral areas **68**
  corpus callosum 7, 38, **69,**
    164
  electrical activity mapping 51
  electroencephalogram **87**
  epilepsy 92–94
  frontal lobe 13, 52, **104**
  hemispheres. *See*
    hemispheres of cerebral
    cortex
  imaging techniques **50–51,**
    170
  minimal dysfunction 136,
    154–155
  occipital lobe **170**
  parietal lobe 19, **176,** 185
  prefrontal lobes **185**
  reticular activating system
    197–198
  temporal lobe **227**
  thalamus **228**
  traumatic injury. *See*
    traumatic brain injury
  Wernicke's area 11, 13, 14,
    34, **240**
brain stem 277
Broca, Paul Pierre **52**
Broca's aphasia 13, **52,** 163
Broca's area 14, **52,** 159, 240
Brown v. Board of Education of
  Topeka **52–54**
Bruininks-Oseretsky Test of
  Motor Proficiency **54**
Buckley Amendment 60, 99

C
cadmium 55, 129
California Achievement Test **55,**
  167, 220

camp facilities 253
cancer therapy and learning
  disabilities 129
carbamazepine 47, 48
case history **55**
categorical classroom 70, 157,
  163, 204, 278
Cattell Sixteen Primary Factor
  Inventory 179, **210**
central auditory processing
  disorder 33, 55
central deafness 33, 55, 63, 110
cerebellum 19, **55**
cerebral cortex **55–56**
  hemispheres. *See*
    hemispheres of cerebral
    cortex
cerebral dysfunction 136
cerebral palsy 9, **56–57,** 62, 63,
  150, 254
channels, sensory **57,** 156
chelation therapy in lead
  poisoning 126
Child Attention Profile 44, **57**
Child Behavior Checklist **57**
childhood disintegrative disorder
  38, **57–58,** 180, 198
child psychiatrist **58**
Children and Adults with
  Attention Deficit Hyperactivity
  Disorder (CHADD) 224
child study committee **58,** 141,
  195, 214
chorea 229
chromosomal abnormalities 150
  Angelman syndrome 10
  Down syndrome 78, 150
  fragile X syndrome 15,
    103–104, 150
  Rett syndrome 198
chunking strategy for memory
  enhancement **58**
Civil Rights Act of 1964 9, 171
classroom
  ability grouping **1**
  academic classes **2**
  categorical grouping 70,
    157, 163, 204, 278
  full inclusion **104**
  general education **105–106**

learning centers **127**
least restrictive environment
  141
mainstreaming **146–147**
management strategies and
  techniques **58**
and resource room 135,
  196–197
self-contained 135, 197,
  202, **203–204**
  modified **156**
cleft lip and palate 62
clinical observation **58**
closure in information processing
  and perception **58,** 116
cloze procedure test **58**
Code of Federal Regulations **58**
coding **58–59**
  ACID profile **4**
  decoding. *See* decoding
  encoding **90**
  Gallistel-Ellis Test of Coding
    Skills **105**
cognition **59,** 65, 66, 277
  metacognition **152–153**
  social **210**
cognitive ability **59,** 277
  brain trauma 51–52, 232
  executive functions **95–96,**
    185, 245, 246
  higher functions **111**
  inferential thinking **115–116**
  and self-concept 203
  thinking skills **228**
  written expression disorder
    245, 246
cognitive-behavioral therapy 27,
  48, 127
cognitive development stages **66,**
  103, 148, 183, **185, 205–206**
cognitive style **59,** 277
cognitive therapy in obsessive-
  compulsive disorder 170
college **59–62**
  accommodations provided
    3–4, 139
  admission testing 1, 8–9, 61,
    201–202
coma in brain trauma 232
communication delay **62,** 124

communication disorders **62–64,** 72, 83, 124
  autistic spectrum disorders 39, 40, 62
  mixed receptive-expressive language disorder 74, **155–156**
  national association 254
comorbidity **64**
compensatory strategies 17, **64,** 277
comprehension **64,** 147
  analogies 9
  background knowledge 43
  cognitive ability 59, 152
  concept imagery disorder 65–66
  decoding compared 71
  dyslexia 82
  hyperlexia 112
  listening 64, **143**
  reading *See* reading, comprehension
  syntax 224–225
compulsion **64.** *See also* obsessive-compulsive disorder
computers
  and assisted instruction **64–65**
  and assistive technology 17–19, 64, 135–136
  Kurzweil reading machine **121–122**
  speech synthesizer/screen readers 18, 121–122, 202, **217–218**
  spell checker programs 18, **218–219**
  voice recognition software 18, **237–238**
  word prediction software 18, **243**
  word processing software 18, **243–244**
concentration **65**
concepts **65–66,** 277
Concerta. *See* methylphenidate
concrete operational stage **66,** 148, 183
concrete thinking **66**

conduct disorders 11, 22, 25, **66–67,** 172
conductive hearing loss 63, 110
confidentiality of student records 60, 67, 99, 277
configuration of words **67,** 277
Connors Rating Scales 44, **67,** 89
constructional apraxia **67**
constructional dyspraxia 84
consultations **86,** 197
context clues **67–68**
continuum of services **68**
contralateral brain areas **68**
contrecoup brain injury 231
control, locus of 31, 126–127, 144
  external 97, 177
  internal 119–120, 144
convergence **68**
convergent retrieval memory **68**
coordination **45, 68, 98, 109,** 277
  dyspraxia 84
  nonverbal learning disabilities 164
  visual motor **236**
copying
  far point **99**
  near point **161**
corporal punishment **68–69**
corpus callosum 7, 38, **69,** 164
corrective reading **69**
counseling 27, 30, 88
court cases 4, **52–54**
criterion-referenced tests **69–70,** 168, 219
cross-categorical grouping **70,** 204, 278
cross dominance **70,** 278
cues **70**
  contextual **67–68**
  decoding 205
  direction sense 77
  miscue analysis **155**
  semantic **205**
  and word attack skills 67, 242
cultural factors **70,** 88, **157,** 211
cumulative files **70,** 278
cursive writing **70,** 186
Cylert (pemoline) 26, **177**

D
deafness **110–111.** *See also* hearing, problems
decoding **71,** 240, 278
  background knowledge 43
  cues 205
  error analysis 94
  pseudoword **186–187**
  reading comprehension 193, 194
  and word attack skills 242
defensiveness, tactile **226**
delay
  communication **62,** 124
  language 124
dementia **71**
depression **71–72,** 89, 96, 126
  attention deficit hyperactivity disorder 24, 25, 64, 71
  autistic spectrum disorders 15, 39, 41
  bipolar disorder **45–49**
  Landau-Kleffner syndrome 123
  nonverbal learning disabilities 165, 166
  obsessive-compulsive disorder 169
  occupational therapy 171
  oppositional defiant disorder 172
  perfectionism 179
  stimulant drug side effect 222
developmental disabilities 5, 6, **72–74,** 94, 255–256
Developmental Disabilities Assistance Bill of Rights Act 6, **72–73**
Developmental Disabilities Council **72–73**
developmental disorders
  apraxia of speech 72, 234, 235
  arithmetic and mathematics 2, 72, 132, 133
  articulation 62, **72,** 132, 138
  expressive language **73,** 132
  not otherwise specified 133
  pervasive. *See* pervasive developmental disorders

developmental disorders *(continued)*
  reading 2, **73,** 132–133
  receptive language 62, **74,**
    132, 155–156
  sensory integration problems
    207
  speech and language **74,**
    132
  spelling **74**
  verbal dyspraxia 84
  writing 2, **74,** 132, 133
developmental lag **73,** 75, 278
developmentally appropriate
  practice **73**
dextroamphetamine 16, 26,
  74–75, 102, 221
diagnosis of learning disabilities
  75–76, 129–133, 165
*Diagnostic and Statistical Manual of
  Mental Disorders* 66, **75–76,**
  132, 180, 198
  attention deficit hyperactivity
    disorder 6, 20, 23, 67
  autism 36
  bipolar disorder 47
diagnostic teaching approach **76**
diet
  attention deficit hyperactivity
    disorder 28, **76,** 99–100,
    148
  autistic spectrum disorders
    41
  Feingold 76, **99–100**
  phenylketonuria 180, 181
  Prader-Willi syndrome
    184–185
differential diagnosis **76**
digit span and ACID profile **4**
dioxins **76–77,** 90, 91
direct instruction approach **77,**
  96, 147, 227, 232
direction, sense of **77,** 278
disability 109
  developmental 5, 6, **72–74,**
    94, 255–256
  language **124, 216**
  learning **127–139**
  multiple disabilities **158**
  national associations 255–259
discipline **68–69,** 119

disclosure of disability in college
  admission 61–62
discrepancy between potential
  and achievement 2, 4, 14, **77**
  dyslexia 81–82
  eligibility for special
    education services 4, 77,
    87, 138–139, 141–142
  legal definition of learning
    disability 115, 133, 137,
    138, 141–142
discrete trial teaching 37, 40, **77**
discrimination 278
  auditory **31–32,** 33–34,
    116–117
  objective left-right **169**
  visual 116, 157, **236**
discrimination against persons
  with disabilities 142, 171, 195
disinhibition **77–78,** 117, 278
disintegrative disorder in
  childhood 38, **57–58,** 180, 198
distractibility 78, 278
divergent retrieval memory 68
dominant hemisphere **70, 78,**
  136, 278
dopamine 21–22, **78,** 163, 229
Down syndrome 15, 36, 63,
  78–79, 150, 259
dressing dyspraxia 84
due process hearing **79–80**
Dursban **80,** 90, 92
dysarthria 62, **80**
dyscalculia 2, 14, 72, **80–81,** 106,
  128, 176
dysfluency 62, **81,** 102
dysgraphia 81, 128, 245,
  246–247
dyskinesia, tardive 212, **226–227**
dyslexia 2, 73, **81–83,** 128,
  132–133, 192
  accuracy of tests 4
  alexia compared 8
  angular gyrus activity 11
  auditory integration training
    32
  auditory processing disorder
    34
  brain research 50, 55
  comorbid conditions 64

corpus callosum 69
developmental lag compared
  73
dysphonia **83–84**
educational therapist 86
genetic factors 106
historical aspects 136
Individuals with Disabilities
  Education Improvement
  Act 115
national associations
  259–260
Orton-Gillingham approach
  106, 174–175
receptive language skills 194
and written expression
  disorder 245
dysnomia **83,** 97
dysphasia **83**
dysphonia **83–84, 212–213**
dyspraxia **84,** 198, 207–208
dyssemia **84**
dystaxia **84**
dystonia 229

E
early childhood assessment **85**
early intervention programs
  85–86, 109–110, 120, 142, 190
educable mentally handicapped
  86, 151
education agencies **144, 221**
educational consultant **86**
educational evaluation **86,**
  94–95, **113–114**
educational psychologist **188**
educational therapist **86**
Education and Handicapped Act
  Amendments of 1986 215
Education Department General
  Administrative Regulations **86**
Education for All Handicapped
  Children Act of 1975 **86–87,**
  109, 115, 214, 215, 216
  autistic spectrum disorders
    42
  Down syndrome 79
elaboration process **87**
electrical activity mapping of
  brain 51

electroconvulsive therapy in
    bipolar disorder 48–49
electroencephalogram **87**
eligibility committee
    (multidisciplinary team) 158,
    185–186, 195, 214
eligibility for services **87,** 88,
    115, 196
        discrepancy between
            potential and achievement
            4, 77, 87, 138–139,
            141–142
        evaluation 95, 215
emotional-behavioral tests **89**
emotions 6, 52, **87–90,** 278
employment issues 3, 9, 30, 139
encoding process **90**
English as a Second Language
    45, 90
Enright Diagnostic Inventory of
    Basic Arithmetic Skills **90**
environmental factors **90–92.**
    See also toxins, environmental
epilepsy **92–94**
episodic memory **94,** 144–145
errors **94,** 186, 204
        insertions **117,** 278
        inversions **120,** 278
        reversals 199, 278
        substitution 72, **224**
        transposition **231**
evaluation **94–95,** 134–135, 137.
    See also assessment
exclusion concept in learning
    disability definition 137
executive functions **95–96,** 185,
    245, 246
experiential learning **96**
explicit direct instruction 96
explicit memory **96**
expository writing **96–97,** 194
expressive language 33, 52, **97**
        disorders 62, **73, 97,** 138
            and receptive language
                disorder 74, 155–156
            specific language
                disability 216
            speech and language
                disorder 74, 132
            writing disorder 74, 97

expulsion from school 29
externalization **97,** 144
extrinsic phonics **98**
eye-foot coordination **98**
eye-hand coordination **98, 109**

F
face recognition in prosopagnosia
    7
Family Educational Rights and
    Privacy Act 60, **99**
family history **99,** 128
family service plan,
    individualized 56, **114**
family therapy **99**
far point copying **99**
fears 12, 147, 178
Federal Register **99**
Feingold diet 76, **99–100**
fetal alcohol effect 7, 91–92,
    100
fetal alcohol syndrome 7, 91–92,
    100–101, 129, 150, 261
field independent/dependent
    cognitive styles 59
figurative language **101**
figure-ground discrimination
    101–102
        auditory **31–32,** 33, 34, 102,
            117
        visual 116
files
        confidential 60, **67,** 99, 277
        cumulative **70,** 278
fine motor skills **102,** 164, 166,
    207, 236–237
finger agnosia **102,** 106, 176
finger spelling communication
    method 63–64
flame retardant chemicals 90,
    91
fluency **102**
        dysfluency **81,** 102
        fluent aphasia 13, **102**
        nonfluent aphasia 13, **163**
        stuttering therapy 223
fluoxetine **102–103**
folic acid in pregnancy 152
foods. *See* diet

formal operational stage **103,**
    148, 183
fragile X syndrome 15, 36,
    103–104, 150, 261–262
free appropriate public education
    104, 115, 138, 141, 142, 215
frontal lobe 13, 52, **104**
full inclusion **104**
functional magnetic resonance
    imaging of brain 51

G
Gall, Franz Joseph **105**
Gallistel-Ellis Test of Coding Skills
    105
gender differences **105**
        antisocial personality
            disorder 11
        Asperger's syndrome 15
        attention deficit hyperactivity
            disorder 21
        autism 35
        brain injury 231
        childhood disintegrative
            disorder 57
        dyslexia 81
        fragile X syndrome 103
        Rett syndrome 198
general education **105–106,** 195
genetic factors **106,** 128, 150
        Angelman syndrome 10
        attention deficit hyperactivity
            disorder 21, 106
        autism 36, 38
        bipolar disorder 46
        borderline personality
            disorder 50
        fragile X syndrome 103–104,
            150
        phenylketonuria 180
        Prader-Willi syndrome 184
        Rett syndrome 198
        Williams syndrome 241
Gerstmann's syndrome 7, **106,**
    176
giftedness **106,** 213, 216
Gillingham, Anna **106,** 174
        Orton-Gillingham approach
            106, **174–175**
global aphasia 13, **107**

government agencies **144, 221, 267–268**
  Office of Civil Rights **171,** 267–268
  Office of Special Education Programs **171,** 268
grade equivalent scores **107**
Grandin, Temple **107**
grapheme **107,** 181
graphic organizer **107,** 147
graphomotor ability **107**
graphophonemic knowledge **107**
Gray Oral Reading Test-Diagnostic **107**
gross motor skills 6, **108,** 164, 207
guided reading **108**

H
hand-eye coordination **98, 109**
hand gestures in cued speech 70
handedness 78, 124
handicap **109**
handwriting **70,** 107, 186
  cursive **70,** 186
  dysgraphia 81, 128, 245, 246–247
  printed **186**
haptic sense **109**
hard neurological signs **109**
head injury with brain trauma 231
Head Start **109–110**
hearing **31–35, 110–111**
  auditory integration training **32–33,** 35, 37
  auditory processing 31, 32, **33–35,** 55, 64, 130
  communication disorders 62, 63–64
  and discrimination ability **31–32,** 33–34, 102, 116–117
  Down syndrome 78–79
  learning disability 130
  and memory 33, 35, 117
  problems 63–64, 70, **110–111**
    central loss 33, 55, 63, 110
    conductive loss 63, 110
    mixed loss 63, 110

national associations 254–255
sensorineural loss 63, 110
special education services 110, 213, 214
hearing aids 63, 64
helplessness, learned **126–127**
hemispheres of cerebral cortex 55, 69
  cross or mixed dominance **70**
  dominant **78,** 124, 136
  right hemisphere learning disorders 163
higher order thinking and cognitive functions **111**
holistic assessment **111**
home instruction 197
hotlines **271–272**
hyperactivity 7, **111,** 123
  Angelman syndrome 9, 10, 11
  attention deficit hyperactivity disorder **20–30.** *See also* attention deficit hyperactivity disorder
hyperkinesis **111,** 136
hyperlexia **111–112**
hypersensitivity 39, 40, 226
hypoactivity **112**

I
ideation 84, **113**
illiteracy **113,** 139, 143
imagery disorder **65–66**
implicit memory **113**
impulsive behavior 12, **113,** 155
  attention deficit hyperactivity disorder 20, 23, 24, 25, 30, 113
  disinhibition **77–78,** 117, 278
inattention **113**
  attention deficit hyperactivity disorder 20–21, 23, 24
independent educational evaluation **113–114**
individualized education program **114,** 115, 135, 215
  autistic spectrum disorders 42

brain trauma 51, 231
cerebral palsy 56–57
child study committee 58
college 60
eligibility 87
emotional disturbance 89
evaluation 86, 94, 95, 214
free appropriate public education **104**
interim alternative educational setting 119
itinerant teachers 120
least restrictive environment 141
mainstreaming 146
minimum competency testing 155
nonverbal learning disabilities 165–166
referral process 195
remedial programs 196
resource room instruction 197
self-advocacy skills 203
transition plan 231
individualized education program committee **114,** 119
individualized family service plan 56, **114**
individualized reading instruction **114–115**
Individuals with Disabilities Education Improvement Act 86–87, 114, **115,** 138–139, 141–142
  accommodations requirements 3
  Americans with Disabilities Act compared 9
  attention deficit hyperactivity disorder 28–29
  autistic spectrum disorders 42
  brain trauma 231
  cerebral palsy 57
  classification of learning disabilities 132
  college admission 59–60
  continuum of services **68**
  due process hearing 79–80

eligibility assessment 95, 115, 138–139, 141–142, 215
emotional disturbance 89
free appropriate public education **104,** 115, 138, 142
hearing problems 110
independent educational evaluation 113
least restrictive environment 141, 214
multidisciplinary team approach 158
Office of Special Education Programs 171
Rehabilitation Act of 1973 compared 195, 196
state education agencies 221
transition plan 231
inferential thinking **115–116**
information processing **116–117**
   auditory 31, 32, **33–35,** 116–117, 140
   kinesthetic **121,** 140
   perceptual 178
   sensory channels **57**
   sensory integration **206–208**
   visual 116, 140, 236–237
inhibition 77–78, **117**
initial blend of consonant sounds **117**
insertion of words or letters **117,** 278
institutional placement 197
integration, sensory **206–208**
intelligence **117–119,** 128, **158–160**
intelligence quotient 5, 103, **118–119,** 134
   borderline intellectual functioning 49–50
   mental retardation 150, 151, 154
intelligence tests 1, 14, 118, **119,** 149–150, 151
   Stanford-Binet Intelligence Scale 16, 118, 119, **220,** 239
   Wechsler Adult Intelligence Scale 4, 118, **239**

Wechsler Intelligence Scale for Children 1, 4, 14, 16, 119, **239**
Wechsler Preschool and Primary Scale of Intelligence—Revised **239–240**
interim alternative educational setting **119**
internalization **119–120,** 144
interpersonal intelligence 159
interventions
   early **85–86,** 109–110, 120
   referral process 185–186, **195,** 214
intrapersonal intelligence 159
invented spelling **120**
inversion of letters or numbers **120,** 278
itinerant teacher **120,** 197, 278

K

Kaufman Test of Educational Achievement **121**
Key Math Diagnostic Arithmetic Test-Revised **121**
kinesthetic intelligence 158–159
kinesthetic learning **121,** 140, 278
Kurzweil reading machine **121–122**

L

Landau-Kleffner syndrome **123–124**
language **74, 124,** 132
   aphasoid **13**
   English as a Second Language 45, 90
   expressive. *See* expressive language
   figurative **101**
   learning disability 127, 130–131
   mixed receptive-expressive language disorder 74, **155–156**
   oral **173,** 194
   pragmatic **185**
   receptive. *See* receptive language

specific language disability **216**
   written **247**
language-based learning disorders 164
laryngeal dystonia 212
lateral preference **124**
laterality **124,** 136, 278
lateralization 124
laws. *See* legal issues
lead exposure 90, 91, **124–126,** 129
   and attention deficit hyperactivity disorder 22, 91
   and mental retardation 152
   national associations 262
learned helplessness **126–127**
learning **139–141**
   atypical **31**
   auditory 130, 140
   experiential **96**
   kinesthetic **121,** 140, 278
   lifetime education **142**
   metacognitive skills **152–153**
   motor **177**
   multisensory 83, **160,** 174–175, 234
   Orton-Gillingham approach 106, 174–175, 234
   readiness **190–191**
   visual 107, 140, 147
   whole language approach **240–241**
learning centers **127**
learning disability **127–139**
   diagnosis **75–76,** 129–133, 164–165
   discrepancy between aptitude and achievement. *See* discrepancy between potential and achievement
   information resources **275–276**
   legal issues *See* legal issues
   national associations 262–263
   nonverbal **163–166**
   perceptual **177**
   specific language learning disability 216

learning disability *(continued)*
symptoms 129–133,
164–165
treatment options and
outlook 133–139,
165–166
least restrictive environment
105–106, **141,** 146, 204, 214,
216
legal issues 137, 138–139,
141–142. *See also specific laws*
Americans with Disabilities
Act **9**
Assistive Technology Act of
2004 **19**
blindness criteria 141
Code of Federal Regulations
58
Developmental Disabilities
Assistance Bill of Rights
Act **72–73**
discrepancy between
potential and achievement
115, 133, 137, 138,
141–142
Education for All
Handicapped Children Act
of 1975 **86–87**
Family Educational Rights
and Privacy Act **99**
Federal Register **99**
free appropriate public
education **104,** 142
Individuals with Disabilities
Education Improvement
Act **115**
least restrictive environment
141
mainstreaming 146
Office of Civil Rights **171,**
267–268
Office of Special Education
Programs 171, 268
referral process 195
Rehabilitation Act of 1973
195–196
special education services
214–215
specific learning disabilities
216

transition plan 231
United States Code **233**
letters
insertion errors **117,** 278
inversion errors **120,** 278
names and sounds 192
orthographic awareness **173,**
174
recognition **142**
reversal errors **199,** 278
sound/letter/word retrieval
211
transposition errors **231**
lifetime education **142**
limbic system **142,** 144
lindane 90, 92, **142–143**
linguistics **143,** 159, 208, **211**
lip reading 70
listening 64, **143,** 173, 194
literacy **143,** 154, 191
and illiteracy **113,** 139, 143
lithium in bipolar disorder 47, 48
local education agency **144**
locus of control 31, 126–127, 144
external 97, 177
internal 119–120, 144
logical-mathematical intelligence
159
long-term memory **144–145,**
149, 199
and recall **194**
retrieval **198,** 210
semantic knowledge **205**
look-say reading instruction
model 43
low-birth-weight infants **49**
Lowe syndrome 263

M

magnetic resonance imaging of
brain 51
mainstreaming 5, 62, **146–147,**
216
maladjustment, social **210**
mania in bipolar disorder **45–49**
mapping 64, 107, **147**
margin notes **147**
mastery of skills **147,** 175
mathematics **147–148.** *See also*
arithmetic and mathematics

maturation **148**
mean score **148**
meaning-based instruction **148**
measles-mumps-rubella vaccine
39
megavitamins and ADHD **148**
memory 58–59, 62, 131, **149**
auditory 33, 35, 117
cognitive functions 59, 96
concentration **65**
cues or prompts 70
dementia **71**
dyslexia 83
dyspraxia 84
elaboration process **87**
episodic **94,** 144–145
explicit **96**
frontal lobe functions 104
hyperlexia 112
implicit **113**
information processing
model 117
long-term. *See* long-term
memory
mnemonic devices 70, 156
nonverbal 165, **166**
procedural 144–145
recall **194**
retrieval **68, 198, 219**
reverbalization strategy
199
semantic 94, 144–145, **205**
short-term 145, 149
source **211**
verbal **236**
visual 116, 209, **236**
writing process 245
mental age **149–150**
mental retardation 73, 95,
150–152
anoxia 11
autism 35, 36, 39
borderline intellectual
functioning 49–50
cerebral palsy 56, 150
childhood disintegrative
disorder 57–58
Down syndrome 78, 150
Dursban exposure 80

educable mentally
    handicapped **86,** 151
fetal alcohol exposure 7,
    101, 150
fragile X syndrome 103–104,
    150
Individuals with Disabilities
    Education Improvement
    Act 115
intelligence tests 119, 150,
    151
learning disability compared
    128
mild 86, 151, **154**
multiple disabilities 158
occupational therapy 171
phenylketonuria 150, 152,
    180, 181
Prader-Willi syndrome 184
mercury exposure 39, 90, 91,
    151, **152**
metacognition **152–153**
methylphenidate 11, 16, 41,
    153–154, 221, 222
    attention deficit hyperactivity
        disorder 20, 25–26, 102,
        153–154
Metropolitan Achievement Test
    153, 167, 220
micrographia 7
micro-uniting **154**
mild mental retardation 86, 151,
    154
Millon Clinical Multiaxial
    Inventory **154,** 179
mind maps 107, 147
minimal brain dysfunction 136,
    154–155
minimum competency testing
    155
Minnesota Multiphasic
    Personality Inventory 154,
    155, 179
miscue analysis **155**
mixed receptive-expressive
    language disorder 74, **155–156**
mnemonic devices **70, 156**
modalities
    learning **140**
    sensory 57, **156**

molds, toxic black 90, 92, **156**
monitoring 20, **204**
morpheme **156**
morphology of words 156–157,
    222
motivation 31, 126–127, 144, **157**
    external sources 97, 177
    internal sources 119–120, 144
motor cortex 52
Motor Free Visual Perception Test
    157
motor planning **157,** 185
motor sequencing 45, **157,** 208
motor skills 131, 133, **157,** 164,
    166
    Angelman syndrome 10–11
    Bender Visual-Motor Gestalt
        Test **45**
    Bruininks-Oseretsky Test of
        Motor Proficiency **54**
    cerebral palsy 56
    coordination *See*
        coordination
    Down syndrome 79
    dyspraxia 84
    fine **102,** 164, 166, 207,
        236–237
    graphomotor ability 107
    gross 6, **108,** 164, 207
    low-birth-weight infants 49
    perceptual-motor skills
        177–178, 237
    sensory integration
        dysfunction 207–208
    and visual perception 157,
        236–237
    written expression disorder
        245, 246
multicategorical classroom **157**
multicultural assessment **157**
multidisciplinary team **158**
    referral process 185–186,
        195, 214
multifactored evaluation **158**
multiple disabilities **158**
multiple intelligences **158–160**
multisensory learning and
    teaching 83, 106, **160,**
    174–175, 234
music 37, 158

N
naming ability 13, 83, 97
narrative text reading
    comprehension 194
National Association of School
    Psychologists 1, 189
National Institute of Mental
    Health 50, 137–138
National Joint Committee for
    Learning Disabilities 136, 137
national organizations **250–266**
    hotlines **271–272**
naturalistic intelligence 160
near point vision **161**
needs assessment **161**
negative reinforcement of
    behavior **161**
neurobiology **161**
neurological assessment **109,**
    161, 211
neurological disorders **161**
neurological impress reading
    instruction method **161–162**
neurologist **162**
neurology **161–163,** 206
neuropsychology 16, **162–163,**
    206
neurotransmitters 21–22, 78,
    163, 229
noncategorical grouping **163**
nonfluent aphasia 13, **163**
nonphonetic words **163**
nonsense words and pseudoword
    decoding 186–187
nonverbal learning disabilities
    64, **163–166**
nonverbal memory **166**
norm-referenced tests 70,
    166–168, 190, 219–220
normalization **166**
norms **168**
nutrition *See* diet

O
objective left-right discrimination
    169
obsessive-compulsive disorder
    41, **169–170**
    and attention deficit hyper-
        activity disorder 64, 169

obsessive-compulsive disorder
  (continued)
    and perfectionism 178
    and Tourette's syndrome
      169, 229, 230
occipital lobe 170
occupational therapy 166,
  170–171
    Angelman syndrome
      10–11
    autism 37
    cerebral palsy 56
    sensory integration
      dysfunction 206, 208
Office for Civil Rights 171,
  267–268
Office of Special Education
  Programs 171, 268
oppositional behavior 171–172
oppositional defiant disorder 22,
  25, **172–173**
oral language 173, 194
oral reading 173, 224
organicity 173
organizational strategies and
  problems 131, **173, 213, 227**
organophosphate pesticides 80,
  90, 92
orientation, spatial 213
orthography 173–174
Orton, Samuel Torrey 106, 136,
  174
Orton-Gillingham approach 106,
  174–175, 234
outcomes assessment 175

P
palsy, cerebral 9, **56–57,** 62, 63,
  150, 254
parapnasias 176
parent skills training 176
    attention deficit hyperactivity
      disorder 27–28
    autistic spectrum disorders 40
    cerebral palsy 56
    conduct disorder 67
    emotional and behavioral
      disorder 88
    stuttering 223–224
parietal lobe 19, **176,** 185

pattern recognition 176
PCBs (polychlorinated biphenyls)
  90, 91
Peabody Picture Vocabulary Test-
  Third Edition **176–177**
pedagogy 177
pemoline 26, **177**
percentile **177,** 221
perception **177–178,** 236–237
    auditory 31, **33**
    brain trauma 52
    closure **58**
    and motor skills **177–178,**
      237
    space **211–212**
    tactile **226**
    visual **236–237**
perfectionism **178–179**
performance assessment 16,
  69–70
perseveration 179, 278
personality disorders **11–12, 50**
personality tests 179
    Millon Clinical Multiaxial
      Inventory **154,** 179
    Minnesota Multiphasic
      Personality Inventory 154,
      155, 179
    Sixteen Primary Factor
      Inventory 179, **210**
pervasive developmental
  disorders 15, **179–180**
    auditory processing disorder
      34
    autism 35, 38, 179, 180
    not otherwise specified 38,
      179, 180, 198
Pervasive Developmental
  Disorders Screening Test-II **180**
pesticide exposure 80, 90, 92,
  142–143
phenylketonuria 150, 152,
  180–181
phobia, math **147**
phonemes 31, 49, 71, **181–182,**
  183, 192
phonetics 15, 163
phonics **98, 182–183,** 191, 224
    whole language approach
      compared 240, 241

Phonological Awareness Test
  192
phonology 7, **183,** 192
phrenology 105
Piaget, Jean **183**
    cognitive development
      theory 66, 103, 148, 183,
      185, 205–206
Picture Exchange
  Communication System 40
planning, motor **157,** 185
play activities 28, 36
Plessy v. Ferguson 53
polybrominated diphenyl ether
  flame retardants 91
polychlorinated biphenyls 90,
  91
portfolio assessment 16–17, **184**
positive reinforcement of
  behavior **184,** 230
positron emission tomography of
  brain 51
Prader-Willi syndrome **184–185,**
  263
pragmatic language and skills
  185
praxia **185**
praxis **185**
prefrontal lobes **185,** 278
pregnancy 128–129, 150, 152
    alcohol use 7, 22, 91–92,
      100–101, 128, 129, 150
    bipolar disorder therapy 48
    Down syndrome 78, 79
    Dursban exposure 80, 92
    lindane exposure 142–143
    mercury exposure 91
    phenylketonuria 181
prematurity 207
preoperational stage of cognitive
  development 148, 183, **185**
pre-referral process **185–186**
pretest **186**
print disabilities **186**
printing instruction **186**
problem solving 17, 59, 62, **68,**
  186
procedural memory 144–145
program specialist **186**
proofreading **186**

proprioceptive system **186**
prosody **186**
prosopagnosia 7
Prozac (fluoxetine) **102–103**
pseudoword decoding **186–187**
psychiatrist **58, 187**
psychological evaluation 16, **162, 187**
psychologists 1, **187–189,** 214
    neuropsychologist **162–163**
psychomotor tests 278
psychotherapy 27, 30, 48, 170
punishment, corporal **68–69**

R
raw score **190,** 220
readability **190**
readiness **190–191,** 278
reading 81–83, 127–128, 131, 132–133, **191–194**
    accuracy of tests 4, 191–192
    active **4–5, 219**
    alexia 7, **8**
    basal readers **43**
    comprehension 64, 190, 191, **193–194**
        achievement tests 4
        active reading techniques 5
        cloze procedure test **58**
        context clues **67–68**
        Gray Oral Reading Test-Diagnostic **107**
        instructional level 117
        monitoring **64**
        morphological awareness 156–157
    contextual **68**
    corrective **69**
    decoding process 71
    developmental disorder 2, 73, 132–133
    dyslexia 81–83, 132–133. *See also* dyslexia
    guided **108**
    hyperlexia **111–112**
    individualized instruction **114–115**

instructional level **117**
Kurzweil reading machine **121–122**
language processing disabilities 124
letter recognition 142
linguistic teaching approach 143
literacy 113, 143, 191
look-say instruction 43
margin notes 147
miscue analysis 155
neurological impress instruction 161–162
oral **173,** 224
Orton-Gillingham approach 106, 174–175
phonics instruction **182–183,** 191
print disabilities **186**
readiness 190
receptive language skill 194–195
reciprocal reading/teaching **195**
sight words **209–210**
whole language teaching approach 182, 191, 240–241
word configuration cue 67
reasoning, mathematics 14, 132
recall **194**
receptive language 97, **194–195**
    disorders 62, **74,** 132
        and expressive language disorder 74, 155–156
        specific language disability 216
reciprocal reading/teaching **195**
referral process 185–186, **195,** 214
reflex tests **195**
regular education classes **195**
Rehabilitation Act of 1973 3, 9, 142, **195–196**
    attention deficit hyper-activity disorder 28–29, 142, 196
    college admission 59, 60
    Down syndrome 79

reinforcement of behavior 44, **161, 184,** 230
reliability of tests **196**
remedial programs 17, 135, 196–197
resource room instruction 135, **196–197**
reticular activating system **197–198**
retrieval memory **68, 198, 210**
Rett syndrome 38, 180, **198–199,** 264
reverbalization strategy **199**
reversal errors **199,** 278
Rh disease 152
rhetorical patterns **199**
Ritalin (methylphenidate) 11, 16, 41, **153–154,** 221, 222
    attention deficit hyperactivity disorder 20, 25–26, 102, 153–154
rule-governed behavior **200**

S
saliency **201**
scale scores **201**
scatter in subtest scores **201**
Scholastic Aptitude Test 1, 14, 61, 119, **201–202**
school psychologist 1, **188–189,** 214
screen reader programs 18, **121–122,** 202, **217–218**
screening tests **180, 202**
    Down syndrome 79
    lead poisoning 125–126
    phenylketonuria 152, 180
script (cursive writing) **70,** 186
second language, English as **45, 90**
secretin in autistic spectrum disorders 41
segregated other facility 197, **202**
seizures 41, **92–94**
    Angelman syndrome 9, 10, 11
    Landau-Kleffner syndrome 123, 124
    Rett syndrome 198–199
selective attention **202**

self-advocacy skills **203**
self-concept **203,** 204, 210
self-contained classroom 135, **156,** 197, 202, **203–204**
self-correction of errors **204**
self-efficacy **204**
self-esteem 139, 203, **204,** 206
    emotional disturbance 89
    externalization 97
    internalization 119
    intrapersonal intelligence 159
    locus of control 144
    perfectionism 179
self-monitoring 20, **204**
self-regulation **204–205**
semantics **205**
    memory 94, 144–145, **205**
sensorimotor stage of development 148, 183, **205–206**
sensorineural hearing loss 63, 110
sensory avoiders 207
sensory channels **57,** 156
sensory diet in occupational therapy 206
sensory impairment 36, **206**
sensory integration 32, 37, 40, **206–208**
sensory seekers 207
separate but equal doctrine 52–54
sequencing skills **208**
    auditory 33, 34, **35**
    linguistic 208
    motor 45, **157,** 208
    spatial **213**
    temporal-sequential organization problems **227**
serotonin in obsessive-compulsive disorder 169
shaken baby syndrome **208–209,** 231
short-term memory 145, 149
sight words **209–210,** 244
sign language 63–64
Simon-Binet intelligence tests 118

simultaneous retrieval memory **210**
Sixteen Primary Factor Inventory 179, **210**
social skills 131, 163, 165, **210**
    and antisocial behavior **11–12,** 66, 67, 172
    Asperger's syndrome 15–16, 38
    attention deficit hyperactivity disorder 27
    autism 35, 36, 37, 39
    childhood disintegrative disorder 57
    emotional and behavioral disorder 87, 88–89
    hyperlexia 112
    interpersonal intelligence 159
    pragmatic language 185
social worker **210–211**
sociocultural factors **157,** 211
socioeconomic status **211**
sociolinguistics **211**
soft neurological signs **211**
sounds **211,** 217
    blending **49, 117,** 192, **211**
    and letter name knowledge 192
    phonemic awareness **181–182,** 192
source memory **211**
Southeastern Community College v. Davis 4
space perception **211–212,** 213
spasmodic dysphonia **212–213**
spatial relationships 116, 159, 211–212, **213**
    acalculia 3
    agraphia 7
special education services 127, 135, **213–216**
    accommodations 3, 214
    atypical learner 31
    autistic spectrum disorders 40, 41–42
    brain trauma 231
    communication disorder 62
    confidentiality 67

continuum of **68**
due process hearing 79–80
dyslexia 82
educational consultant specialty 86
eligibility 4, **87,** 95, 115, 141–142
emotional and behavioral disorder 88, 89
evaluation 94–95, 214
fetal alcohol syndrome 100
fragile X syndrome 104
free appropriate public education **104**
full inclusion **104**
gender differences 105
hearing problems 110, 213, 214
individualized education program 114
itinerant teachers **120**
low birth weight 49
mainstreaming 146, 147
national associations 264
nonverbal learning disabilities 166
Office of Special Education Programs **171**
Prader-Willi syndrome 184
referral process 185–186, **195,** 214
segregated other facility 197, 202
social maladjustment 210
specific language disability **216**
specific learning disability **216**
speech 62, 63, **74,** 132, **216–217**
    aphasia **13,** 52
    aphemia **13**
    apraxia **13–14,** 72, 234–235
    articulation **14–15,** 62, **72**
    blending of sounds **49, 117,** 192, **211**
    cued **70**
    Down syndrome 78–79
    dysarthria **80**
    dysphasia 83
    dyspraxia 84

fluency 102

language processing disability 124

national associations 264–265

oral language **173,** 194

screen reader/synthesized speech technology 18, 121–122, 202, **217–218**

stuttering 62, 102, 217, **222–224,** 265

voice recognition software 18, 237–238

speech-language pathologist 14, **217**

speech-language specialist 15, **217**

speech-language therapy 37, 56

speech synthesizer/screen readers 18, 121–122, 202, **217–218**

spell checker programs 18, **218–219**

spelling **74, 218–219**

assistive technology 18, **218–219**

dysphonia 83–84

invented **120**

linguistic teaching approach 143

orthography 173–174

Orton-Gillingham approach 174–175

phonics instruction **182–183**

proofreading 186

sight-word approach **209**

written expression disorder 245

SQ3R active reading method **219**

standard deviation **219**

standard scores **220–221**

standardized tests and scales 4, 5–6, 16, **219–220**

aptitude 14

diagnostic 75, 134

percentile values 177

scale scores 201

Stanford Achievement Test 167, 219, **220**

Stanford-Binet Intelligence Scale 16, 118, 119, **220,** 239

stanine (standard nine) scores **220–221**

state education agency **221**

stereotypy 229

stimulant drugs 74–75, **221–222**

strabismus 278

strategy instruction 5, **222**

Strattera (atomoxetine) **19–20,** 25

Strauss syndrome 136

stress management in attention deficit hyperactivity disorder 28

structural analysis **222**

study skills **222,** 224

stuttering 62, 102, 212, 217, **222–224,** 265

subdural area 278

substitution errors 72, **224**

support groups 27, **224**

survival skills 224

suspension from school 29, 119

syllabication **224,** 244

symbols **211, 224**

syntax **224–225,** 278

synthesized speech technology 18, 121–122, 202, **217–218**

T

tactile sensations 109, **226,** 278

talent and giftedness 106, 216

tardive dyskinesia 212, **226–227**

task analysis **227**

temporal lobe **227**

Test of Adolescent and Adult Language—Third Edition **228**

Test of Auditory Comprehension of Language—Revised **228**

Test of Language Competence—Expanded Edition **228**

Test of Language Development **228**

Test of Phonological Awareness 192

thalamus 43, **228**

thematic maturity **228**

thimerosal 39, 91

thinking 131, **228**

brain injury 51–52, 232

concrete thinking **66**

higher order **111**

inferential **115–116**

thyroid disorders 152

tics **157, 228,** 229, 230

token economy **228**

touch sense 109, **226,** 278

Tourette's syndrome 75, 154, 222, **229–230,** 265

and attention deficit hyperactivity disorder 22, 229, 230

and autism 36

and obsessive-compulsive disorder 169, 229, 230

and oppositional defiant disorder 172

toxins, environmental 22, 80, 129, 151, 152

cadmium 55, 129

dioxins **76–77,** 91

Dursban **80,** 92

flame retardants 91

lead *See* lead exposure

lindane 92, **142–143**

mercury 39, 90, 91, 151, **152**

molds 90, 92, **156**

polychlorinated biphenyls 91

tracking

ability grouping **1**

reading process **230**

transition plan 60, 61, **230–231**

transposition errors **231**

traumatic brain injury **51–52, 231–232**

eligibility for services 95, 115

national organizations 253

nonverbal learning disability 164

sensory integration problems 207

shaken baby syndrome **208–209,** 231

trisomy 21 (Down syndrome) 15, 36, 63, **78–79,** 150, 259

tutoring 135, **232**

U

United States Code **233**

universal access/design 3, **233**

V

vaccines with mercury content 39, 91
VAKT instruction method **234**
validity of tests **234**
valproate therapy in bipolar disorder 47, 48
ventricles of brain 278
verbal apraxia 13–14, 72, **234–235**
verbal dyspraxia, developmental 84
verbal memory **236**
vestibular disorders 266
Vineland Adaptive Behavior Rating Scale 6, **236**
Vineland Social Maturity Scales 150
vision 157, 170, **236–237**
  and agnosia 7
  discrimination ability 116, 157, **236**
  far point **99**
  and learning style 107, 140, 147
  and memory 116, 209, **236**
  and motor skills 45, 116, **236–237**
  near point **161**
  and spatial information 64
  training 37, **236**
visual-auditory-kinesthetic-tactile (VAKT) instruction method **234**
vitamins 28, 148, 152
vocabulary **143,** 157, 176–177, 193, 194
vocational education 266

voice 62, 63, 212–213
voice recognition software 18, **237–238**

W

Wechsler Adult Intelligence Scale 4, 118, **239**
Wechsler Individual Achievement Test **239,** 246
Wechsler Intelligence Scale for Children 1, 4, 14, 16, 119, **239**
Wechsler Preschool and Primary Scale of Intelligence—Revised **239–240**
Wernicke's aphasia 13, 240
Wernicke's area 11, 13, 14, 34, **240**
whole class ability grouping 1
whole language approach 182, 191, **240–241**
Williams syndrome **241,** 266
Woodcock-Johnson assessment system 1, 14, 16, **241–242,** 246
Woodcock Reading Mastery Test Revised 192
word attack skills 67, **242–243**
word blindness 136
word configuration **67,** 277
word deafness 33–35, 243
word-finding ability 11, 13, 83, 97, 211, 243
word prediction software 18, **243**
word processing software 18, **243–244**
word recognition 209–210, 222, 224, **244**

  and word attack skills 242–243
word retrieval **211,** 244
writing 131, 132, **244–247**
  agraphia **7**
  cursive **70,** 186
  developmental disorders 2, **74,** 132, 133
  disorder of written expression 97, **244–247**
  dysgraphia 81, 128, 245, 246–247
  dysphasia 83
  expository **96–97,** 194
  language processing disability 124
  literacy 113, 143
  narrative 194
  printed 186
  process approach **244**
  rhetorical patterns 199
  thematic maturity **228**
  word processing software 18, 243–244
written expression disorders 97, **244–247**
  dysgraphia 81, 128, 245, 246–247
written language **247**

Y

Yopp-Singer Test of Phoneme Segmentation 192

Z

zone of proximal development **248**